FORENSIC MEDICINE AND TOXICOLOGY

VOLUME 2: TOXICOLOGICAL EVIDENCE, REPRODUCTIVE FORENSICS, AND ETHICAL PRACTICE

Mohamed Amine Kerdoun

ALLIED HEALTH PRESS

Forensic Medicine and Toxicology

Volume 2: Toxicological Evidence, Reproductive Forensics, and Ethical Practice

Author: **Mohamed Amine Kerdoun**

Allied Health Press
4164 Lakeshore Road
Burlington ON L7L 1A4
Canada
www.alliedhealthpress.com
Email: orders@arclereducation.com

ISBN: 978-1-77956-843-4

Allied Health Press publishes wide variety of books and eBooks. For more information about Allied Health Press and its products, visit our website at www.alliedhealthpress.com

ABOUT THE AUTHOR

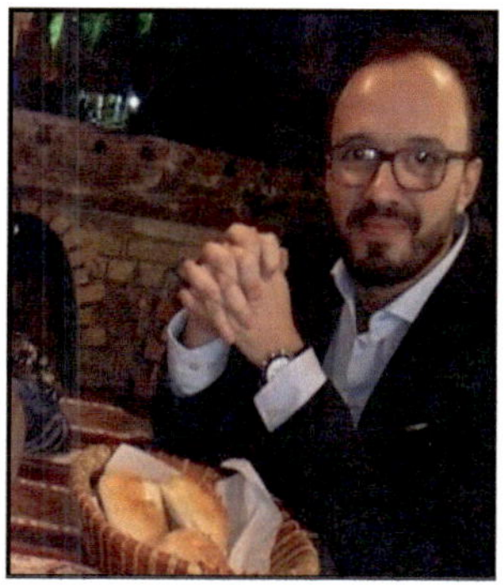

Amine Kerdoun, PharmD, PhD, is an associate professor of Toxicology at the Faculty of Medicine, Kasdi Merbah University in Ouargla, Algeria. A specialist in medical and environmental toxicology, he brings over a decade of academic, clinical, and regulatory experience to his work. Dr. Kerdoun holds a Doctorate in Medical Sciences with a focus on toxicology, along with degrees in pharmacy and specialized medical studies from leading Algerian institutions. His research focuses on chemical risk assessment, heavy metals, endocrine disruptors, and cosmetic safety, with numerous peer-reviewed publications in international journals. A respected educator and scientific communicator, Dr. Kerdoun combines rigorous toxicological expertise with a commitment to public health protection and regulatory excellence across global frameworks.

Brief Table of Contents

Getting Started with This Book

Chapter Openers

A list of Chapter Outline is presented providing a brief Introduction to what will be covered in the chapter.

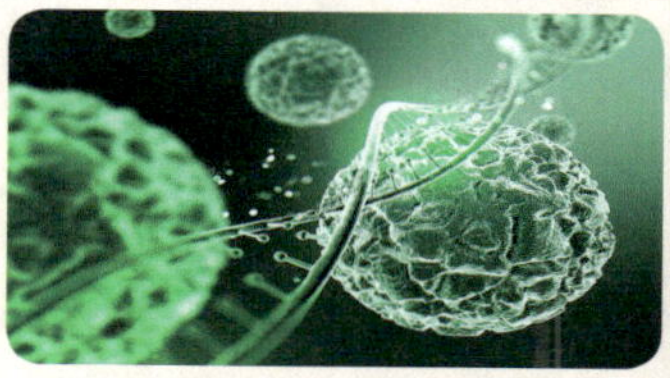

Introduction

Often referred to as the science of life, biology is a broad field of study aimed at comprehending the several kinds of life on Earth, from tiny creatures to sophisticated multicellular entities. Comprising several subfields, including molecular biology, ecology, and evolutionary biology, each of which advances our knowledge of living systems, this field clarifies the mechanisms controlling life events, including development, reproduction, and interaction with the surroundings, which is the central goal of biology. Moreover, biology fills in the void between the natural sciences and medicine by offering a necessary understanding of health, illness, and the interactions between organisms and their environments. Dealing with urgent global issues such as climate change, biodiversity loss, and new diseases depends on an awareness of these complex biological interactions, therefore highlighting the critical part biology plays in modern civilization. Fundamentally, biology explores and tests ideas about the living world using the scientific method. Through methodical observation and experimentation,

LEARNING OBJECTIVES

After studying this chapter, you will be able to:

1. Discuss the scientific method in biology;
2. Explain the cell theory;
3. Discuss the genetics and heredity;
4. Evolution and natural selection;
5. Focus on ecology and ecosystems;
6. Learn about human biology;
7. Evaluate the plant biology;
8. Explain the microbiology;
9. Focus on current trends in biology.

1.1. The Scientific Method in Biology

Learning Outcome

1. Describe the steps of the scientific method;
2. Focus on hypothesis formation;
3. Learn about experimental design.

Learning Outcomes

The beginning of each section of every chapter contains a set of Learning Outcomes that inform students of concepts they should understand. These outcomes help students understand what they should be able to do if they have mastered the material in that section.

Test Your Knowledge

Throughout each chapter, Test Your Knowledge cues you to note which topics have been covered and to self-test your understanding of the material presented.

Test Your Knowledge

1. Explain why correlation does not imply causation in scientific experiments.
2. How does the scientific method help reduce the influence of personal opinions in research?

Chapter Summary

The Summary Section appear at the end of each chapter and summarize main concepts covered throughout the chapter. These points provide key concepts in an engaging and meaningful way.

Summary

The investigation of biological principles highlights the importance of a comprehensive view of life by reflecting the intricate interactions that occur within living systems. The complexity of biology goes beyond individual species or systems, as this essay highlights; it also includes the interactions that mold ecosystems and affect biodiversity. Researchers can conduct in-depth analyses of metabolomic data using sophisticated technologies like MetaboAnalyst, which offer insights into the molecular mechanisms underlying these interactions. As demonstrated by the developments in MetaboAnalyst, for example, the integration of diverse omics data promotes a thorough understanding of metabolic pathways and helps identify important biological markers necessary for research on development and disease (Chong et al., 2018). Additionally, the phenomenon of ecological invasions is a key component of biological research and a vital field of study. The introduction of non-native species into unfamiliar habitats has significant ramifications and calls for multidisciplinary management strategies. Examining the origins and effects of these biological incursions, invasion science has become a crucial field that highlights the need to comprehend ecological dynamics and community interactions. As interest in biological invasions increases, new findings are emerging that put conventional ecological theories and practices to the test. The importance of incorporating various scientific viewpoints is shown by this developing discipline, which also highlights how invasive species shape ecosystems and advances our knowledge of ecological resilience (David et al., 2013). When taken as a whole, these discoveries from invasion science and metabolomics highlight the value of multidisciplinary biology research. Fostering cross-disciplinary collaboration and utilizing technological breakthroughs to improve our comprehension of intricate biological interactions are crucial as we look to the future of biological research. In addition to deepening our understanding of the complexities of life, this method lays the groundwork for tackling urgent environmental issues. Future studies can ensure the continued relevance of biology in a world that is constantly changing by acknowledging the interconnection of biological systems and opening the door to creative solutions that support sustainability and biodiversity conservation. We might imagine a thorough comprehension of life that serves both academia and society at large through ongoing investigation and integration of scientific knowledge.

Knowledge Assessment

The chapter includes material designed to review and reinforce each content. It includes Critical Thinking Questions to help test of your understanding of information presented in the chapter and Short answer Questions to review your understanding of the key concepts presented in the chapter.

Critical Thinking Questions

1. **Who is known as the "Father of Modern Biology"?**
   a. Aristotle
   b. Charles Darwin
   c. Gregor Mendel
   d. Louis Pasteur
2. **What is the basic unit of life?**
   a. Atom
   b. Molecule
   c. Cell
   d. Organism
3. **Which branch of biology studies the interaction of organisms with their environment?**
   a. Genetics
   b. Ecology
   c. Physiology
   d. Botany
4. **Which macromolecule is the main source of energy for living organisms?**
   a. Proteins
   b. Lipids
   c. Carbohydrates
   d. Nucleic acids
5. **DNA is primarily responsible for which function in living organisms?**
   a. Energy production
   b. Protein synthesis
   c. Storing genetic information
   d. Regulating body temperature

Short Answer Questions

1. What is biology, and why is it important to study biology?
2. What are the three main domains of life, and how are they different from one another?
3. Define homeostasis and give an example of how it works in living organisms.
4. What is the cell theory, and why is it fundamental to biology?
5. How do autotrophs and heterotrophs differ in the way they obtain energy?
6. What is the scientific method, and how is it applied in biological research?
7. Discuss how biology helps address global challenges such as climate change, disease, and food security.
8. Explain the levels of biological organization from the smallest unit to the largest. Provide examples at each level.
9. Describe the relationship between structure and function in biology, giving specific examples from cells or organs.
10. How has the discovery of genetics shaped our understanding of inheritance and variation among organisms?

Supplementary Materials

Key Terms: A list of key terms is given for quick reference

KEY TERMS FROM THIS CHAPTER

Annotation enrichment analysis
Cell theory
Ecosystems
Microbiology
Plant biology
Biological structure
Cellular structure
Genetics
Natural selection
Cell
Ecology
Human biology
Organism

Further Resources: Recommendations for additional readings, websites, and multimedia resources.

References

1. Argelaguet, R., Velten, B., Arnol, D., Dietrich, S., Zenz, T., Marioni, J. C., Buettner, F., et al. (2018). Multi-omics factor analysis—A framework for unsupervised integration of multi-omics data sets. *Molecular Systems Biology, 14*. https://doi.org/10.15252/msb.20178124.
2. Bacher, S., Blackburn, T. M., Essl, F., & Genovesi, P. (2017). *Socio-Economic Impact Classification of Alien Taxa (SEICAT).* https://core.ac.uk/download/286567949.pdf (accessed on 8th March 2025).
3. Barnett, R., Brace, S., Cucchi, T., & Dobney, K. (2013). *Divergent Evolutionary Processes Associated with Colonization of Offshore Islands.* https://core.ac.uk/download/20664364.pdf (accessed on 8th March 2025).

Detailed Table of Contents

CHAPTER 5

Corrosive Poisons 113

CHAPTER 6

Metallic Poisons 139

CHAPTER 9

CHAPTER 11

Medical Ethics and Professional Conduct 283

CHAPTER 12

Consent in Medical Practice 313

LIST OF FIGURES

LIST OF ABBREVIATION

AAS	Atomic Absorption Spectrophotometry
AAS	Atomic Absorption Spectroscopy
AChE	Acetylcholinesterase
ACMD	Advisory Council on the Misuse of Drugs
AIMS	Ambient Ionization Mass Spectrometry
AMI	Acute Myocardial Infarction
BAC	Benzalkonium Chloride
BAC	Blood Alcohol Concentration
BBB	Blood-Brain Barrier
CNV	Copy Number Variation
CPD	Continuous Professional Development
CS	Chemical Submission
CWA	Chemical Warfare Agent
CZ	Cetirizine
DBS	Dried Blood Spots
DFSA	Drug-Facilitated Sexual Assault
DNT	Developmental Neurotoxicity
EBP	Evidence-Based Practice
ECG	Electrocardiographic
EDX	Energy-Dispersive X-Ray
EV	Extracellular Vesicle
FGM	Female Genital Mutilation
FGM/C	Female Genital Mutilation and/or Cutting
FISH	Fluorescent in Situ Hybridization
FSL	Forensic Science Laboratories

GBD	Global Burden of Diseases
GC	Gas Chromatography
GC-MS	Gas Chromatography-Mass Spectrometry
GDPR	General Data Protection Regulation
GHB	Gamma-Hydroxybutyrate
GMP	Good Manufacturing Practice
HCl	Hydrochloric Acid
HPLC	High-Performance Liquid Chromatography
HRMS	High-Resolution Mass Spectrometry
HZ	Hydroxyzine
IAFM	Indian Academy of Forensic Medicine
ICP-MS	Inductively Coupled Plasma Mass Spectrometry
IGG	Investigative Genetic Genealogy
IQ	Intelligence Quotient
ISAG	International Society for Animal Genetics
ISSR	Inter Simple Sequence Repeat
JDTC	Juvenile Drug Treatment Courts
LC-MS/MS	Liquid Chromatography-Tandem Mass Spectrometry
LC-MS-MS	Liquid Chromatography Paired with Tandem Mass Spectrometry
LSI-R	Level of Service Inventory-Revised
MIP	Molecularly Imprinted Polymer
MRT	Moral Reconation Therapy
MS	Mass Spectrometry
NFLIS	National Forensic Laboratory Information System
NGS	Next-Generation Sequencing
NPS	New Psychoactive Substances
NSO	Novel Synthetic Opioids
OP	Organophosphate Pesticide
PAD	Psychiatric Advance Directive
PCC	Poison Control Centers
PCP	Phencyclidine
PCR	Polymerase Chain Reaction
PFAS	Polyfluoroalkyl Substances
PGPR	Plant Growth Promoting Rhizobacteria
PSS	Peer Support Service

PVT	Performance Validity Test
RFLP	Restriction Fragment Length Polymorphism
ROS	Reactive Oxygen Species
SARC	Sexual Assault Referral Centre
SCRA	Synthetic Cannabinoid Receptor Agonist
SDM	Shared Decision Making
SDS	Safety Data Sheets
SEM	Scanning Electron Microscopy
SMAC	Spacecraft Maximum Allowable Concentration
SNP	Single Nucleotide Polymorphism
SRH	Sexual and Reproductive Health
START	Short-Term Assessment of Risk and Treatability
STR	Short Tandem Repeats
SVT	Symptom Validity Test
TLC	Thin Layer Chromatography
TTT	Training the Trainer
UHPLC	Ultra-High-Performance Liquid Chromatography
VAWH	Violence Against Women's Health
WBE	Wastewater-Based Epidemiology
XAI	Explainable AI
XRF	X-Ray Fluorescence

PREFACE

Toxicology and forensic medicine utilize medical science to address questions raised in legal and investigative contexts. The field unites clinical practice, laboratory science, and the judicial system to understand causes of injury, illness, and death. This book focuses on cases and situations where evidence from the human body and its reaction to injury or poisoning can help answer questions regarding responsibility, intent, and care. The readers will learn how medical results guide inquiry into sexual violence, reproductive health issues, mental health assessments, poisoning in all its forms, trends in misuse of substances, and the application of biotechnology in identification. These subjects highlight the diversity of problems professionals encounter when operating at the intersection of health and law.

Within this volume of *Forensic Medicine and Toxicology*, every chapter focuses on a specific branch of practice, providing thorough descriptions of the principles, procedures, and equipment used by practitioners. Based on prevailing standards, research evidence, and case illustrations, the book offers well-defined instruction on the collection, interpretation, and presentation of medical and toxicological evidence.

The first chapter investigates sexual offences with medical examination of victims and suspects, documentation of injuries, interpretation of trace evidence, and expert testimony in the courtroom. It describes how the timing of assault must be established, consent issues examined, and sensitive examinations conducted with respect for the person and for the law. The second chapter addresses reproductive health in forensic settings—evaluating assertions of virginity, monitoring pregnancy, and conception timing, and analyzing delivery outcomes. Techniques for determining gestational age and differentiating between spontaneous and induced deliveries are explained comprehensively.

The third chapter introduces forensic psychiatry, discussing competency assessment procedures, criminal responsibility evaluations, violence risk appraisal, and the application of standardized rating scales. It covers legal concepts of insanity and diminished capacity, and discusses the ethical issues that arise when psychiatric evidence impacts legal decisions. The fourth chapter introduces general toxicology and describes principles of toxin absorption, distribution, metabolism, and excretion. It outlines sampling methodologies, laboratory analyzes, and interpreting concentration data in blood, urine, and tissues.

The subsequent four chapters examine categories of poisons. The fifth chapter deals with corrosive chemicals—alkalis and acids—and states their action on the skin, mucous membrane, and organs. Emergency management, sampling of gastrointestinal contents, and distinguishing between chemical burns and other types of damage are covered in the guidance. The sixth chapter is on metallic toxins like lead, mercury, arsenic, and thallium. It provides information on routes of exposure, clinical features, analytical techniques for detecting them, and criteria for determining toxicity. The seventh chapter addresses neurotoxic agents—organophosphates, certain industrial chemicals, and plant neurotoxins—describing the mechanisms by which they disrupt nerve function and the laboratory tests used to establish exposure. The eighth chapter considers cardiotoxic and miscellaneous poisons, including abused drugs that impair cardiac conduction, as well as less frequently encountered substances that cause diverse systemic effects.

The ninth chapter covers substance abuse, describing the techniques for the detection of alcohol, illegal drugs, and prescription drugs in biological samples. It provides procedures for interpreting screening and confirmatory tests, postmortem redistribution considerations, and methods for quantifying impairment. The tenth chapter discusses DNA fingerprinting and biotechnology, describing molecular methods applied to human identification, paternity testing, and genetic marker analysis in wildlife forensics. The book describes laboratory quality controls, chain-of-custody requirements, and reporting standards.

The last two chapters are about professional practice. Chapter 11 addresses medical ethics and professional behavior, covering topics such as confidentiality, informed consent, conflict of interest, and reporting obligations. It offers case illustrations of ethical problems and guidelines for resolving them. Chapter 12 looks at consent in clinical practice, highlighting how competent consent is secured, recorded, and contested within the forensic context. It addresses consent to examination of minors, incapacitated adults, and in cases where consent is granted by legal guardians or under court order.

The text is intended for forensic pathologists, toxicologists, psychiatrists, and laboratory scientists who need an updated reference for casework and expert testimony. It will also benefit medical examiners, coroners, and clinicians who have medicolegal issues in emergency and hospital practice. Law enforcement officers and lawyers can benefit from clear, easy-to-understand descriptions of medical and scientific techniques when preparing for investigations or court proceedings. Forensic science students and postgraduate trainees in forensic professions will find helpful the applied advice, step-by-step procedures, and end-of-chapter review questions. By covering both theoretical principles and practical methods, this book aims to facilitate correct, trustworthy, and ethical practice across the diverse careers that comprise the discipline of forensic medicine and toxicology.

SEXUAL OFFENCES IN FORENSIC MEDICINE AND TOXICOLOGY

1

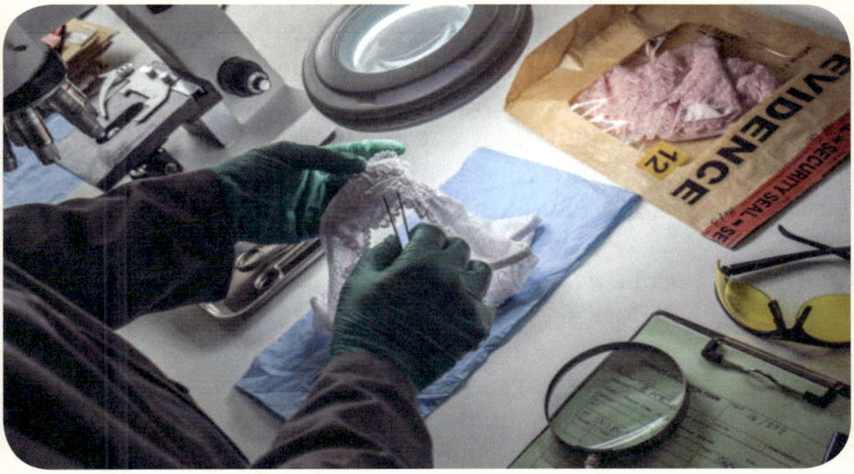

LEARNING OBJECTIVES

After studying this chapter, you will be able to:

1. Identify types of sexual offences
2. Explain forensic examination in sexual offences
3. Learn toxicology in sexual offences
4. Identify the legal framework and challenges

Introduction

Forensic science and sexuality blend in ways that have long fascinated us. We tend to laud intimacy, but its shadowy counterpart—sexual crimes—causes many legal and medical professionals to grope in the dark. In most instances, the waves from sexual violence strike victims and communities forcefully; their impact appears in unanticipated guises. Some recent reports have raised disquieting figures that emphatically point toward greater forensic inquiry. For instance, case studies of intimate partner violence in Bangladesh identify the importance of increasing efforts in forensic medicine and toxicology (Roy et al., 2023). Artificial intelligence is becoming a part of the equation, raising the possibility of improved assessments and better-targeted interventions in these complex cases, and opening the way to more straightforward understanding and prevention protocols (Piraianu et al., 2023). Overall, an examination of sexual offences from a forensic perspective is still something both timely and essential.

Definition of Sexual Offences

Legal frameworks for sexual offenses are complicated and require careful examination—it is not simply definitions but how each detail is handled. In forensic medicine and toxicology, it is essential to have clear definitions, as they directly guide how evidence is collected and subsequently analyzed. Law enforcement and healthcare professionals are also frequently allied, working in cooperation that blurs boundaries but where each maintains distinct ground. Take Sexual Assault Referral Centers (SARCs) for instance—they kick off investigations by providing healthcare and support while diligently gathering forensic evidence, and in numerous cases, they actually get things underway. Each stage of an investigation—from that initial response through to ultimate court proceedings—is governed by legal frameworks that categorize different crimes into tidy boxes; this even extends to instances such as drug-facilitated sexual assault (DFSA), which typically requires specialized forensic approaches (Dawnay et al., 2023). In the majority of cases, the manner in which we delineate sexual offences not only determines legal results but also ends up shaping the very approaches forensic teams use to reconstruct a case (Markwerth et al., 2020) (Figure 1.1).

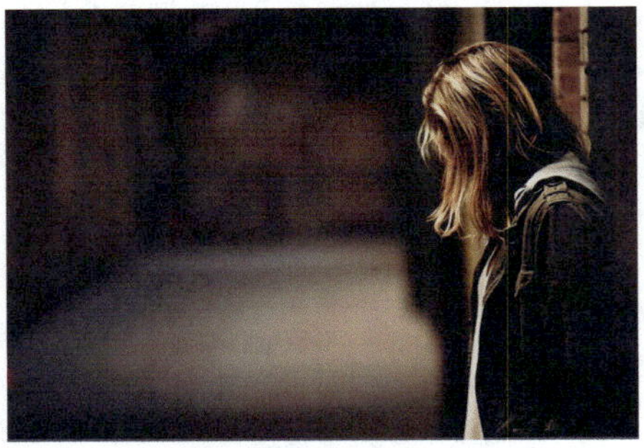

Figure 1.1. Sexual offences.

Source: Sanity.io. (n.d.). *Person Leaning Against a Wall in a Dimly Lit Urban Environment*. https://cdn.sanity.io/images/akxw9u2m/production/16b01f686c0a074e13c345cc15da4d30aeb7b792-6000x4000.jpg?w=2048&fm=webp.

Importance of Forensic Medicine in Sexual Offences

Sexual crimes are not merely a matter of identifying the suspect—meticulous documentation of injuries and other details in forensics has a massive influence on determining court verdicts and dictating how survivors are assisted. Thorough records of injuries can actually help a victim's credibility in court, as unambiguous physical evidence tends to increase the chances of a conviction. Generally speaking, studies suggest that while DNA evidence is essential to confirm an assault, visible injuries tend to carry more weight in legal settings—especially in areas like South Africa, where non-intimate partner rapes are alarmingly frequent (Cupido et al., 2014). Looking back at past practices sheds valuable light on today's approaches; a peek into historical records shows that earlier methods of understanding sexual crimes still inform now. A reading of past medical and legal reports in England is illustrative of how physicians have, over the years, married changing concepts with legal definitions of sexual offenders, paving the way for more sophisticated, individualized intervention to these serious crimes (Weston et al., 2025).

Role of Toxicology in Sexual Assault Cases

Sexual assault cases can be messy—they take a combination of biological evidence and chemical residues, with toxicology generally being the key to the whole thing. When victims become incapacitated due to alcohol or drugs, reports from toxicology become instrumental in reconstructing what occurred and how bad the assault was. Forensic toxicology tends to be good at identifying substances that impair one's judgment or prevent them from being able to provide consent clearly, which in most instances corroborates the account given by the victim. Waiting for a very long time to have a medico-legal examination has been known to result in missing out on such key evidence, such as semen or traces of drugs remaining in the body, hence confusing the criminal justice process (Kumar et al., 2014). Moreover, whereas a potency test for the suspect is still necessary under Indian law, its need is mostly contested today because contemporary legal standards no longer require unique acts to qualify a case as rape (Jaiswal et al., 2016). Overall, this changing legal landscape effectively illustrates the importance of toxicology in aiding the provision of justice for victims (Figure 1.2).

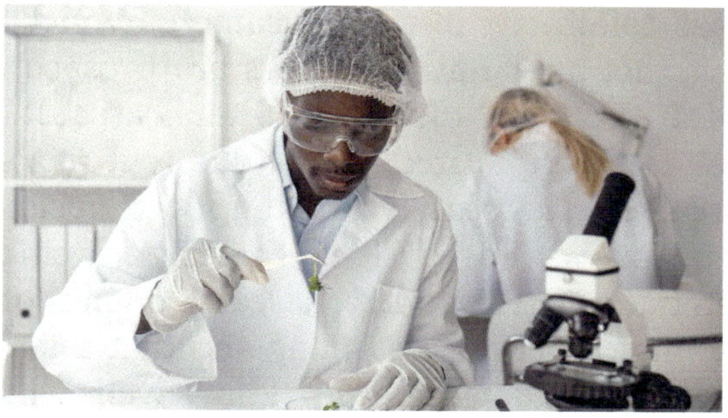

Figure 1.2. Role of toxicology in sexual assault cases.

Source: LinkedIn. (n.d.). *Scientist Examining Plant Sample in Laboratory.* https://media.licdn.com/dms/image/v2/D4D12AQEv_ouHXoKbZQ/article-cover_image-shrink_720_1280/article-cover_image-shrink_720_1280/0/1732287164693?e=2147483647&v=beta&t=U8Ws0x2Fgd_io1Ys8f8vHd3aLoH4Hpk2UhHssqgc8fo.

Overview of the Legal Implications

DNA helps a great deal in handling cases of sexual offence. In Zambia, for instance, there isn't always a consistent pattern in gathering forensic proof, which actually hinders prosecutors from constructing a case. Examining previous cases reveals that DNA data is rarely utilized, despite the fact that it often supports witness accounts and narrows down the suspects in most situations (Makasa et al., 2017). Between 2010 and 2012, only 39% of defilement cases reached court, with convictions hitting an all-time low of just 13%. Over in South Africa, although they place a high premium on recording physical injuries, they still manage to find that without DNA as evidence, it is nearly impossible to establish that there was a sexual act, and this contributes to the knotted problem of consent (Cupido et al., 2014). Overall, these hybrid methods fairly clearly indicate a demand for improved forensic procedures toto enhance judicial results in sexual offence cases genuinely.

Historical Context of Sexual Offences

Forensic medicine evolved in ways that altered our understanding of sexual offences while reflecting shifts within society and the law. In the past, such offences were often dismissed or misrepresented, leaving victims without the assistance they actually needed. Following the war, forensic journals exhibited an intriguing shift – a decline in fields such as forensic psychiatry and psychology. In contrast, interest in forensic genetics and scientific examinations skyrocketed (Wirth et al., 2022). This shift, in the majority of instances, indicates how the discipline included increased use of scientific techniques and emerging technology, so that work to analyze sexual crimes was much more complex. Between 1970 and 1990, research in sexual medicine split further, suggesting an increasing awareness of subtlety that is reflected in growing global contributions to forensic literature (Schmeling et al., 2023). Overall, this snapshot of the past highlights both the entrenched difficulties and the gradual improvement in the way sexual offences are investigated today.

Current Trends in Sexual Offences

Patterns of substance misuse have altered radically, and these are an unanticipated driving force for much of today's sexual offending. Emerging psychoactive substances are appearing in ways that confuse our traditional notions of drug use while changing the character of associated criminal activity. The Advisory Council on the Misuse of Drugs (ACMD) has, for instance, highlighted that drugs such as mephedrone appear to be associated with increased sexual violence and episodes of skewed decision-making among those consuming them. Similarly, the expansion of new benzodiazepines takes us into new territory—these are drugs vulnerable to abuse and linked to sexual crime, and they unmistakably demand urgent legislative action. Overall, the combination of drug abuse and sexual violence represents a serious issue in fields like forensic medicine and toxicology, calling for a multidisciplinary public health response to reduce risks and improve victim support in an ever-changing environment.

1.1. Types of Sexual Offences

Learning Outcome

1. Understand rape and its legal definitions
2. Discuss sexual assault and harassment
3. Know child sexual abuse
4. Explain consent and its complexities
5. Learn statutory rape laws
6. Identify online sexual offences
7. Focus on human trafficking and sexual exploitation
8. Describe domestic violence and sexual offences
9. Know cultural variations in defining sexual offences

Sexual crimes are not an easy issue—they exist in so many different guises, and forensic medicine and toxicology units often have to intervene to sort out the mess. Research tends to indicate that young women, particularly those from poorer backgrounds, are most affected; many of the cases involve victims aged between 11 and 20 (Rani et al., 2020). It is noteworthy to observe that almost all reported cases—approximately 97%—have victims who already knew the perpetrator (Patra et al., 2015), only increasing the intricacies of consent and coercion. Crimes such as abduction with rape appear quite frequently, suggesting there is indeed a need to educate vulnerable groups about their rights under the law and the true meaning of such acts. When you actually go deep into these particular categories of offences, you begin to notice the knotted social arrangements involved—and that, in most instances, requires superior, more anticipatory preventive tactics.

1.1.1. Rape and Its Legal Definitions

Legal definitions of rape become entwined in ways that alter how offenders are prosecuted and victims are cared for. Sexual assault in itself is a complicated affair—different regions perceive and treat it in their own peculiar manners, so it is difficult to assign a single methodology (Figure 1.3). Research often shows that many victims are young and that a lot of cases occur in places they know well, which hints that these painful events usually take place among close people (Bhoi et al., 2017).

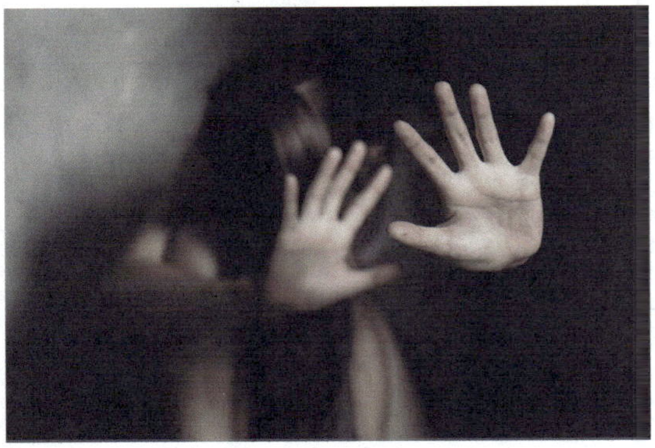

Figure 1.3. Sexual assault itself is a tricky issue—different places see and handle it in their own odd ways, so it is hard to pin down one single approach.

Source: Lawsuit Legal News. (2023). *Rideshare Sexual Assault Lawyer.*

In the context of forensic medicine, it is clear that having straightforward guidelines is crucial, as these rules form the basis for the medical checks carried out by certified doctors (Malik, 2017). Strong legal principles benefit more than just convictions; they create a sense of community where victims can more easily come forward. Briefly, taking a revised glance at and fine-tuning these definitions remains a pivotal step if we are to actually achieve justice in sexual offense cases.

1.1.2. Sexual Assault and Harassment

Sex crimes nowadays are so complex that we actually have to go into all their various facets—this is particularly the case for topics related to forensic medicine and toxicology (Figure 1.4). Of particular concern is a new trend, Drug-Facilitated Sexual Assault (DFSA); in this, psychotropic drugs are utilized to incapacitate victims enough that they cannot resist sexual abuse.

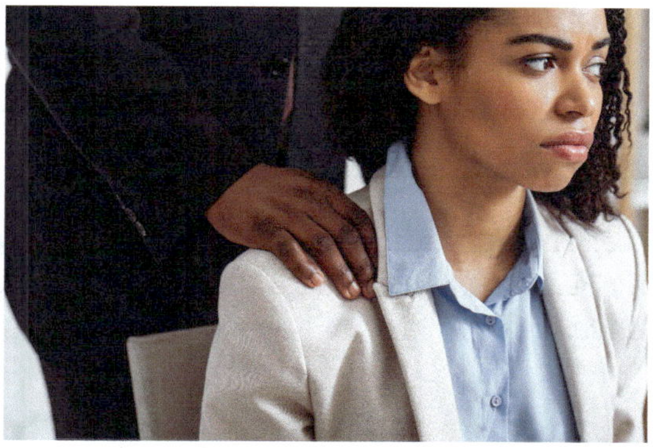

Figure 1.4. Sexual assault and harassment.

Source: Inspired eLearning. (2021). *Sexual Harassment vs. Sexual Assault.*

Also referred to by some as Chemical Submission (CS), the strategy demonstrates how manipulative these crimes are—criminals exploit the volatile situation brought about by the drugs. To be fully aware of DFSA is not just to follow the frequency with which these incidents have increased, but to appreciate who becomes the victim and who the perpetrators are, more often than not. There are evident clinical indications that can lead towards potential victimization, making the urgent conduct of toxicology tests immediately when symptoms of CS arise very significant (Alías et al., 2017). Ultimately, by investigating forensic information, the medical fraternity can play a crucial role in addressing pressing social issues.

1.1.3. Child Sexual Abuse

Child sexual abuse is a challenging subject that merits more than a cursory glance—it challenges us to delve deep into such areas as forensic medicine and toxicology (Figure 1.5). In most instances, knowing how frequently these abuses are committed and what they do is of significant importance because they severely impact the physical and emotional well-being of young victims.

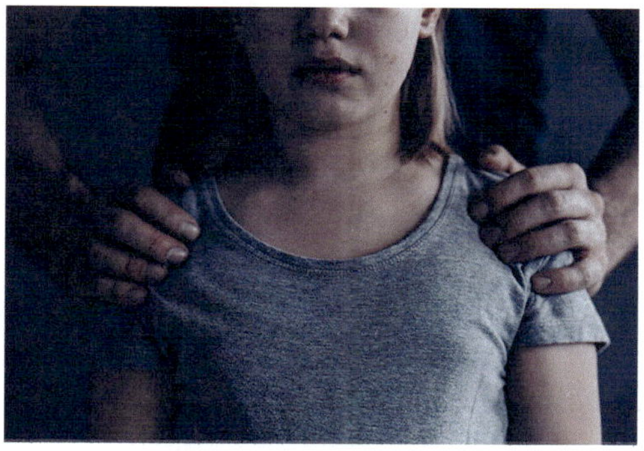

Figure 1.5. Child sexual abuse.

Source: Child Protection Company. (2018). *Child Sexual Abuse.*

Recent research in forensic genetics, as reported in several studies, has largely altered the approach to collecting and analyzing evidence in sensitive matters (Schmeling et al., 2023). Meanwhile, it appears that there has been a decline in forensic psychiatry research over recent decades despite the continued mental aftermath of child sexual abuse remaining in the limelight for researchers (Wirth et al., 2022). By interlacing evidence from both forensic science and psychological understanding, professionals are gradually constructing intervention measures that not only address immediate health concerns but also help pave the way for long-term recovery. This blended method—and yes, it is far from ideal—actually emphasizes that cooperation among various fields is crucial when addressing such a complex issue.

1.1.4. Consent and Its Complexities

Sex crimes are not so simple a yes or no—these are a tangled web of consciousness, desire, and consent, which tends to get confused frequently, particularly with children and other vulnerable populations. Research informs us, in most instances, that most young victims do not even have a picture of what truly constitutes consent; for example, research indicates merely 67% appear to understand much about rape (Rahman et al., 2024). This is not simply a narrow gap—it interferes with their capacity for informed decision-making and makes them vulnerable to coercion and manipulation. Matters become even further knotted when the offenders happen to be relatives or known individuals (Roy et al., 2023), introducing yet another turn in the theme of consent and victimization. All of these areas of overlap indicate, quite strongly, the necessity for improved, more direct educational programs to explain consent. Meeting these challenges is therefore essential if we wish to make our communities safer for all.

1.1.5. Statutory Rape Laws

Sexual offenses against children are a complicated matter that truly calls for a strict legal system, one that considers squarely the concepts of consent and exploitation. Statutory rape statutes, for instance, tend to shield adolescents who cannot yet provide actual informed consent. In most instances, any sexual activity with them is considered criminal regardless of the circumstances. There is a good bit of back-and-forth on whether these rules work as intended, especially when you check out the startling figures on sexual offences; some reports even point to distressingly high rates that hint at a public health crisis affecting vulnerable groups like women and children (Gitanjali et al., 2011). In countries like Zambia, the lack of proper prosecution of cases of defilement serves as a testament to why enforcing such laws is crucial if we desire a legal system that truly prioritizes the protection of victims and accountability (Figure 1.6).

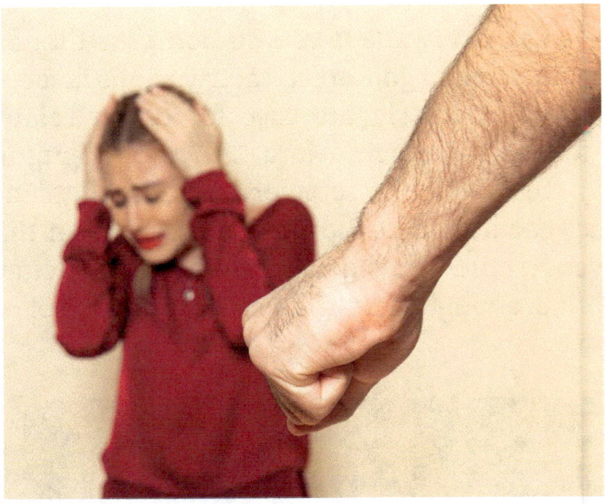

Figure 1.6. Statutory rape laws.

Source: The Fernandez Firm. (2023). *Front View Young Female in Red Shirt Suffers from Physical Violence.*

1.1.6. Online Sexual Offences

Online sexual crimes have become increasingly complex as online platforms proliferate at dizzying rates. Perpetrators manipulate trust and operate under the veil of anonymity, committing crimes such as cyberstalking, online grooming, and sending explicit content without permission. Such acts usually cause profound psychological damage to victims—a nightmare complicated further by difficulties in accurately documenting and prosecuting these offenses. Consider, for example, DFSA; in most cases, the combination of toxicology and forensic medicine becomes essential, as proper investigations can provide the information regarding which drugs were used to render victims incapacitated in the real world as well as online (Amzat et al., 2023). In most instances, there is a strong appeal for professional expertise—developing solid training materials for forensic nurses, for example, can significantly aid them in navigating these complex matters and assisting victims more effectively (Yesodharan et al., 2022).

1.1.7. Human Trafficking and Sexual Exploitation

Human trafficking is a challenging puzzle that is not only difficult for law enforcement to figure out, but also throws curveballs at people working in forensic medicine and toxicology (Figure 1.7). Victims do serious physical injury and heavy psychological damage, which typically means every forensic screen requires a close, sometimes even patient, examination of what they are actually experiencing.

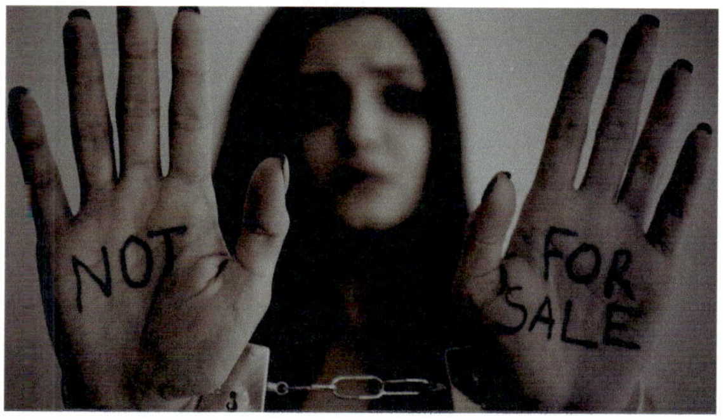

Figure 1.7. Human trafficking.

Source: Santa Clara Valley Transportation Authority. (2022). *Sex Trafficking Lawyers.*

In most cases, sexual exploitation creeps into the equation with forensic examination—this is particularly crucial when specialists are attempting to reconstruct definite evidence of abuse or identify the substances that may have been utilized to coerce an individual. A thorough examination can at times reveal traces of drug use, and these clues can contribute significantly to knowing how the abuse occurred.

Forensic specialists, quite frankly, must be aware of how signs of trafficking and exploitation show up both on the body and in a person's behavior; these clues often overlap in unexpected ways. Recent reports (Tennessee Bureau of Investigation, 2017) suggest that, in most cases, forensic experts and social services must joincollaborate to support survivors and address the aftermath of these troubling issues.

1.1.8. Domestic Violence and Sexual Offences

Drugs spoil the works of home life with their own kind of messing with domestic violence and sexual crimes in a manner that disturbs the entire scenario. Drugs are frequently blamed for ratcheting up violent acts and driving people towards criminal activities, which only creates already weak home situations even more dangerous (Sharma et al., 2019).

Women and children, especially, end up locked into these perpetuating cycles of abuse—alcohol/drug problems only lead to more negative patterns repeating themselves. Oftentimes, being under the influence majorly screws up one's normal thinking processes, so bad decisions result in critical consequences such as rape, a crime that, sadly, appears on the increase in the world overall (Gitanjali et al., 2011). There is also a knotted web of social stigma and a paucity of support structures, whereby incidents often come to light late and, consequently, medical tests and legal procedures become disorganized. Speaking in general, an easy, no-nonsense understanding of all these forces is quite vital to forensic workers endeavoring to contain and mitigate the effects of domestic violence and sexual crime (Figure 1.8).

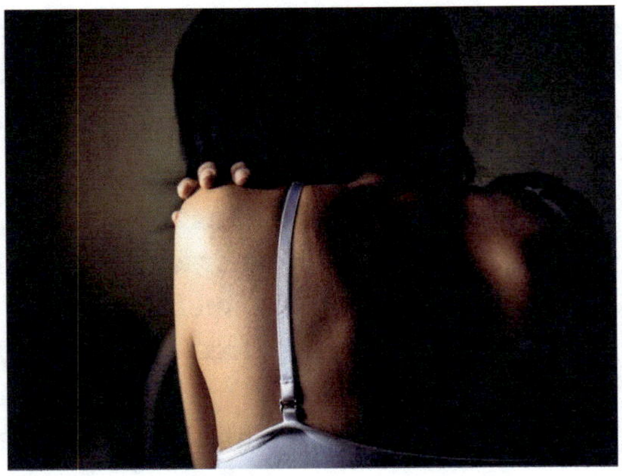

Figure 1.8. Domestic violence and sexual offences.

Source: Shutterstock. (n.d.). Sexual assault survivor. *Patch*. https://patch.com/img/cdn20/shutterstock/22880692/20190708/062252/styles/patch_image/public/shutterstock-617496536__08182222777.jpg.

1.1.9. Cultural Variations in Defining Sexual Offences

Various communities perceive sexual crimes in ways that tend to confuse legal systems and forensic examinations. Cultural norms, religious principles, and ordinary attitudes ultimately determine what constitutes a criminal offense – and, in most instances, this determines whether victims report cases and how promptly authorities intervene. Consider marital rape: in one community, it is regarded as a non-crime, while in another, it is punished as a serious crime that merits actual legal repercussions. This sort of dichotomy, in general, effectively conveys that a more culturally attuned response in forensic toxicology and medicine is required—after all, the legal terminology we employ tends to dictate how evidence is collected and investigations are conducted. And research (such as studies on AAS abuse and its connection with risk behaviors) also reveals that cultural narratives may have a profound impact on both the frequency and the public attitudes towards such crimes (Lood, 2021; Kennedy et al., 2023).

Test Your Knowledge

1. What are the different types of sexual offences recognized under forensic and legal frameworks?
2. What is statutory rape, and how is it different from other forms of rape?

1.2. Forensic Examination in Sexual Offences

Learning Outcome

1. Explain the role of forensic medical examiners
2. A thorough collection of evidence from victims
3. Describe the chain of custody in forensic evidence
4. Understand the importance of a timely medical examination
5. Focus on the use of DNA evidence in sexual offences
6. Learn psychological evaluation of victims
7. Discuss documentation and reporting procedures
8. Identify challenges in forensic examinations
9. Explain case studies highlighting forensic findings

For sexual crimes, there is an interconnected set of difficulties that requires more than a single strategy, but a combination of various methods. A good forensic interview looks beyond DNA and physical evidence—it also examines the emotional and social consequences that linger after the act. Current research suggests that these medical exams are crucial in reconstructing what actually occurred, even under less-than-ideal conditions.

However, inadequate legal directives regarding forensic work can sometimes hinder the proper utilization of this information in court. Redesigning forensic labs—perhaps restructuring them to be more accessible and effective—could unlock the maximum value from expert opinion in these investigations. Overall, the gradual, continuous development we're seeing in forensic procedures demonstrates an actual dedication towards refining techniques that maintain legal investigations both strong and equitable (Schmeling et al., 2023).

1.2.1. Role of Forensic Medical Examiners

Sexual offenses pose a network of challenges that require the applied expertise of forensic medical examiners (Figure 1.9). These professionals conduct thorough examinations to gather physical evidence, which, in most cases, plays a critical role in determining the outcome of an investigation. In Zambia, for example, a study (Makasa et al., 2017) found that although sexual abuse occurs at high rates, forensic DNA analysis has played only a limited role in matching identities or supporting witness testimonies. This modest use of forensic methods not only suggests that such techniques are frequently undervalued but also underscores the pressing need for standardized clinical protocols. As Clinical Forensic Medicine evolves, examiners —experts in integrating precise medical reports with legal knowledge —clearly demonstrate why expertly trained professionals are invaluable in upholding both the integrity and effectiveness of sexual offence investigations (Barrett, 2025).

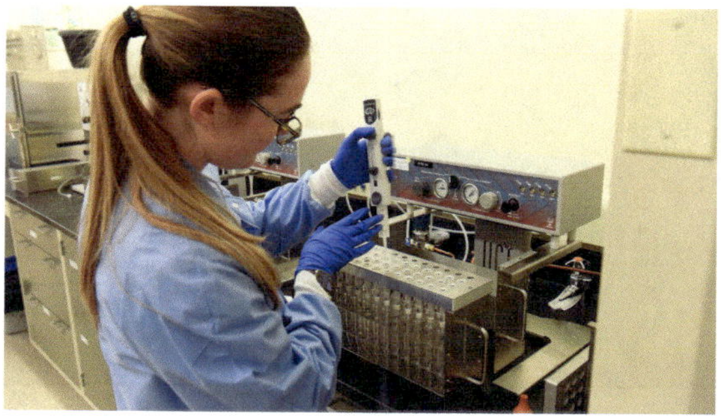

Figure 1.9. Role of forensic medical examiners.

Source: Defense Health Agency. (n.d.). *Forensic Toxicology Laboratory Testing*. https://dha.mil/-/media/Project/Images/ForTox.JPG.

1.2.2. Collection of Evidence from Victims

Sexual crimes leave a lot of mess, and one significant aspect of cleaning things up is rapidly gathering evidence from victims—one step that is actually central to forensic medicine and toxicology (Figure 1.10). Statistics typically indicate that the majority of the victims tend to be young and predominantly within the ages of 15 to 25 years, and by and large, most of them are unmarried and from poorer backgrounds (Samad et al., 2023). And occasionally, when evidence is not collected within 48 hours, matters become even more complicated – details provided about penetration do not typically correlate with what is found in the lab, which subsequently complicates the process of bringing offenders to court (Samad et al., 2023). It also usually happens that the perpetrator is familiar to the victim, providing yet another emotional and psychological burden that they may not be prepared to face. In total, having a structured, albeit somewhat loose, method of evidence gathering not only enhances legal systems but also demands improved social sensitivity and safeguards.

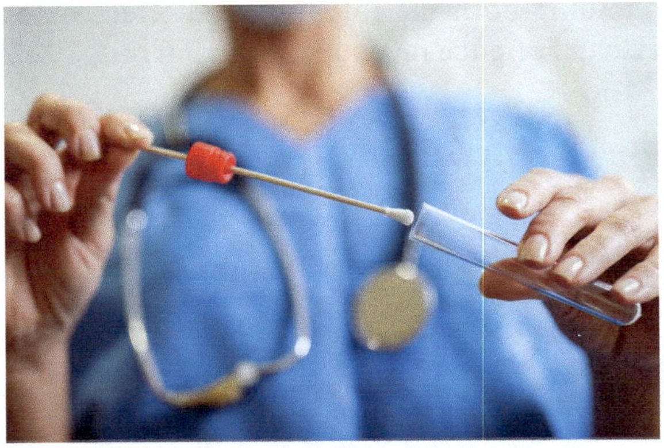

Figure 1.10. Collection of evidence from victims.

Source: Taylor & Ring. (2024). *The Role of Forensic Nurses in Sexual Assault Cases.*

1.2.3. Chain of Custody in Forensic Evidence

Forensic evidence relies heavily on maintaining the chain of custody – without that detailed record, anything collected during a sexual offense investigation may not stand up in court. Consider this: in cases like DFSA, having those potentially toxic samples (blood, urine, etc.) appropriately processed truly comes into play, since even the most minor error can ruin the entire outcome. More often than not, emergency doctors and forensic groups must collaborate closely; if they make even a slight miscalculation, vital biological information can be lost, rendering the evidence useless for future use. A well-documented chain not only increases the credibility of the evidence but also enhances the overall credibility of the investigative process – providing victims with appropriate care and ensuring that justice is served (Marc, 2008; Malik, 2017). In total, adhering to stern evidence-handling procedures is fundamentally crucial in forensic medicine in handling sexual crimes.

1.2.4. Importance of Timely Medical Examination

Following a sex crime, obtaining medical attention immediately really counts. Quick examinations are not only about repairing injuries—they also catch vital clues before they're gone. In instances where physical injury is apparent, early tests can catch DNA evidence that might tip the balance for both identification and prosecution of the perpetrator. Research indicates that most cases, particularly those of defilement, often remain in the courts since there is insufficient concrete evidence; for instance, one study cited that there were only 14 cases that were upheld by forensic samples, which, of course, resulted in fewer convictions (Makasa et al., 2017). Rapid checks do not only document bodily impacts but also provide some badly needed psychological comfort to sufferers, assisting them in initiating the healing process (Rural Support Programs Network, 2019). Provided that medical treatment is delayed, however, the opportunity to gather valuable evidence diminishes drastically, ultimately hindering a fair judicial process (Figure 1.11).

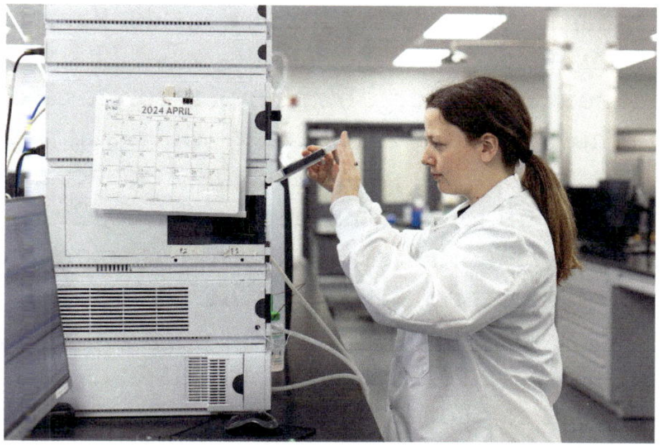

Figure 1.11. Importance of timely medical examination.

Source: Center for Forensic Science Research and Education. (2024). *Laboratory Toxicology Research*.

1.2.5. Use of DNA Evidence in Sexual Offences

With sexual offences, you tend to find a motley crew of agencies collaborating—each contributing their role to ensure forensic evidence is gathered and analyzed with care. DNA evidence becomes a genuine fulcrum in such instances, employed to target suspects and substantiate allegations in ways that, for the most part, cannot be ignored. It all typically begins at Sexual Assault Referral Centers (SARCs), where expert staff step in to assist victims promptly while collecting biological samples with utmost care. Such hands-on interventions clearly demonstrate how effective forensic work can drive justice forward – consider the advancements in DNA profiling that aided the exoneration of wrongly accused individuals in Ghana (Amankwaa et al., 2019). The entire journey—from collecting evidence to putting it forth in court—is scrutinized, in general, and that puts pressure on everyone to construct a solid setup combining legal, medical, and scientific understanding to keep DNA analysis on course in cases of sexual assault (Dawnay et al., 2023).

1.2.6. Psychological Evaluation of Victims

Sexual crimes have a profound psychological impact that not only disrupts the process of healing but also clouds the legal process that follows. Survivors might end up coping with a hand-me-down assortment of things such as anxiety, depression, and even symptoms of post-traumatic stress disorder—in some cases all at once, in others migrating later. Research tends to indicate that many of these individuals fail to follow through on the care they require, perhaps due to stigma or the availability of resources; only about one in three receives adequate support after assault (Choi et al., 2019). It should be kept in mind that factors such as someone's age or the extent to which they were involved with the perpetrator can actually influence the way recovery goes and the possibilities of receiving assistance. Researchers also observed that aggressive and paranoid behavior—characteristics commonly seen among offenders—may resonate with the harsh environments in which the incidents take place (Emamhadi et al., 2012). Overall, detailed psychological assessments do appear to have an important role to play, not only in facilitating survivors' return to recovery but also in influencing action to avoid subsequent issues in forensic settings.

1.2.7. Documentation and Reporting Procedures

In forensic toxicology and medicine, good record-keeping is absolutely critical when dealing with sexual offenses. Precise files are the foundation for legal actions – they ensure that evidence is stored safely, thoroughly analyzed, and on hand when required. Sometimes, adhering to standard procedures is more difficult than anticipated, particularly in extreme circumstances such as armed conflicts. On a general note, it is evident that clinical competence is of great importance; numerous medical students demonstrate varying levels of competency in forensic methods applied to these cases (Shrestha et al., 2022). Thorough note-taking not only paves the way for an unbiased investigation, but it also reveals loopholes in the legal guidelines that regulate forensic operations. Overall, sound reporting practices, when they are properly functioning, enhance the credibility of forensic findings and ultimately contribute to driving forward the pursuit of justice for victims of sexual offenses (Figure 1.12).

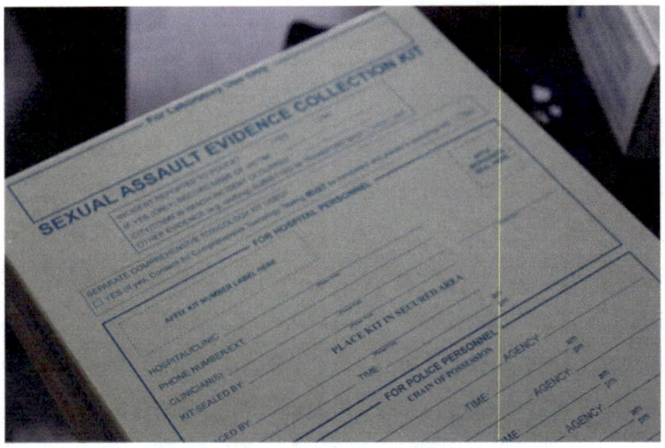

Figure 1.12. Accurate files serve as the bedrock for legal moves – they help ensure that evidence is kept safe, carefully examined, and available when needed.

Source: Greenfield, R. (2023). Sexual assault evidence collection kit. *MassLive*.

1.2.8. Challenges in Forensic Examinations

Forensic medicine, particularly in the case of sexual offence, has numerous stumbling blocks to deal with. Merging medical work with detective-like focus is the essence of serving justice. Still, such indispensable fusion is often relegated to an afterthought—most places present evidence collection protocols that simply fail to meet the standards (Verma et al., 2023). Consider Zambia, for instance: as a general rule, there is a vast gulf between the large number of reported cases and how few ever reach court, which suggests entrenched problems in managing evidence and standing up for victims (Makasa et al., 2017). Cases frequently rely on witness memory rather than forensic DNA—when taken at all, often done so poorly—that not only depresses conviction rates but also clearly demonstrates the need for conventional, uniform protocols. Overall, addressing these lingering issues is crucial if forensic tests are ever to become more dependable and produce fairer results in such sensitive cases.

1.2.9. Case Studies Highlighting Forensic Findings

Case studies provide us with a true window into the operational realities of probing sexual crimes. A survey from Himachal Pradesh, for instance, revealed that about 68.56% of cases constituted either blatant coercion or what can be labeled as dubious consensual encounters – and, all things being equal, delays in medico-legal examinations habitually ruin the timely collection of essential biological samples such as spermatozoa and semen (Kumar et al., 2014). Back in Mumbai, studies determined that the majority of victims were young, unmarried women aged 16 to 20; however, interestingly enough, the perpetrator was most often someone that they knew (Haridas et al., 2016). Each of these instances quietly alludes not just to the disturbing rate of sexual violence but also to how important it is to obtain forensic evidence collected promptly—something which actually comes into play for legal results in cases of sexual assault.

Test Your Knowledge

1. What is the primary aim of a forensic examination in a case of alleged sexual assault?
2. What is the significance of conducting a forensic exam within 72 hours of the alleged offence?

1.3. Toxicology in Sexual Offences

Learning Outcome

1. Explain the role of toxicology in sexual assault cases
2. Identify common drugs used in sexual crimes
3. Perform detection of drugs in biological samples
4. Know the impact of alcohol on consent
5. Learn interpretation of toxicology reports
6. Know the limitations of toxicological analysis
7. Describe the legal implications of toxicology findings
8. Focus on case studies involving toxicology
9. Define future directions in forensic toxicology

Sexual crimes have a lot of underlying layers, and an understanding of toxicology helps in exploring such cases to a great extent. Analyzing victims' samples most of the time will reveal the presence of alcohol or drugs - elements that could have facilitated an assault or even caused it. In many cases, research has shown that postponing medico-legal tests can compromise the opportunity to identify crucial evidence, such as sperm cells or biochemical markers that indicate unwanted interactions (Kumar et al., 2014). It also happens that victim profiles often reveal they are pretty young—sometimes underage in many instances—which usually requires rapid, thorough toxicology tests (Haridas et al., 2016). In general, the incorporation of toxicology into forensic medicine not only advances the quest for justice among victims but also reveals larger issues presented by sexual violence to our societies.

1.3.1. Role of Toxicology in Sexual Assault Cases

Toxicology usually finds itself being that silent hero in sexual assault cases. It supplies the critical proof that truly determines the instances of way go—on both the investigative and later judicial levels. By identifying substances such as drugs and alcohol within a victim's body, these tests to support allegations that an individual was too intoxicated to consent, which, as one may observe, is paramount in many legal jurisdictions. Occasionally, when biological samples are not gathered promptly or properly, the entire case suffers. Research has established that a significant number of cases fail because forensic samples are not utilized optimally (Haridas et al., 2016). Additionally, when witness statements are somewhat incongruous or when evidence is almost non-existent, toxicology can serve as that crucial piece of corroborative evidence, potentially enhancing the chances of prosecution and even conviction (Makasa et al., 2017). Altogether, integrating toxicological evidence into sexual offence investigations is crucial to ensuring justice is served and that legal proceedings remain robust (Figure 1.13).

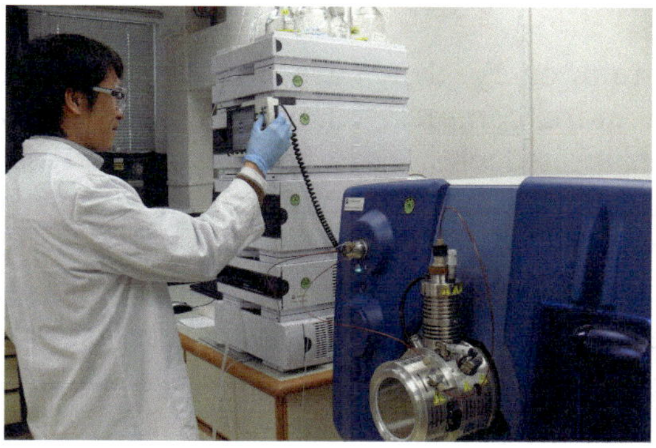

Figure 1.13. Toxicology often ends up being that unsung hero in sexual assault investigations.

Source: Government Technology Lab. (n.d.). *Fire Safety Design and Fire Testing*. https://www.govtlab.gov.hk/images/content/about_us/fsd/fts-1.jpg.

1.3.2. Common Drugs Used in Sexual Crimes

Drug use combined with sexual offenses is an emerging public health problem that truly deserves some scrutiny. Numerous studies broadly indicate that psychoactive drugs—particularly benzodiazepines and ethanol—are commonly used when offenders use them to incapacitate victims. One cross-sectional study in Cordoba, for instance, reported that all the victims were female and that a majority of cases were associated with individuals who were already familiar from social encounters. Ethanol was a predominant factor (Ruano-Segado et al., 2022). Khyber Medical College research also indicated that benzodiazepines emerged as the leading drug in such cases, highlighting their seemingly eerie power to incapacitate someone (Nadeem et al., 2024). The big picture is quite scary – the frequent abuse of these drugs not only makes forensic activity more difficult but also emphasizes the necessity for more societal awareness and aggressive prevention measures to combat this ongoing issue.

1.3.3. Detection of Drugs in Biological Samples

Contemporary drug use has become more and more complex, challenging us to create sophisticated methods for testing for the presence of drugs in biological material, particularly for sexual offenses. Today, with such a diverse assortment of psychoactive substances (including some entirely novel ones), it is pretty clear that accurate detection is crucial to maintaining both justice and public safety. In the majority of instances, the Advisory Council on the Misuse of Drugs (ACMD) emphasized that all should collaborate, even going as far as to recommend that vendors be partially responsible for establishing the safety of their merchandise. Laboratories in places such as Quebec have been at the forefront with new analysis methods for detecting these substances (Cimon et al., 2014). These technologies not only assist in determining what is available in a specimen but also increase the general capability of forensic examinations related to sexual crimes, ultimately aiding legal procedures and increasing victim protection. It can be said that whenever new challenges are faced, our approach must also continue to change (Figure 1.14).

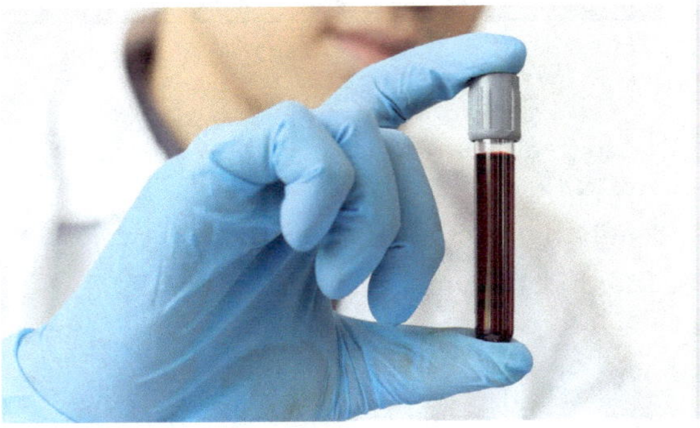

Figure 1.14. Detection of drugs in biological samples.

Source: LeBeau Forensic Toxicology Consulting. (2024). *Untitled Design 6.* https://lebeau-toxicology.com/wp-content/uploads/2024/06/Untitled-design-6.webp.

1.3.4. Impact of Alcohol on Consent

Sexual consent matters become complicated when alcohol is involved. When a person has been drinking, her or his capacity to utter a clear, voluntary yes suffers—a whole set of moral and legal problems follow. Alcohol makes people fuzzy in their thinking, decreases their self-discipline, and even makes it more difficult for a person to identify where their boundaries are, which makes it difficult to affirm that consent exists. Combining alcohol and sex only introduces another level of complexity for forensic analysis, causing it to become difficult at times to determine if an experience was actually consensual or not. There has been several studies into these unclear scenarios; for instance, one thorough survey of sexual assault investigations reveals that police and healthcare professionals must collaborate to gather and evaluate evidence (Dawnay et al., 2023). This type of collaborative work is particularly valuable in situations involving alcohol, as determining whether there was consent can sometimes be deceptively nuanced and frequently needs careful examination of the entire context of events (Schmeling et al., 2023).

1.3.5. Interpretation of Toxicology Reports

Sex crimes are plagued with issues, and toxicology reports have a significant role in revealing what truly happened. Such reports inform us whether alcohol, drugs, or other chemicals were present in the equation—things that could have clouded a victim's clear capacity for consent. Usually, the tests in the laboratory detect traces that can actually determine the course of a case. Adding DNA evidence to a case adds more credibility to a victim's testimony, strengthening the case as a whole. Studies usually demonstrate that, for the majority of cases, an intelligent combination of forensic evidence can increase prosecution rates—particularly in those regions where cases tend to go underreported and convictions are low, such as Zambia, where barely a small fraction of cases ever see the inside of a courtroom (Makasa et al., 2017). And as more new psychoactive substances (NPS) emerge, it is increasingly crucial for forensic practitioners to stay on top of toxicology so that legal practices can respond to such new challenges (Figure 1.15).

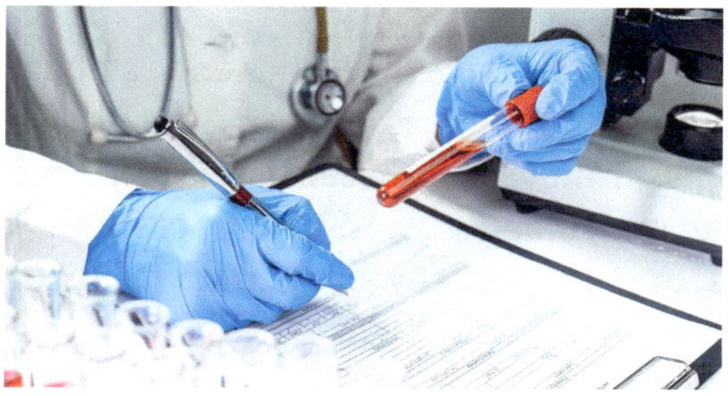

Figure 1.15. Interpretation of toxicology reports.

Source: American Academy of Forensic Sciences. (n.d.). *AdobeStock_319612966*. https://www.aafs.org/sites/default/files/styles/og_image/public/media/images/AdobeStock_319612966.jpeg?itok=tAekZVrE.

1.3.6. Limitations of Toxicological Analysis

Forensic analysis of sexual crimes meets actual difficulties when it deals with toxicology, and these challenges can determine court verdicts in ways that are not always predictable. Identifying and quantifying the mixture of biological and chemical compounds is essential—but individual differences in metabolism, the precise time frame over which drugs were administered, and natural degradation of evidence all combine to complicate matters. Several reviews suggest that groups comprising healthcare professionals, forensic specialists, and others should collaborate, and this collaboration—although necessary—may occasionally lead to misinterpretations at various points (Dawnay et al., 2023). In retrospect, changes in political and scientific ideology tend to alter the quality of toxicological results, which in turn restricts the effectiveness of forensic analysis in obtaining justice (Wirth et al., 2022).

1.3.7. Legal Implications of Toxicology Findings

Sexual crimes can be a genuine mess, so having a legal system that blends in chemical test results is rather crucial to prosecution. In most jurisdictions, discovering drugs or alcohol in victims or defendants tends to change the way everyone interprets issues of consent and blame. For instance, toxicology can determine whether someone was too intoxicated to consent, which tends to invalidate any claim of voluntary consent. Consider Zambia—there are just so many abuse cases there that really identify the reasons we need to incorporate forensic testing into legal practice; the testing supports victims' claims and tightens up cases in court (Makasa et al., 2017). In South Africa, although recording physical injuries is essential for convictions, conducting comprehensive DNA and toxicology tests is equally important, particularly with the high number of rapes that are not committed by intimate partners (Cupido et al., 2014). Overall, the use of this type of evidence does more than create a stronger case for prosecution; it enhances the overall balance and equity of the judicial process (Figure 1.16).

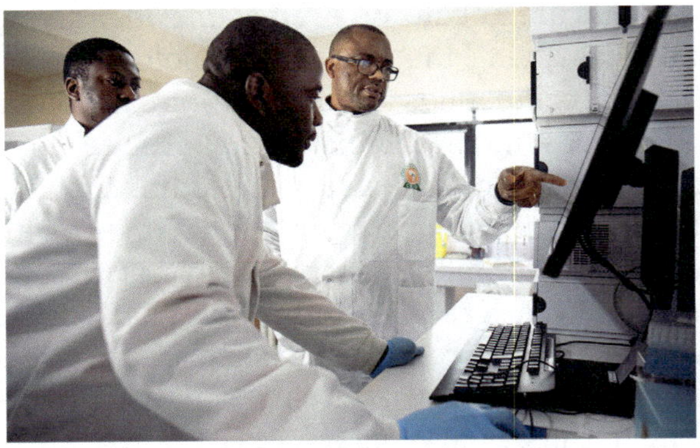

Figure 1.16. Sexual offences can be a real tangle, so having a legal system that mixes in chemical test results is pretty essential for prosecution.

Source: Gates Notes. (2023). *Charles Wendi Malaria Research*. https://images.gatesnotes.com/12514eb8-7b51-008e-41a9-512542cf683b/7c5c194c-b9f2-4434-a0b8-7f0debc41b0a/Charles-Wondji-malaria-research-2400px_by_1500px-001.jpg?w=1400&h=900&fit=clip&fm=jpg&q=75.

1.3.8. Case Studies Involving Toxicology

Drug-facilitated crimes are a dirty business, and we need to get our hands dirty with hands-on toxicology experiments, particularly in the case of sexual crimes in forensic medicine. In general terms, a closer examination of such cases reveals how complicated things can become. One of the more recent studies, for instance, examined 40 alleged victims and discovered that many of them had been incapacitated using drugs such as diazepam, a substance all too frequently used to knock individuals out to facilitate predatory behavior. Surprisingly, motives were not solely based on abuse; robbery and sexual misconduct blended to underscore a concerning intersection between substance abuse and violent activity (Rahimi et al., 2021). The same report also pointed out, in the majority of situations, an increase in incidents of intentional poisoning—highlighting just how vital toxicology is for both catching perpetrators and assisting survivors (Maples et al., 2023). Such studies, following the same trends with offender action, appear to open the door to intervention as well as legislative adjustments intended to curb such activities.

1.3.9. Future Directions in Forensic Toxicology

Sex crimes introduce a great deal of dirty details that compel us to advance forensic toxicology so we can scoop up and examine evidence more effectively. Scientists now employ cutting-edge techniques—tools such as mass spectrometry (MS) and high-performance liquid chromatography—that capture a wider range of substances, including new and emerging drugs and novel psychoactive substances that might otherwise go undetected. This change is significant because alcohol tends to appear in such instances, tampering with a victim's memory and complicating the investigation further (Wall, 2025).

Even some experts recommend establishing standard procedures for taking biological samples from victims because this can typically make toxicology results more credible and consequently actually contribute to bringing justice (Argo et al., 2018). Ultimately, through embracing these scientific advances, forensic toxicology may not only make the case stronger in sexual offence cases but also reveal new lines of approach to comprehend the finer, usually underrated roles that some substances play in both victimization and perpetration.

Test Your Knowledge

1. Name two common "date rape" drugs used in drug-facilitated sexual assaults (DFSA).
2. Why is timing critical when collecting toxicological samples from a suspected DFSA victim?

1.4. Legal Framework and Challenges

Learning Outcome

1. Give an overview of laws governing sexual offences
2. Explain the role of law enforcement in sexual offence cases
3. Learn victim rights and protections
4. Identify challenges in prosecuting sexual offences
5. Know the impact of public perception on legal outcomes
6. Describe international laws and conventions
7. Focus on advocacy and support for victims
8. Discuss reforms in legal frameworks
9. Understand case law examples and their implications

Sexual crimes are a lot of complexities that need a robust legal framework, but in all honesty, enforcing and revising these laws is a real challenge. Recently, with the emergence of brand NPS, there is a clear indication that reforms need to move in and address these issues head-on. The ACMD even goes so far as to recommend that sellers bear more of the responsibility in demonstrating compliance—a step many believe would help alleviate the risks associated with these drugs. Further, locations like Indonesia expose an apparent lacuna in the law on some crimes like necrophilia, which indicates a broader problem of regulatory steps failing to safeguard both our social values and personal dignity (Isnawan et al., 2024). Since our society and the drugs that we come in contact with continuously evolve, it becomes relatively straightforward that the responses by law should not merely be reactive; they must look ahead and provide more comprehensive safeguards against the novel challenges in sexual offences.

1.4.1. Overview of Laws Governing Sexual Offences

Blending medicine with the law actually upsets the way sexual offences are dealt with. Today, legislation is designed to deliver justice – it aims to address crimes that infringe upon individual liberty and the sanctity of our bodies (Figure 1.17).

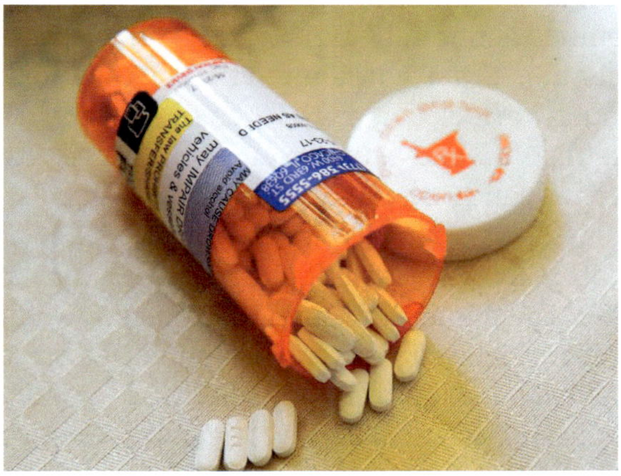

Figure 1.17. Mixing medicine with the law really shakes up how sexual offences get handled.

Source: RVO Health. (2022). *Bottle for Prescription and Pills*. https://media.post.rvohealth.io/wp-content/uploads/2022/08/bottle-for-prescription-and-pills-thumbnail.jpg.

Legal practices and forensic medicine often combine, and at times, in a somewhat careless manner, to cohesively gather evidence that ultimately influences court rulings. In most instances, our justice system relies on those medical observations to determine innocence or guilt (Verma et al., 2023). And then there is the surprise of the quick evolution of substances such as new psychoactive drugs, which only complicate the legal waters and force law enforcement and public health to confront new challenges. Overall, the constantly changing nature of sexual offence laws demands frequent reconsideration and adjustment to keep pace with contemporary issues of justice.

1.4.2. Role of Law Enforcement in Sexual Offence Cases

Sexual offense cases tend to become actual mazes, with shocking turns from gathering evidence to hearing a case out in court. Police are right in the middle of it all, and often, the manner in which officers conduct an investigation really makes a difference in how matters turn out. To cut it short, acquiring good training in forensic methods is not only unnecessary—it is entirely essential. Legal guidelines dictate that police should work closely with forensic specialists to establish a solid foundation of evidence. That sort of hands-on collaboration is particularly important, especially when you consider the emotional and psychological hurdles that are also thrown into the equation. Some knowledge of forensic psychology, combined with a street-smart understanding of scientific evidence methods, can enhance investigations, ensuring that victims receive justice while all parties' rights receive equal consideration (Wirth et al., 2022). Overall, combining strict law enforcement with practical forensic expertise is paramount in successfully pursuing these delicate cases.

1.4.3. Victim Rights and Protections

Forensic medicine combined with legal regulations provides an avenue to truly safeguard victims of sexual crimes (Figure 1.18). Examining the way victims and their perpetrators are connected reveals, in the majority of instances, that improved victim protection measures are necessary—this concept arises repeatedly. We know from research that survivors tend to suffer from heavy social and psychological loads, in addition to that of sexual violence trauma, making it even more imperative to obtain timely psychiatric assessments (Şair et al., 2022). Some studies even note that a significant majority of survivors fall into certain age ranges, with many being unmarried and residing in both large cities and rural areas (Bhoi et al., 2017). All of this appears to point to the urgent need for policies that prioritize victims' welfare, getting them immediate medical attention, mental health assistance, and legal aid. By blending education and awareness in a more active manner, society can better protect vulnerable individuals and create an atmosphere in which their rights are familiar—and, ultimately, enforced.

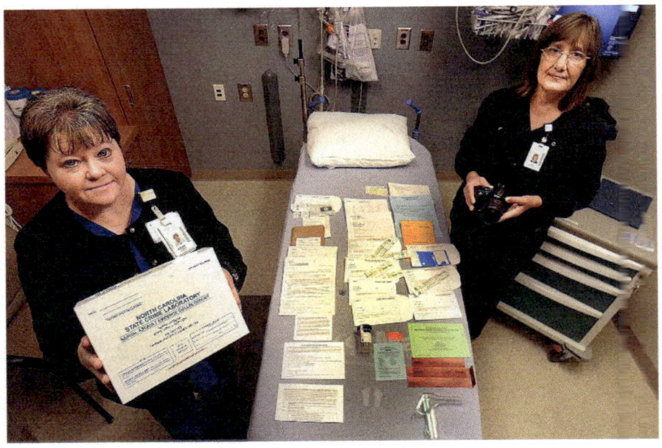

Figure 1.18. Forensic medicine teamed up with legal rules opens a pathway to really protect victims of sexual offenses.

Source: North Carolina Health News. (2019). *Day 3 SANE Nurses.* https://i0.wp.com/www.northcarolinahealthnews.org/wp-content/uploads/2019/03/Day-3-SANE-Nurses-photo.jpg?fit=3300%2C2186.

1.4.4. Challenges in Prosecuting Sexual Offences

Prosecuting sexual crimes is entwined with a range of impediments that frequently hold back actual justice for survivors. Perhaps the biggest obstacle is the severe stigma attached to sexual violence that can quietly influence public opinion and even judicial rulings. In retrospect, as Adler et al. (2020) illustrate, euphemistic language and hidden codes have too frequently concealed what actually occurred—contributing to a culture of silence and muddled comprehension. Root problems in both the legal and medical communities, as described by the Rural Support Programs Network (2019), indicate an acute need for new guidelines that prioritize survivors' dignity. When law enforcement officials and medical professionals are not adequately trained, investigations can get derailed, adding unnecessary barriers to successful prosecution. In the end, tackling these challenges requires a complete rethink of our current methods so that survivors feel supported and genuine justice can be achieved.

1.4.5. The Impact of Public Perception on Legal Outcomes

Public opinion, shaped by day-to-day social attitudes, significantly impacts legal judgments—particularly in cases involving sexual crimes (Figure 1.19). Court trials often take place amidst a mix of cultural narratives and media vignettes that quietly influence the way communities perceive things. These perceptions can influence not only juries but also law enforcement officials and even judges, sometimes creating bias that either supports or undermines a victim's testimony. For instance, if victims are stigmatized, they may be reluctant to report cases, resulting in a loss of valuable forensic data required in court. According to some research, when the community supports initiatives to fight sexual crimes, police tend to have additional finances and access to superior resources for forensic services, ultimately improving investigation results (Voce et al., 2022). All in all, understanding and dealing with these public perceptions is essential to maintaining our legal framework equitable and fair in sexual offense cases (Suvitha et al., 2024).

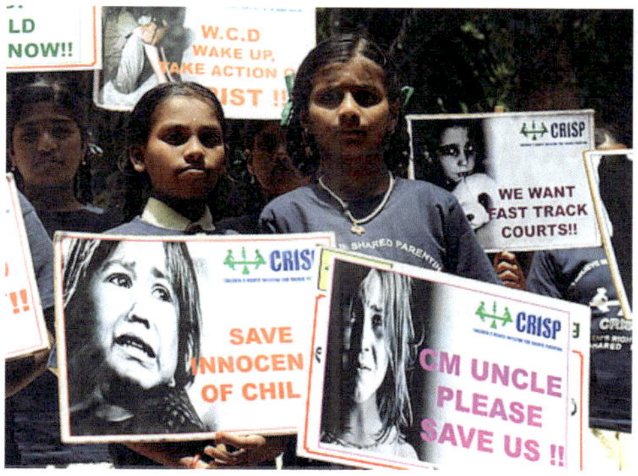

Figure 1.19. Public opinion, molded by everyday societal views, massively influences legal decisions—especially in sexual offense cases.

Source: The New Indian Express. (2014). *Bangalore Rape Case.* https://media.assettype.com/TNIE%2Fimport%2F2014%2F7%2F23%2F7%2Foriginal%2FBangaloreRape1EPS.jpg?w=480&auto=format%2Ccompress&fit=max.

1.4.6. International Laws and Conventions

International laws and forensic procedures have a special relationship when dealing with sexual crimes. In most cases, these regulations are closely tied to forensic procedures, creating a complex system that not only guides investigations but also provides ongoing support to victims throughout the legal process. Forensic medicine—in all its ethical importance—keeps a careful eye on gathering evidence, especially when survivors, a particularly vulnerable group, are involved. Sometimes issues crop up unexpectedly: research ethics may fall a bit short, and data handling practices can get messy; this lack of standardized guidelines has, in some cases, cast doubt on the legitimacy of findings (D'Souza et al., 2019). In general, a closer examination of these legal frameworks is crucial because they essentially regulate the way the forensic work is carried out and highlight most significant medical ethics (Malik, 2017). Overall, combining these aspects not only appears to be necessary for the development of our justice system but also necessary for the treatment of victims with fairness.

1.4.7. Advocacy and Support for Victims

Sexual crimes can be very complex, and therefore, victims must have a healthy, practical support and advocacy network. Victims should be able to feel deeply heard and understood—even when they're facing the mazes of confusing, sometimes overbearing disciplines of forensic medicine and toxicology—so that their own, individual experiences are not lost in a medical shuffle. A compassionate, authentic setting can mitigate the brutal trauma that these crimes impose, allowing survivors to confront legal challenges with a little more assurance and clarity. During times such as the COVID-19 pandemic, when gender-based violence increased exponentially, it has become glaringly apparent that such advocacy is urgently required. Even some reports indicate a dramatic increase in abusive actions and violence against women, emphasizing the imperative for preventive measures and accessible support systems (Rathod et al., 2023). By strengthening these support systems, society can strive towards healing and justice, making survivors not just heard but also provided with the support they require on their torturous path to healing (Suvitha et al., 2024).

1.4.8. Reforms in Legal Frameworks

Legal frameworks and medical concepts have blended for centuries, influencing how we speak about sexual crimes (Figure 1.20). See how sexual consent rules have evolved—there was usually a time when medical professionals arrived with recommendations that mattered but weren't necessarily easy to come by. Instead of a single, overbearing medical figure telling them what to do, there was plenty of give-and-take among various groups within society. Such give-and-take—albeit sometimes messy—meant that medical advice was generally sought for subtlety rather than employed in an effort to impose a rigid agenda. Meanwhile, being sensitive to age adds a further layer of nuance to the way we perceive sexual offences, particularly when looking at who the victims were. When scholars delve into these complex relationships, they tend to discover older factors that, by and large, continue to leave their mark on legal arrangements today, suggesting that reform is still an urgent requirement (Bates et al., 2015; Shapiro et al., 2019).

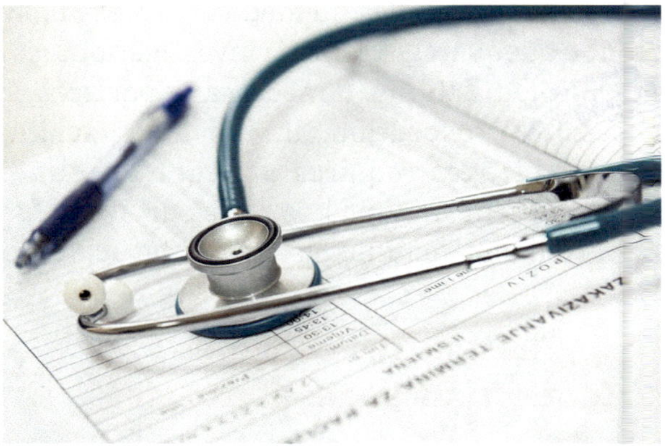

Figure 1.20. Legal systems and medical ideas have been mixing for ages, shaping the way we talk about sexual offences.

Source: iPleaders. (2021). *Evaluation of Medical Evidence*. https://blog.ipleaders.in/wp-content/uploads/2021/08/evaluation-of-medical-evidence-1.jpg.

1.4.9. Case Law Examples and Their Implications

Considering case law actually highlights how sexual offenses are accompanied by a complex web of issues, particularly in forensic practice. According to one report, out of 4288 medicolegal cases, sexual abuse constituted a significant, though smaller, portion of the bigger picture in forensic medicine (Zarif et al., 2023). Yet another study, overall, discovered that young people—typically those between 11–20 years of age—appear to carry the most significant burden, more often involving acquaintances and even scenarios in which consent clouds legal waters (Rani et al., 2020). The findings here imply that legal officials and forensic experts must join forces, sharpening reporting systems and updating legal policies to better protect vulnerable groups. Overall, everyday case law not only identifies emerging patterns in sexual crimes but also provokes continuous, sometimes grubby, discussions of protection and the sort of education that could actually make a difference.

Test Your Knowledge

1. What is the value of having a legal system to deal with sexual offences?
2. Define consent in the context of sexual offences in the law.

SUMMARY

Sexual crimes viewed through the lens of forensic medicine and toxicology present unexpected revelations on how the investigation is shifting and suggest profound social waves. Forensic science today tends to be moving toward contemporary gimmicks such as DNA analysis, which, in the majority of instances, implies that our legal standards have to play catch-up. There has also been an appreciable increase in research on forensic genetics (Wirth et al., 2022), which forces us to adopt practices even more rooted in hard science, and, as honest as it is, it's difficult not to notice. You also get word of disagreements on drug policy (Tham, 2021) that appear to illustrate just how entwined cases become when the abuse of alcohol or drugs becomes an issue. In general terms, it seems that upcoming laws and studies need not only to roll with these technological developments but also to grapple with the numerous social considerations at stake, so prevention and justice sound fully-rounded—and, I should say, a bit more human in methodology.

Sexual crimes are not straightforward, demanding the cross-pollination of ideas from forensic medicine and toxicology that does not always proceed along the direct line. Recently, new psychoactive drugs have been appearing increasingly in these instances, which indicates that drug taking is evolving and bringing with it an entire new range of hazards. The ACMD noted that, although efforts had been made to reduce harms from drugs such as mephedrone, an overarching, comprehensive strategy remains necessary. A glance back at historical forensic literature also indicates an increase in the use of forensic genetics. This method has become a linchpin in identifying and prosecuting sexual crimes (Fracasso et al., 2023). Overall, these pieces of evidence indicate that professionals from various disciplines truly need to collaborate, bringing both medical procedures and legal approaches up to date to catch up with the disordered complications that poisonous factors introduce into sexual crimes.

KEY TERMS FROM THIS CHAPTER

- Chemical submission
- Consent
- Emotional health
- Human trafficking
- Offenders
- Sexual assault
- Sexual exploitation
- Toxicology
- Child sexual abuse
- Domestic violence
- Harassment
- Medical community
- Rape
- Sexual crimes
- Temptation
- Victims

CRITICAL THINKING QUESTIONS

1. **What is the primary role of forensic toxicology in sexual assault cases?**
   a. To confirm the identity of the perpetrator
   b. To detect drugs or alcohol that may have been used to facilitate the crime
   c. To determine the manner of death
   d. To evaluate the physical injuries of the victim
2. **Which of the following substances is most commonly associated with drug-facilitated sexual assault (DFSA)?**
   a. Alcohol
   b. Gamma-hydroxybutyrate (GHB)
   c. Heroin
   d. Methamphetamine
3. **Which of the following is a key forensic test performed on semen found at a sexual assault crime scene?**
   a. Blood typing
   b. DNA profiling
   c. Urinalysis
   d. Microbial culture
4. **In the forensic examination of a sexual assault victim, which of the following is most important for the proper handling of biological evidence?**
   a. Securing the crime scene
   b. Collecting all biological evidence and maintaining the chain of custody
   c. Taking photographs before performing an examination
   d. Performing an autopsy immediately after the examination
5. **Which of the following drugs is often involved in cases of alcohol-induced sexual assault, making the victim unconscious or less able to resist?**
   a. Cocaine
   b. Rohypnol
   c. Methadone
   d. MDMA

Short Answer Questions

1. What are the key forensic procedures involved in the examination of sexual assault victims?
2. How does toxicological analysis help in sexual assault cases, especially in drug-facilitated sexual assault (DFSA)?
3. Explain the role of semen analysis in the forensic investigation of sexual assault cases.
4. What are the potential toxicological substances that can be used to facilitate a sexual assault, and how are they detected?
5. How do forensic experts collect and preserve biological evidence such as semen, saliva, or hair during a sexual assault investigation?
6. What role does DNA profiling play in forensic investigations of sexual offences?
7. How can alcohol and drugs impair a victim's ability to recall the assault and affect the forensic investigation?

Answers to Critical Thinking Questions

1. (b); 2. (b); 3. (b); 4. (b); 5. (b)

REFERENCES

1. Adler, A., Angelozzi, A., Appignanesi, L., Archer, D., et al. (2020). *"Monstrous and Indefensible"? Newspaper Accounts of Sexual Assaults on Children in 19th-Century England and Wales.* https://core.ac.uk/download/288394165.pdf (accessed on 9th May 2025).
2. Advisory Council on the Misuse of Drugs. (2011). *Consideration of the Novel Psychoactive Substances ('Legal Highs').* https://core.ac.uk/download/1643031.pdf (accessed on 9th May 2025).
3. Alías, A., Boubeta, A. R., Isorna, M. F., McCartan, K., et al. (2017). *Drug-Facilitated Sexual Assault and Chemical Submission.* https://core.ac.uk/download/323893412.pdf (accessed on 9th May 2025).
4. Amankwaa, A. O., Amoako, E. N., Bonsu, D. N. O., & Banyeh, M., (2019). Forensic science in Ghana: A review. *Forensic Science International Synergy, 1*, 151–160. https://doi.org/10.1016/j.fsisyn.2019.07.008.
5. Amzat, J., Kanmodi, K. K., Aminu, K., & Egbedina, E. A. (2023). Drug-facilitated sexual assault in Africa: A scoping review of empirical evidence. *Public Health Challenges, 2.* https://doi.org/10.1002/puh2.119.
6. Argo, A., Milone, L., Nardello, R., Piscionieri, C., et al. (2018). *Medico-Legal Procedures Related to Sexual Assault: A 10-Year Retrospective Experience of a Daphne Protocol Application.* https://core.ac.uk/download/153520564.pdf (accessed on 9th May 2025).
7. Barrett, M. E. (2025). *Historical Development and Contemporary Dilemmas of a Police Surgeon.* https://core.ac.uk/download/16414494.pdf (accessed on 9th May 2025).
8. Bates, V. L. (2015). *'Not an Exact Science': Medical Approaches to Age and Sexual Offences in England*, 1850–1914. https://core.ac.uk/download/12826778.pdf (accessed on 9th May 2025).
9. Bhoi, S. B., Shirsat, K. B., Meshram, S., Waghmare, S., & Rizwan. (2017). Profile of sexual offences: A 4-year retrospective study at tertiary care hospital of Western Maharashtra. *Medico-Legal Update, 2*, 17–21. https://www.semanticscholar.org/paper/79fb22bd8f5ee7ec7bd2738584c2fbc484231941 (accessed on 9th May 2025).
10. Choi, E. S. (2019). *The Care of the Sexual Assault Patient.* https://core.ac.uk/download/232776434.pdf (accessed on 9th May 2025).
11. Cimon, D., Desharnais, B., & Dicaire, C., (2014). *One Hundred Years of Forensic Sciences in Quebec: The Evolution of Scientific Techniques Since 1914.* https://core.ac.uk/download/323460649.pdf (accessed on 9th May 2025).
12. Cupido, D., (2014). *The Assessment of the Utility and Impact of Sexual Assault Evidence Collection Kits (SAECKs) as DNA Evidence in Suspected Cases of Rape.* https://core.ac.uk/download/185389790.pdf (accessed on 9th May 2025).
13. D'Souza, H., Shetty, P. H., Rao, J., Shetty, S., & Bhagavath, P., (2019). Research ethics in forensic medicine—The Indian scenario: Problems and suggestions. *Indian Journal of Forensic Medicine & Toxicology.* https://www.semanticscholar.org/paper/f46c748380434f716f6d886393d6d60c5ca87b0a (accessed on 9th May 2025).
14. Dawnay, N., & Sheppard, K., (2023). From crime scene to courtroom: A review of the current bioanalytical evidence workflows used in rape and sexual assault investigations in the United

Kingdom. *Science & Justice, 63*, 206–228. https://doi.org/10.1016/j.scijus.2022.12.006.

15. Emamhadi, M., & Jalilvand, M., (2012). *Can Psychopathic Traits Predict Homicidal Behavior in Male Murderers?* https://core.ac.uk/download/483635392.pdf (accessed on 9th May 2025).
16. Fracasso, T., Pfeiffer, H., Schmeling, A., Wirth, I., et al. (2023). From Deutsche Zeitschrift to International Journal of Legal Medicine—100 years of legal medicine through the lens of journal articles: Part 3: *Zeitschrift für Rechtsmedizin—Journal of Legal Medicine* from 1970 to 1990. *International Journal of Legal Medicine, 37*, 567–579. https://core.ac.uk/download/586717646.pdf (accessed on 9th May 2025).
17. Gitanjali, D., (2011). *A Study on Victims of Sexual Offences.* https://core.ac.uk/download/235663920.pdf (accessed on 9th May 2025).
18. Haridas, S., & Nanandkar, S. D. S. (2016). *Medicolegal Study of Alleged Rape Victim Cases in Mumbai Region.* https://core.ac.uk/download/483635498.pdf (accessed on 9th May 2025).
19. Isnawan, F., (2024). *Protection of the Dignity of the Corpse: A Study on the Criminalization of Necrophilia Reviewed from the Maqashid Syariah.* https://core.ac.uk/download/642806204.pdf (accessed on 9th May 2025).
20. Jaiswal, A. K., Kumar, G. S., Pooniya, S., Raheel, A., et al. (2016). *Potency Test of a Rape Accused in India: Rationale, Problems and Suggestions in Light of the Criminal Law (Amendment) Act, 2013.* https://core.ac.uk/download/pdf/82646788.pdf (accessed on 9th May 2025).
21. Kennedy, B., Bugeja, L., Olivier, J., Koppel, S., Dwyer, J., & Ibrahim, J., (2023). A population-based cross-sectional study examining homicides among community-dwelling older adults in Victoria, Australia: A study protocol. *PLoS ONE, 18*, e0292837. https://doi.org/10.1371/journal.pone.0292837.
22. Kumar, S. P., Rana, A., Singh, A., Sehgal, A., Kumar, S., Sharma, R., et al. (2014). *A Study of Sexual Assaults in Northern Range of Himachal Pradesh.* https://core.ac.uk/download/483635474.pdf (accessed on 9th May 2025).
23. Lood, Y., (2021). *Testosterone use and Abuse: Methodological Aspects in Forensic Toxicology and Clinical Diagnostics.* Linköping University medical dissertations. https://doi.org/10.3384/diss.diva-173146.
24. Makasa, I., (2017). *Evaluating the Role of DNA Evidence in Sexual Offence Cases in Zambia Between 2007 and 2014.* https://core.ac.uk/download/185391727.pdf (accessed on 9th May 2025).
25. Malik, A., (2017). *Forensic Medicine v/s Forensic Pathology: A Difference that Everyone Should Know* (Vol. 23). Annals of King Edward Medical University. https://www.semanticscholar.org/paper/9a429755655f8bcdb596ea4dbbfe3aee5e1dffc0 (accessed on 9th May 2025).
26. Maples, A. C. (2023). *Timing is Everything: State-by-State Analysis of the Collection of Lawfully owed DNA from Offenders.* https://core.ac.uk/download/567889898.pdf (accessed on 9th May 2025).
27. Marc, B., (2008). Current clinical aspects of drug-facilitated sexual assaults in sexually abused victims examined in a forensic emergency unit. *Therapeutic Drug Monitoring, 30*, 218–224. https://www.semanticscholar.org/paper/55beb26970fc82b6249f009e01228ae92464ef1e (accessed on 9th May 2025).

28. Markwerth, P., Bajanowski, T., Tzimas, I., & Dettmeyer, R., (2020). Sudden cardiac death—Update. *International Journal of Legal Medicine, 135*, 483–495. https://doi.org/10.1007/s00414-020-02481-z.

29. Nadeem, F., Wasif, M., Ahmad, I., Ali, S. A., Shazia, S., & Khan, O., (2024). Prevalence and pattern of injury in sexual assault cases presented at Khyber Medical College Peshawar. *Journal of Ayub Medical College, Abbottabad: JAMC, 36*(3), 518–521. https://www.semanticscholar.org/paper/d908ec7a4695f22b76a02b083dc83c04d5c8219b (accessed on 9th May 2025).

30. Patra, A. P., Shaha, K. K., Rayamane, A. P., & Mohanty, S., (2015). Victimology of alleged rape cases: A three-year institution-based cross-sectional study. *Indian Journal of Forensic and Community Medicine, 2*, 203–213. https://www.semanticscholar.org/paper/382a0e4cf2cc91a6b02e820458657bdd2a190d1b (accessed on 9th May 2025).

31. Piraianu, A., Fulga, A., Musat, C., Ciobotaru, O., Poalelungi, D. G., Stamate, E., Ciobotaru, O., et al. (2023). Enhancing the evidence with algorithms: How artificial intelligence is transforming forensic medicine. *Diagnostics, 13*. https://www.semanticscholar.org/paper/295dc873de03e817e0355e6b7789baf235e4e83d (accessed on 9th May 2025).

32. Rahimi, M., & Salari, M. M., (2021). *Criminal Poisoning: A Hospital-Based Survey in an Academic Center of Iran.* https://core.ac.uk/download/483635756.pdf (accessed on 9th May 2025).

33. Rahman, F., Ahmed, H., Ray, D., Chowdhury, M. A., & Mahmud, S., (2024). Awareness of sexual violence, status of temptation and consent among children experiencing sexual violence. *Journal of Shaheed Suhrawardy Medical College*. https://www.semanticscholar.org/paper/28f399c10c2a8282e250a34ac0ccc69855d26975 (accessed on 9th May 2025).

34. Rani, S., Chinmayi, Y., & Arun, M., (2020). A study on the socio-demographic profile of the victims of sexual offences: A retrospective study. *Medico-Legal Update, 20*, 569–573. https://www.semanticscholar.org/paper/cfbd9fd9d5a34356c04f704a96d241b32172e13a (accessed on 9th May 2025).

35. Rathod, V., & Simon, R., (2023). Effect of COVID-19 lockdown on crimes against women in India. *Deleted Journal, 15*, 1–9. https://doi.org/10.51767/jsw1501.

36. Roy, A., Tasnim, Z., & Nargis, F., (2023). Investigating unnatural deaths linked to sexual assault: A forensic analysis. *Asian Journal of Medicine and Health*. https://www.semanticscholar.org/paper/9e5cfcb790a9e7ebe4f6499d7557831f860d3154 (accessed on 9th May 2025).

37. Ruano-Segado, J., Sáez-Rodríguez, J., Girela-López, E., & Beltran-Aroca, C. M. (2022). *What is the Prevalence of Alleged Drug-Facilitated Sexual Assault in the Province of Cordoba?* Cuadernos de Medicina Forense. https://www.semanticscholar.org/paper/24083561e5d6201ff65d1a398953c24fcd3a1620 (accessed on 9th May 2025).

38. Rural Support Programs Network. (2019). *Building Partnerships for Scaling Access to Justice for Survivors of Sexual Violence in Pakistan.* https://core.ac.uk/download/542480767.pdf (accessed on 9th May 2025).

39. Şair, Y., Doğan, B., & Dirlik, M., (2022). The clinical features of victims and offenders admitted to the forensic psychiatry outpatient clinic: A single-center retrospective analysis. *Meandros Medical and Dental Journal*. https://www.semanticscholar.org/paper/f59493af0e3fd21c90b17af7deb9dd4057d546da (accessed on 9th May 2025).

40. Samad, A., Khalid, A., Imran, S., Akhter, N., Bibi, I., & Naz, R., (2023). Sociodemographic characteristics and forensic evidence of sexual assault victims. *Pakistan Journal of Medical and Health Sciences.* https://www.semanticscholar.org/paper/7ef4092efb8ad078d7aba8c1abbf775fdb86bead (accessed on 9th May 2025).
41. Schmeling, A., Fracasso, T., Pfeiffer, H., & Wirth, I., (2023). From Deutsche Zeitschrift to International Journal of Legal Medicine—100 years of legal medicine through the lens of journal articles. *International Journal of Legal Medicine, 137,* 567–579. https://doi.org/10.1007/s00414-023-02949-8.
42. Shapiro, D. L. (2019). *Retrying Leopold and Loeb: A Neuropsychological Perspective.* https://core.ac.uk/download/275753827.pdf (accessed on 9th May 2025).
43. Sharma, A., & Mishra, A. K. (2019). *Management of Drug Abuse Patient Through Ayurveda.* https://core.ac.uk/download/333810060.pdf (accessed on 9th May 2025).
44. Shrestha, S., Gurung, S., & Bhandari, B., (2022). Self-assessment of undergraduate medical students regarding the clinical knowledge in forensic medicine. *Journal of Nepalgunj Medical College, 20,* 10–13. https://doi.org/10.3126/jngmc.v20i2.51832.
45. Suvitha, S., Margaret, A., & Volantine, I., (2024). *A Comprehensive Solution for BSc Nursing Students.* Ana Publishing Private Limited eBooks. https://doi.org/10.47211/book.2024.9788194680468.
46. Tennessee Bureau of Investigation. (2017). *Annual Report 2016–2017.* https://core.ac.uk/download/553361730.pdf (accessed on 9th May 2025).
47. Tham, H., (2021). *Retreat or Entrenchment? Drug Policies in the Nordic Countries at a Crossroads.* https://doi.org/10.16993/bbo.
48. Verma, R. K., Kumar, R., & Verma, R. K. (2023). *Justice Accessibility in Perspective of Juristic Rational Science with Specific Dimension of Medical and Forensic Science.* https://core.ac.uk/download/588467299.pdf (accessed on 9th May 2025).
49. Voce, A., & Sullivan, T., (2022). *What are The Monetary Returns of Investing in Programs that Reduce Demand for Illicit Drugs?* https://doi.org/10.52922/ti78733.
50. Wall, L., (2025). *Under the Influence? Considering the Role of Alcohol And Sexual Assault in Social Contexts.* https://core.ac.uk/download/pdf/30674261.pdf (accessed on 9th May 2025).
51. Weston, J., (2025). *Curing Sexual Deviance: Medical Approaches to Sexual Offenders in England, 1919–1959.* https://core.ac.uk/download/333900675.pdf (accessed on 9th May 2025).
52. Wirth, I., Fracasso, T., Pfeiffer, H., & Schmeling, A., (2022). *From Deutsche Zeitschrift to International Journal of Legal Medicine*—100 years of legal medicine through the lens of journal articles. *International Journal of Legal Medicine, 137,* 279–294. https://doi.org/10.1007/s00414-022-02912-z.
53. Yesodharan, R., Nayak, V. C., Jose, T. T., Palimar, V., & George, A., (2022). The effectiveness of a sexual assault nurse examiner-grounding program (SANE-GP) on knowledge, skill and practice regarding sexual assault examination (SAE) among nurses working in a tertiary care hospital in Udupi district, India: A study protocol. *F1000Research, 11,* 134. https://doi.org/10.12688/f1000research.74978.2.

VIRGINITY, PREGNANCY, AND DELIVERY

2

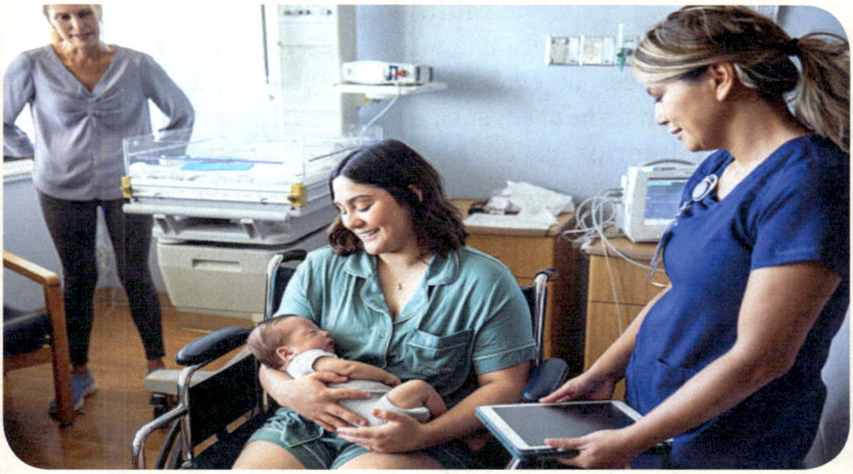

LEARNING OBJECTIVES

After studying this chapter, you will be able to:

1. Understand virginity in a forensic context
2. Focus on pregnancy and forensic investigations
3. Describe delivery and forensic analysis
4. Discuss interconnections between virginity, pregnancy, and delivery

Introduction

Sexual violence discussions today often veer into the complicated cocktail of pregnancy, childbirth, and virginity as encountered in forensic evidence. Virginity stigma usually adds another dose of trauma to victims—particularly when consent becomes complicated during rape. More often than not, the international epidemic of sexual crimes only adds to this pain, with children and women bearing the lion's share of its weight (Gitanjali et al., 2011). Forensic examinations are instrumental in corroborating assault allegations, even if there are no clear-cut injuries; the lack of those does not erase what the victim experienced (Chikadzi et al., 2018). Seeing these factors so clearly is essential not only for the individual healing of survivors but also for informing changes in legal protections in the face of a serious public health crisis. Considering these connected themes actually underscores how deep and tangled the issues are in forensic examinations of sexual offenses.

Definition of Key Terms: Virginity, Pregnancy, Delivery

In handling sexual violence cases, several terms become conflated in a way that impacts legal jurisdictions as well as common understanding (Figure 2.1). Virginity, for instance, tends to be commonly understood as never having had sexual intercourse—a term freighted with varying cultural connotations and iteratively repeated in talk, though constantly shifting from community to community. Then there is the transition from virginity to preparing for pregnancy, a change that occurs through sex that results in conception—a nuance forensic professionals actually notice. Pregnancy itself refers to that state of body condition that comes on after fertilization, and it can precipitate passionate, emotional, or legal disputes, particularly when the assault factor comes into play.

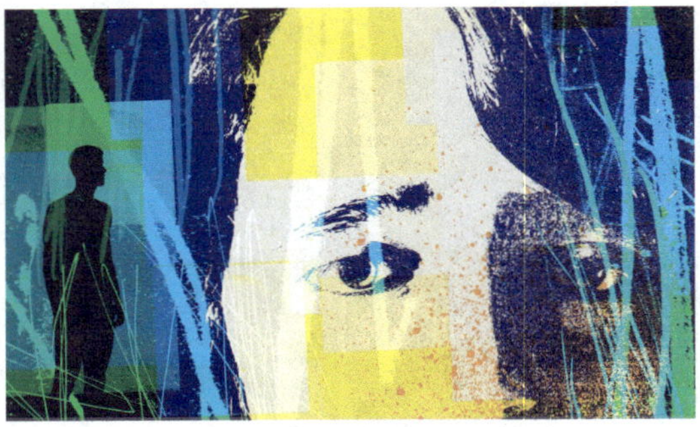

Figure 2.1. When dealing with sexual violence cases, a few key terms end up mixing in ways that affect both legal boundaries and everyday perceptions.

Source: The Guardian. (n.d.). *Day of Atonement.* https://i.guim.co.uk/img/media/6d812f521474765658f0bfaaf52d2a7e907e26f8/0_6_3248_1949/master/3248.jpg?width=1200&quality=85&auto=format&fit=max&s=7bc26b10235cf0089b300a4750e029c8.

And childbirth—delivery—the act of giving birth—not only poses a significant moment in terms of medicine but also appears as proof in investigations, particularly in matters involving child abuse or gender violence; these different definitions, in the majority of instances, contribute to the broader debates witnessed in previous reports (Guyo et al., 2009; Chikadzi et al., 2018).

Importance of Forensics in Understanding these Concepts

Forensics lies at the center of unraveling how virginity, pregnancy, and childbirth get mixed up—particularly in cases that are characterized by sexual assault. Forensic experts apply practical forensic techniques to bring together pieces of evidence that expose what victims have endured; such evidence, in most instances, informs us as to why these matters get so entangled. The CARE Kenya report, for example, reveals that gender and sexuality-based abuse tends to get confused with issues of virginity and reproductive rights, which actually highlights the necessity of recording and investigating such cases for legal reform and for support for the survivors (Guyo et al., 2009). And then there is the continuing sequence of violations documented in the Special Rapporteur's report on gender-based violence in India, revealing the profound difficulties women encounter on a routine basis; here, forensic data speaks not merely in courts of law but also in daily social spheres (Chatterji et al., 2015). Overall, forensics becomes an essential instrument for revealing the complex connections between virginity and reproductive well-being.

Overview of the Relationship Between Virginity and Forensic Evidence

Societal concepts regarding virginity and the dirty manner in which forensic evidence is acquired have a way of blurring into an encounter that really transforms sexual violence cases. Fundamental misperceptions about what exactly constitutes virginity can ruin legal procedures – in a lot of situations, such confusions culminate in victim-blaming as well as warped conceptions regarding consent. Research, for example, has recorded that cultural stigma places additional layers on the trauma of a survivor; one study even identifies high stigma rates in areas such as Kenya's North Eastern Province (Guyo et al., 2009). Despite attempts by legal reforms to play down the significance of a survivor's sexual history, there remain residual attitudes towards rape, which leads to complaints being treated differently because of assumptions about a victim being a virgin (Allen et al., 2018). Overall, these dynamics ultimately impact the reading and presentation of forensic evidence – and, in the end, they have a significant impact on survivors' justice outcomes.

Historical Context of Virginity in Forensic Investigations

Virginity's presence in forensic practice weighs heavily with historical significance that continues to influence the way law and society perceive women's bodies even today (Figure 2.2). Most cultures associate virginity with honor—in a manner that, in the majority of instances, ends up stigmatizing women who have been victims of sexual violence with additional layers of shame. A particularly poignant illustration is provided by the Special Rapporteur on Violence Against Women, who highlights that in India, the combination of deeply ingrained cultural norms and widespread gender-based abuse creates a brutal, almost inescapable reality (Chatterji et al., 2015). Standard law systems, such as English common law, tended to silence the voices of women by forcing them to rely on male representatives in the courtroom, thus making it even more difficult for them to assert justice in cases of sexual crimes (Butler, 2019). All this complicated, entangled history doesn't just affect contemporary forensic procedures—it also ends up informing the way virginity gets interpreted in sexual violence cases, fueling the larger, more current arguments over women's rights and actual autonomy.

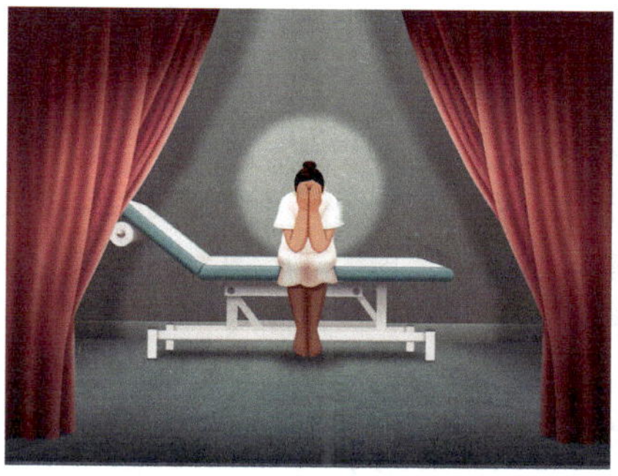

Figure 2.2. Virginity's role in forensic work carries a heavy historical weight that still shapes how law and society view female bodies today.

Source: Afza, N. (2018). *Day of Atonement. The Guardian*. https:// i.guim.co.uk/img/ media/27acaf5f19f0b33c70c8e76ec646fac c2768f6e3/0 _0_3000_1800/master/3000. jpg? width= 1200&height= 900&quality= 85&auto=format&fit= crop&s=7a48ee6da6198 2fcba57e3662f360a0a.

The Role of Pregnancy in Forensic Work

Pregnancy actually complicates forensic work to a large extent, particularly in cases of sexual abuse allegations. It is not all about body development in a case involving a pregnant adolescent—there's a whole legal quagmire to be sorted as well. Consider a 14-year-old female presenting with signs of pregnancy yet possessing an intact hymen (Serbülent et al., 2022). That sort of confusion makes it difficult to determine precisely what happened based solely on physical tests. It appears that pulling together opinions from physicians, lawyers, and even counselors is typically required in order to put things together accurately. Most of the time, the environment in which these cases are investigated—such as our Victim-Friendly System—can also complicate matters due to limited budgets and staff shortages (Chikadzi et al., 2018). Overall, understanding the contribution of pregnancy is critical in developing forensic techniques that really defend and aid those most vulnerable.

Significance of Delivery in Forensic Examinations

Forensic examinations at the time of birth carry a surprising significance in legal conflicts and commonplace arguments about virginity and pregnancy. At times, evidence reveals itself during birth that suggests concealed aspects of a case—particularly when sexual assault is involved and questions of consent and trauma become entwined. Researchers review not just physical evidence—such as bruising or other trauma—but attempt to gauge the residual psychological wounds that a victim suffers. People's perceptions appear to confirm these results; many contend that changes in rape law have not truly shaken free of entrenched gender stereotypes that all too frequently serve to challenge a woman's credibility (Allen et al., 2018). Next are cultural practices such as virginity testing, which continue to fuel debates regarding who gets to make sexual decisions and what is valued in society. Altogether, these types of forensic checks during birth become an integral piece in the grand scheme of gender and sexual rights debates (Mhlongo et al., 2009).

2.1. Virginity in Forensic Context

Learning Outcome

1. Give definition and cultural perceptions of virginity
2. Identify forensic methods to assess virginity
3. Learn the legal implications of virginity in forensic cases
4. Focus on the psychological impact of virginity assessments
5. Explain case studies involving virginity in forensics
6. Learn ethical considerations in virginity examinations
7. Describe the role of medical professionals in virginity assessments
8. Know the limitations of forensic evidence related to virginity
9. Discuss future directions in the study of virginity in forensics

Sexual assault cases are complicated and tend to center around the way society constructs virginity. Virginity in most locations is not merely a status—it is a cultural symbol that affects everything from healthcare to legal reactions. At times, practitioners attempting to assist victims within systems designed to be benevolent to them encounter enormous obstacles; instances of sexual abuse of children, for example, become entangled with historical notions of purity and shame (Chikadzi et al., 2018). Increased rates of sexual and gender violence only compound the need, indicating that we have service models that actually work for those vulnerable, particularly unmarried girls who then bear the brunt of these cultural expectations (Guyo et al., 2009). Forensic professionals in general must understand these dynamics as they are integral to both the investigative process and how these types of cases are processed on a whole basis.

2.1.1. Definition and Cultural Perceptions of Virginity

Virginity's definition has been thumped into the pot of honor, morals, and purity for so long that it is difficult to define what that is specifically. Cultural notions such as these have, throughout history, influenced people's perceptions of themselves and of one another, particularly in the aspects of gender and sexuality. In Egyptian young communities, for instance, virginity is crucial in comprehending sexual and reproductive health (SRH); the Population Council, however, in the majority of cases, operates to respond to these youth demands and ensure that accurate information is within an accessible range (Abdel-Tawab et al., 2013). You also witness a comparable pressure among Korekore women in Zimbabwe, where religious and cultural teachings, in most cases, put on extra layers of pressure that influence women's control over their bodies, making it more challenging to navigate sexual and reproductive rights (Mudzimu et al., 2021). All these varied interpretations of virginity reflect wider social values that, in a rather complicated manner, also shape everything from pregnancy experiences to how delivery is talked about in forensic communities (Figure 2.3).

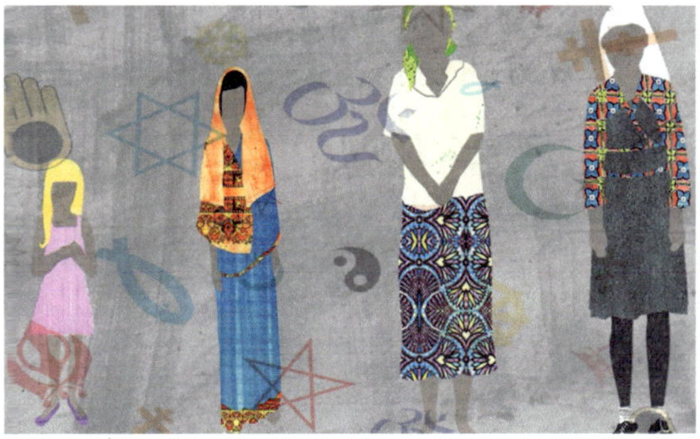

Figure 2.3. Cultural perceptions of virginity.

Source: Free Muslim. (2021). *Virginity Test.* https://freemuslim.org/wp-content/uploads/2021/01/virginity-test--1040x640.png.

2.1.2. Forensic Methods to Assess Virginity

Virginity testing by a forensic means is always tricky; legal impediments and societal pressure have the knack of twisting matters around plenty of times. Most often, physical signs are searched for through medical tests—such as how healthy the hymen and adjacent genital structures appear—to suggest prior sex. However, these physiological signs are not necessarily definitive and are prone to misinterpretation, particularly when age-old cultural traditions, e.g., female genital mutilation (FGM) (Guyo et al., 2009), are involved. It is also noteworthy that the entire process can emotionally drain people who, already stigmatized and threatened by the fear of community reaction, encounter even more challenging situations when legal processes intervene Gitanjali et al., 2011. In general, a delicate touch that combines sound medical expertise with an authentic appreciation of cultural contexts—and, in all honesty, dedication to the protection of survivors' rights—is necessary if justice is going to be respectful of the dignity of all parties involved.

2.1.3. Legal Implications of Virginity in Forensic Cases

Forensic exams now all too frequently charge headlong into complex problems regarding virginity—problems that combine profound cultural conviction with legal challenges in complicated ways that are not necessarily easy to sort out. In sexual violence cases, for instance, the notion of virginity can sometimes influence the perception of witnesses in unexpected ways, even influencing how evidence is treated; sometimes it obscures judgment in ways that we may not at first consider. Judges, physicians, and attorneys are committed to a system that isn't always equipped to handle these subtleties, and that's because ingrained societal stigmas intrude into each step of the process.

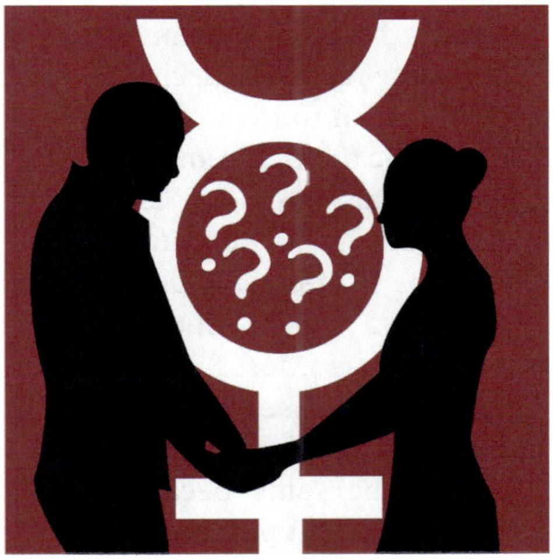

Figure 2.4. Legal implications of virginity in forensic cases.

Source: McIsaac, N. (2021). The value of virginity. *The Quinnipiac Chronicle.*

A recent study on officials who operate in what has been referred to as the Victim-Friendly System in general indicates that most are not adequately trained for handling virginity in instances of child sexual abuse, and this tends to result in miscarriages of justice (Chikadzi et al., 2018). Again, however, it appears that, in the majority of instances, a lack of knowledge regarding survivors' legal rights adds an extra level of complexity, indicating a pressing need for services to coordinate more effectively—findings echoed also in studies of sexual and gender-based violence in Kenya (Guyo et al., 2009) (Figure 2.4).

2.1.4. Psychological Impact of Virginity Assessments

Virgin tests mandated by social expectations tend to affect individuals strongly—women, especially, are on the receiving end of these expectations in both cultural and legal contexts. In most instances, such judgments tend to evoke strong emotions of shame, fear, and incompetence, with most individuals internalizing rigid gender standards and, for the most part, directing that inwardly as self-criticism. Despite recent legal changes that now tend to overlook an individual's sexual past in rape cases, public opinion remains mired in old ideas about female sexuality. This disconnect places survivors in a position where they feel isolated, as if their whole worth depends on them being a virgin (Allen et al., 2018). Additionally, in areas where SRH services are not easily accessible—as research on Afghan women has shown—the psychological load becomes even more cumbersome because of cultural restrictions that inhibit personal autonomy and the freedom to access help, which subsequently results in negative health consequences (Hadi et al., 2016).

2.1.5. Case Studies Involving Virginity in Forensics

These cultural perceptions of virginity have a lasting influence on forensic practice and how evidence is interpreted in sexual assault cases. In parts of Kenya's North Eastern Province, where sexual and gender-based violence is all too prevalent, outdated stigmas associated with virginity have the potential to mess up investigations, particularly when dealing with cases involving vulnerable, young, unmarried girls (Guyo et al., 2009). At times, such embedded notions create an unnecessary double-check on a victim's history, generating more prejudice than light in legal affairs. Although criminal law has done some to limit such prejudice, many outmoded notions persist doggedly, biasing outcomes in investigations. Evidently, in the majority of instances, there is a call for increased education and reform on both forensic and legal levels to ensure sensitive cases receive the fair and meticulous attention they deserve (Allen et al., 2018).

2.1.6. Ethical Considerations in Virginity Examinations

Virginity examinations are more than a routine examination—they reverberate through personal rights and social mores in ways that cannot be brushed aside. Ethical issues, in general, need to be at the forefront, particularly when you think about the dignity and autonomy of individuals who are compelled to undergo these tests. These practices tend to reflect and even uphold outdated beliefs that inappropriately link a woman's value to her sexual history. During discussions about sexual violence, there is always a demand for medical practice that respects survivors fully—a need, perhaps, more starkly felt than ever. Several reports suggest that reforming police procedures and medical practices is crucial to achieving equitable outcomes, with a need for a prompt overhaul of ethical frameworks in healthcare and judicial systems highlighted (Rural Support Programs Network, 2019). Paradoxically, although enhancing secondary prevention can be laudable, it often overlooks primary measures and unwittingly perpetuates victim-blaming cultures (Hailegeorgis, 2019). Overall, reconsidering virginity tests in this broader ethical context is, quite simply, imperative (Figure 2.5).

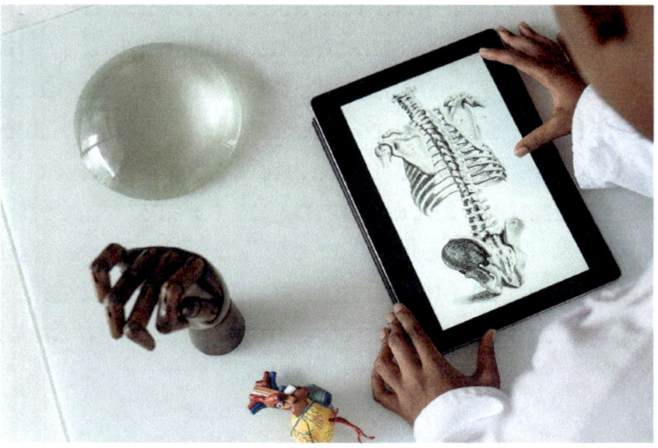

Figure 2.5. Ethical concerns should be front and center, especially when you consider the dignity and independence of those forced to submit to these tests.

Source: New Indian Express. (2024). *New Project*. https://media.assettype.com/newindianexpress%2F2024-09-04%2Fgp2pph8v%2FNew%20Project%20(1).jpg.

2.1.7. The Role of Medical Professionals in Virginity Assessments

Medical practitioners are usually faced with a dilemma where professional ethics conflict with statutory requirements—this conflict particularly comes into sharp relief when they are requested to conduct virginity tests. Such tests raise controversies regarding body autonomy while, in most cases, also raising issues regarding wider cultural perceptions of women's health and rights. In reality, physicians often must balance the demands of cultural expectations against the wisdom of the ageless Hippocratic oath (keep in mind, "do no harm" is not a slogan), and that scale can become quite muddled. At times, the implications are very severe; such evaluations tend to reaffirm negative stereotyping and even perpetuate chronic violence against women's health (VAWH) through the development of stigma and promoting discriminatory treatment of female bodies (Vido, 2020). A closer legal examination, in general, shows an ongoing pattern of human rights concerns throughout various regions, urging medical professionals to reconsider how they work in this process (Vido, 2020). Briefly, the doctor's role here is more than just conducting an examination; it involves a greater responsibility to safeguard the dignity and rights of all individuals.

2.1.8. Limitations of Forensic Evidence Related to Virginity

Determining virginity by forensic evidence is a dirty business that truly cries out for closer examination. Social concepts and cultural perceptions blur in a fashion which makes legal terminology appear to be a pretty long way away from what everyone holds as virginity. This gap makes physical evidence difficult to rely on as clear evidence—generally speaking, the data is not substantial enough. Sometimes the techniques employed to verify virginity are overbearing and can conveniently be misinterpreted, which then raises some pretty complicated ethical dilemmas.

Many forensic specialists have indicated that the tests tend to overlook more substantial issues, such as victim trauma and residual social stigma, thus contributing to the survivors' suffering. Studies on these issues (Chikadzi et al., 2018; Hailegeorgis, 2019) indicate that, in the majority of instances, material and accurate training are woefully inadequate, ultimately compromising the validity of these tests. Ultimately, policymakers need to prioritize improved education and clear ethical standards to address such sensitive situations more effectively.

2.1.9. Future Directions in the Study of Virginity in Forensics

Forensic virginity debates continue to change, but vestiges of ancient myths persist in hanging on to both our judicial systems and common opinion. Some of the previous reforms to rape legislation—aimed at safeguarding victims—have not actually dispelled these ingrained assumptions. In many instances of judicial discourse, claims made by women tend to be dismissed as unfounded (Allen et al., 2018). There are now people who insist that future employment will have more emphasis on public health strategies to debunk these myths, something similar to the processes employed with AIDS or even anti-tobacco campaigns. There is also this strange incident of revirginization, which blends cultural belief with the methods of doing forensics, encouraging us to ask ourselves if our traditional signs of virginity are still valid in today's tests (Güzel et al., 2020). In general, drawing on ideas from sociology, psychology, and law may provide us with a richer, more complex understanding of virginity in forensic science—albeit one that is sometimes a little messy to arrive at (Figure 2.6).

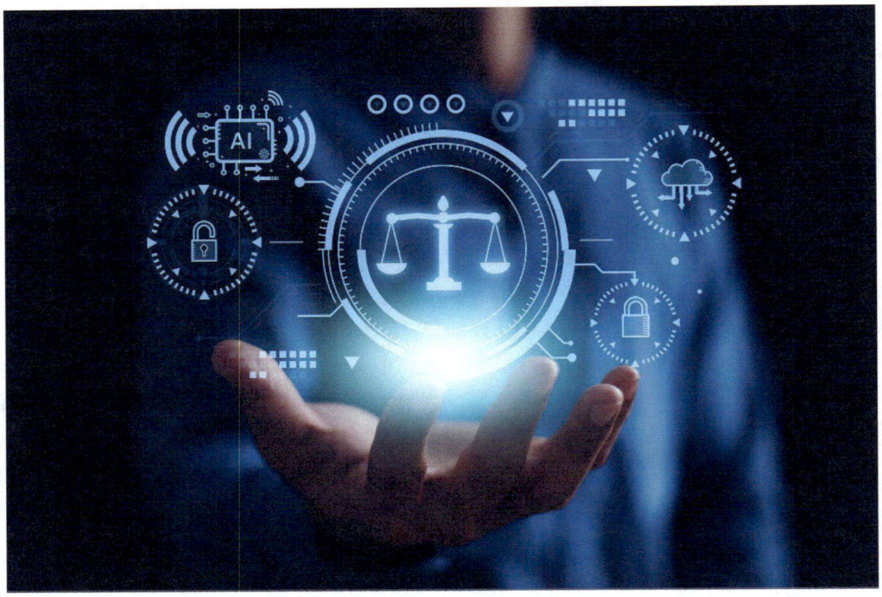

Figure 2.6. Future in the study of virginity in forensics.

Source: Ernst and Young. (n.d.). *EY Indian Real Estate.* https://www.ey.com/adobe/dynamicmedia/deliver/dm-aid--d72deb7a-b24d-443f-8555-08cf0bfbb822/ey-indian-real-estate.jpg?preferwebp=true&quality=85.

Test Your Knowledge

1. Define virginity in a medico-legal context.
2. Can the presence of an intact hymen reliably indicate virginity? Explain briefly.

2.2. Pregnancy and Forensic Investigations

Learning Outcome

1. Define pregnancy in forensic terms
2. Explain forensic indicators of pregnancy
3. Know the role of obstetricians in forensic investigations
4. Describe legal implications of pregnancy in criminal cases
5. Learn case studies involving pregnancy evidence
6. Focus on the psychological effects of pregnancy on victims and suspects
7. Explain ethical considerations in handling pregnancy evidence
8. Identify challenges in proving pregnancy in forensics
9. Know future research directions in pregnancy and forensics

Pregnancy and forensic exams often intersect in ways that ripple through the legal and healthcare fields. Finding a grip on the bodily changes during pregnancy can genuinely be of great assistance to forensic scientists in gathering information about a mother's health and the development of the fetus – something that, in most instances, is the difference-maker. At other times, the discovery of a particular marker or locating DNA within a sample provides timeline clues that have the potential to tip the outcome of a case, particularly regarding violence toward pregnant women. The emergence of forensic nursing illustrates that practitioners must be knowledgeable about the delicate ground of pregnancy-related cases; this involves taking special precautions to preserve evidence as well as maintaining a chain of custody. Shortfalls in these forensic know-hows could result in misinvestigations, so regular, enhanced training within this specialized field is typically a requirement (Coelho et al., 2016).

2.2.1. Definition of Pregnancy in Forensic Terms

Pregnancy is more than a biological process—here, it entwines legal, social, and ethical threads in unexpected ways. In forensic practice, it is usually regarded merely as the fact that there is a fetus in the womb, an item that generally heralds a pivot point for argument over a woman's rights and the fetus's status. In the majority of instances, this same concept is significant in the case of infanticide, where varying perceptions regarding what constitutes pregnancy can influence court verdicts and inform community reactions to out-of-marriage births.

Early records indicate that, for a long time, society has infused our perception of pregnancy; women were often viewed only as mothers—a notion recent research (Oja, 2022) has begun to challenge. Overall, these views remind us that we require an increasingly dynamic vision for pregnancy, one that truly honors women's lived experiences while addressing the moral and legal aspects of reproduction (Lonza, 2002) (Figure 2.7).

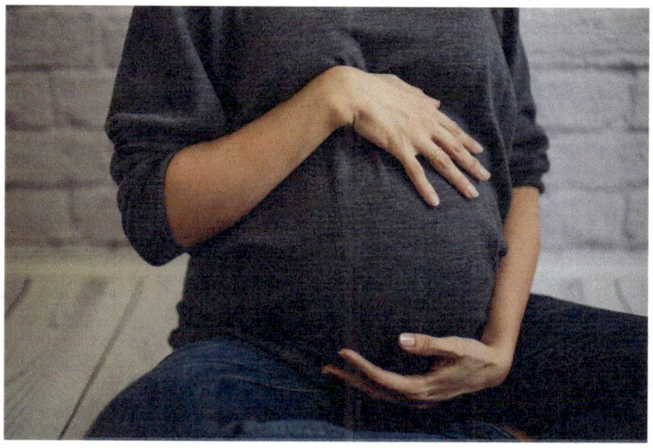

Figure 2.7. Pregnancy.

Source: CloudFront. (n.d.). *Pregnant Woman Holding Her Belly.* https://d1g9yur4m4naub.cloudfront.net/images/Article_Images/ImageForArticle_825_16521914658404888.jpg.

2.2.2. Forensic Indicators of Pregnancy

Pregnancy is not always easy to interpret, particularly when forensic data are involved following events such as sexual violence or cases of virginity. You may observe some corporeal cues—such as an enlarged uterus or a dark line on the belly (linea nigra)—that, in most instances, indicate that a woman had been pregnant at the time of a claimed event. Forensic testing also provides an additional layer by detecting human chorionic gonadotropin (hCG) in body fluids, thereby providing a type of biochemical corroboration that confirms the other indicators. Individual variability in how one feels about being pregnant—and a less-than-optimal understanding of associated health services—can complicate things, however, as observed in countries such as Afghanistan, where prevalent maternal mortality rates related to societal issues also complicate the situation (Hadi et al., 2016). In brief, a cautious, sometimes even chaotic, yet sophisticated methodology is essential for unraveling the facts to facilitate proper legal diagnosis and responsibility (Allen et al., 2018).

2.2.3. The Role of Obstetricians in Forensic Investigations

Obstetricians are increasingly becoming a vital part in forensic practice (Figure 2.8). They are not only involved in everyday medical practice; in most instances, they are the first choice when it comes to solving complicated matters such as virginity, pregnancy, and delivery—particularly in legal proceedings where maternal as well as fetal health come under scrutiny. In many instances, such specialists end up performing in-depth analyses actually to pin down what is medically happening; consider, for example, cases of pregnancy issues, such as when ailments like portal hypertension arise and, in a large majority of instances, increase the risks for both the mother and infant (Pint et al., 2025). Their observation proves helpful with respect to drug use in pregnancy, too; most studies tend to indicate that cannabis use—a developing trend—would be associated with adverse outcomes among infants (Sheedy et al., 2024). Essentially, by opening up the eye to how mothers' behavior may affect forensic findings, obstetricians quietly bridge the gap between clinician practice and the realm of legal investigation.

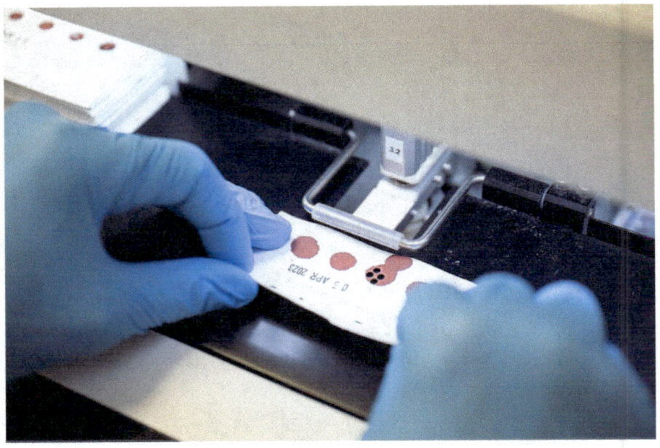

Figure 2.8. Obstetricians are becoming ever more essential in forensic work.

Source: The Royal College of Pathologists. (n.d.). *Newborn Screening Lab Photo.* https://www.rcpath.org/static/320dd667-8384-46d6-916d5639db4cb937/825x550_highestperformance__4a7c7e45a350/Newborn-screening-lab-photo.jpg.

2.2.4. Legal Implications of Pregnancy in Criminal Cases

Legal issues arise when pregnancy complications turn criminal case structures on their head, affecting survivors and the justice system in unpredictable ways. In most jurisdictions, a case's resolution can depend on a survivor's pregnancy specifics—when sexual assault is involved, consent is re-evaluated according to the woman's stage of gestation. Unwanted pregnancies resulting from assault can complicate testimony while increasing the emotional burden on victims. Law often does not explicitly define how to approach these specific circumstances, so survivors are left with less-strengthened protections—particularly in regions where sexual and gender-based violence prevails, as specific Kenyan research has pointed out (Guyo et al., 2009). And, in general, the stigma associated with rape pregnancy can discourage reporting, further complicating the quest for justice and the implementation of current rape laws (Ajagunna et al., 2020) (Figure 2.9).

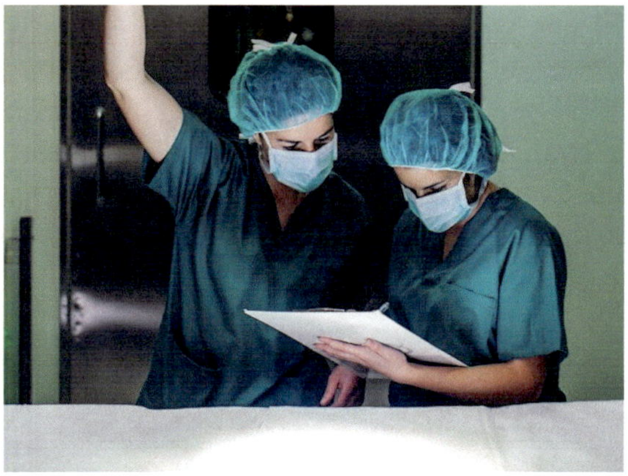

Figure 2.9. Unwanted pregnancies born of assault can muddle testimony while ramping up the emotional toll on victims.

Source: HealthDay. (n.d.). *Nurses in An Operating Room.* https://images.ctfassets.net/pdf29us7flmy/6vNHWNe7pChyceeY2hha6r/4aa91ea9f6bc51ce83237573a2743407/nurses-operating-room.jpeg?w=720&q=100&fm=jpg.

2.2.5. Case Studies Involving Pregnancy Evidence

Stepping back into ancient cases provides us with an engaging glimpse into just how complicated pregnancy evidence can get in court, all tied up with society's understanding of virginity and what is moral. In early modern Venice, for example, courts addressed problematic issues such as illegitimacy and sexual misconduct by mainly relying on the local community's own testimonies to support allegations of rape or seduction. These testimonies – replete with long-standing prejudices – tended to result in unmarried pregnant women not only being legally charged but also subject to personal and social repercussions (Ferraro et al., 2022). Today, studies from Egypt suggest that straightforward information and actual support for youth are crucial in managing SRH, demonstrating that these issues remain relevant (Abdel-Tawab et al., 2013). If you correlate these observations, it is pretty evident that the traditional challenges surrounding demonstrating pregnancy have remained, influencing legal rulings and societal sentiments in ways nobody expected.

2.2.6. Psychological Effects of Pregnancy on Victims and Suspects

Trauma is complicated and multi-layered, particularly when sexual assault results in an unwanted pregnancy. Victims may find themselves struggling with intense anxiety and depression as they must deal not just with the violence but also with the surprise of pregnancy. This experience will at times intensify their feelings of isolation and shame, which will keep them from seeking help or seeking justice. At the same time, suspects can also grapple with their own mental burden—usually worsened when society also hastens to label them with guilt based on outdated perceptions of male control. Lawfully, in most instances, the law has started to pay attention to the suffering of victims but continues to recycle outdated gender conceptions that tarnish women and make their healing process even more challenging (Allen et al., 2018). In regions such as India, in which systemic violence is widespread, the simultaneous impact of trauma and pregnancy is capable of triggering a vicious cycle of harm and victimization (Chatterji et al., 2015).

2.2.7. Ethical Considerations in Handling Pregnancy Evidence

Forensic pregnancy cases tend to be complicated, particularly if sexual violence is part of it (Figure

2.10). In most cases, combining legal obligation with ethical concern creates a genuine dilemma that places professionals in the middle of conflicting rules and their personal sense of empathy. At times, decisions concerning care are influenced by institutional policies and deeply rooted community assumptions, further complicating every case. Consider, for instance, a situation in some Catholic hospitals—EC may be restricted due to religious positions, which results in depriving rape survivors of essential assistance and increasing their trauma (Violi-Satkoske et al., 2008). In most situations, the principles of informed consent and equal access to healthcare services are often distorted in practice. Overall, there is a significant push toward ethical strategies that, in general terms, combine humane care with legal protections, enabling survivors to access the help they require (Chikadzi et al., 2018).

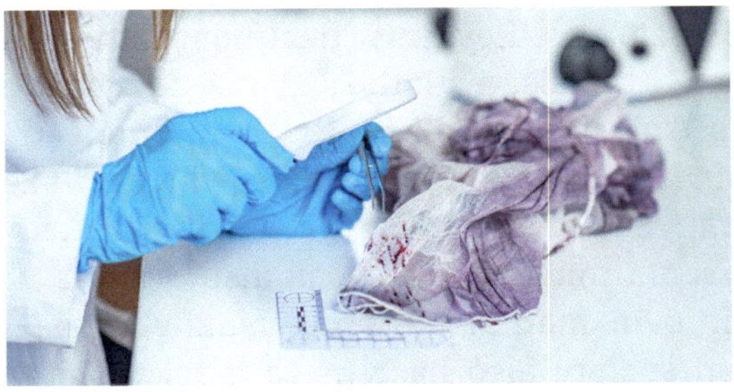

Figure 2.10. Forensic cases around pregnancy evidence tend to get messy, especially when sexual violence is involved.

Source: Forensic Access. (n.d.). *Forensic Access LinkedIn Social Post.* https://www.forensic-access.co.uk/media/g1bibxrc/forensic-access-linkedin-social-post.png?width=750&height=392.5.

2.2.8. Challenges in Proving Pregnancy in Forensics

Forensic science frequently runs into a roadblock when establishing a pregnancy, combining rigid evidence with all forms of legal and social baggage. Experts tend to rely on a combination of physical indicators and psychological clues; however, this type of evidence is often relatively imprecise and makes prosecutors uncomfortable. Cultural notions do not assist either—women are typically understood primarily within the framework of motherhood and reproduction, a perception that is particularly pronounced in the context of reproductive rights (Oja et al., 2022). Historically, cases of infant mortality demonstrate that medical evidence—frequently dodgy at best—has altered legal decisions and even suggested a prejudice in hearing cases of women's experiences (Dixon-Goodall et al., 2017). Overall, the conflict between hard science and changing social realities creates forensic evaluations of pregnancy into a messy, uncertain jigsaw puzzle that resonates through legal cases and reaches into actual lives.

2.2.9. Future Research Directions in Pregnancy and Forensics

Genetics and forensics sometimes combine in ways that can actually alter how we view pregnancy—not merely as a health issue but as something with legal complexities, as well. Sudden changes in technology, particularly in genome sequencing, are prompting us to rethink; in the majority of instances, new research is already suggesting that precise genomic information could unlock family ties as well as identify prenatal afflictions. This additional information can provide researchers with further clues regarding maternal and fetal well-being, presenting information that was not previously obvious. Ethical concerns arise too—concerns regarding who gets to view and utilize our genetic information, for instance, are somewhat tangible when you think about the dangers associated with direct-to-consumer tests on less regulated websites (Ayday et al., 2015; State University, Columbus, 2014). Overall, navigating these issues appears to be crucial if scientists are to effectively integrate genomic advancements with advancements in medicine and forensic practice.

Test Your Knowledge

1. Which hormone is routinely utilized for verifying pregnancy in forensic examinations?
2. Provide two biological specimens used for detecting pregnancy.

2.3. Delivery and Forensic Analysis

Learning Outcome

1. Give a definition of delivery in a forensic context
2. Explain forensic examination of delivery-related evidence
3. Know the legal implications of delivery in forensic cases
4. Describe the role of midwives and obstetricians in forensic delivery cases
5. Learn case studies involving delivery in forensics
6. Know the psychological impact of delivery on victims and families
7. Focus on ethical considerations in delivery-related forensic investigations
8. Identify challenges in forensic analysis of delivery evidence
9. Discuss future trends in the study of delivery in forensics

Confronting SRH services is fraught with challenges—it all makes sense when you notice the convergence of healthcare delivery and forensic audits unexpectedly during maternal health emergencies. Consider Afghanistan as one case; its skyrocketing maternal mortality rate typically reveals a fractured system in which sparse knowledge and persistent social biases give many women fewer options (Hadi et al., 2016). A closer forensic examination of these devastating losses tends to reveal shocking gaps in the delivery of care, suggesting that stronger, more adaptable interventions perhaps may be necessary for the most at-risk. At the same time, as societal attitudes about sexual violence gradually change, tired myths regarding consent and victimhood continue to persist, quietly shaping the way women's health is addressed in forensic contexts (Allen et al., 2018). For the most part, reconsidering both service provision and case analysis ultimately determines policies that can improve women's health outcomes.

2.3.1. Definition of Delivery in a Forensic Context

Delivery is more than the mere act of giving birth. Forensic delivery takes it into an arena much more complicated than mere biology, dealing with legal implications and social consequences that are not necessarily apparent. Virginity and pregnancy cases give us a window into this kind of complexity. Investigators tend to examine the circumstances surrounding a birth, attempting to sort out if consent was truly present or if coercion was a sneaky factor—concerns that tend to trace back to larger cases of gender violence. Consider CARE Kenya's report as an illustration (Guyo et al., 2009). It typically indicates that widespread sexual and gender violence tends to cloud the issue around consent during labor, particularly in the case of unmarried girls. Although legal protections for women have made some advances, entrenched attitudes remain, and it is difficult to obtain justice in most cases, as observed in discussions regarding rape law reform (Allen et al., 2018). On this basis, the concept of delivery in forensics is not simply a clinical one; it represents a complex nexus where biology, law, and social justice intersect (Figure 2.11).

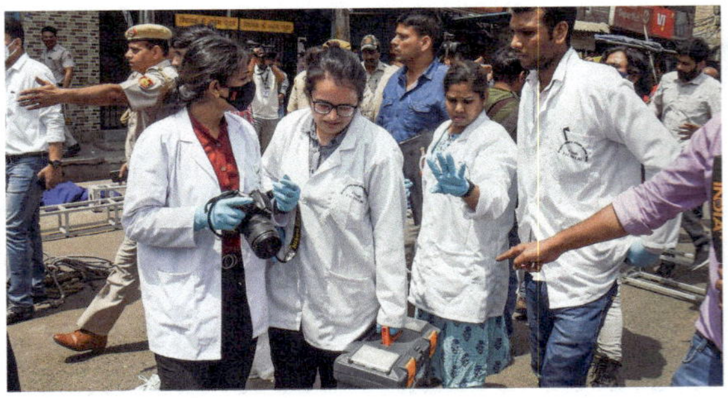

Figure 2.11. In forensic work, it extends into a realm far more complex than biology alone, touching on legal matters and social consequences that are not always apparent.

Source: Deccan Herald. (2022). *The Missing Piece: Forensics in Criminal Investigation.*

2.3.2. Forensic Examination of Delivery-Related Evidence

Pregnancy and delivery can spin a somewhat chaotic puzzle in forensic science, particularly when sexual offenses are involved. In most situations, untangling the sequence of events involves piecing together pieces of evidence that tend to stray from the timeline. Specialists typically immerse themselves in hospital records, interview witnesses, and analyze biological evidence to catch those elusive details, even if the link is not always as clear-cut. They also have to account for the emotional after-effect—surviving women tend to experience a complicated array of feelings after giving birth, which can confuse their accounts somewhat. Research typically indicates that a cautious, gentle-handed strategy towards both medical and mental healthcare not only helps survivors but can also enhance collaboration with law enforcement. Overall, combining vigorous forensic investigation with authentic, compassionate care tends to strip away the trappings and lay bare the true story behind cases that involve pregnancy and delivery (Asadi et al., 2023, 2024)

2.3.3. Legal Implications of Delivery in Forensic Cases

Legal systems and forensic delivery cases intersect in ways both unforeseen and that result in the majority of stakeholders having to navigate a complex web of rules and ethical conundrums. These key players—law enforcement officials and healthcare workers, for example—are ensnared in systems which repeatedly grapple with tight resources and existing problems, according to Chikadzi et al. (2018). In most instances, even the way evidence is collected and interpreted is influenced by issues regarding consent and the responsibility to safeguard vulnerable groups—issues that repeatedly arise. The lingering stigmatization associated with topics such as gender and sexual violence only serves to confuse. Thus, it is imperative for an equally well-coordinated effort that protects the survivors and advocates for their rights in our legal system, as noted by Guyo et al. (2009). Overall, this multifaceted strategy is essential for ensuring that everyone has equal access to justice and support.

2.3.4. The Role of Midwives and Obstetricians in Forensic Delivery Cases

Midwives and obstetricians have evolved into much more than just baby-delivery experts. In forensic cases, they are not simply concerned with the technical process—these individuals are present to keep both mothers and babies safe physically and, for many, emotionally as well. Occasionally, it gets even more complicated. Consider, for instance, cases of female genital mutilation and/or cutting (FGM/C) where surgery may be required; in such cases, their services extend to gathering forensic evidence when necessary. Research tends to indicate that women who have been subjected to FGM/C require a detailed list of all the available surgical procedures so that they can select the care that best suits them (Macher et al., 2021).

In addition, such caregivers are themselves local advocates, closing knowledge gaps and establishing trust, dispelling barriers for those on society's periphery in forensic settings (Farina et al., 2017). Despite a combination of technical responsibilities and investigative activities, they succeed in marrying complex skill with authentic compassion, demonstrating that care in such complex cases is far from routine (Figure 2.12).

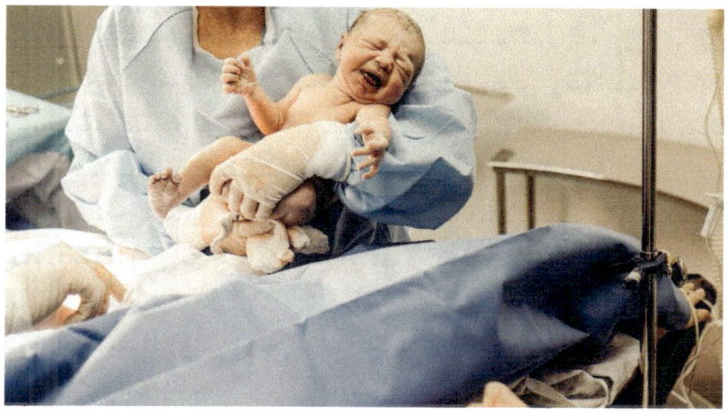

Figure 2.12. The role of midwives and obstetricians in forensic delivery cases.

Source: Borba, J. (2020). Pregnant woman standing next to a man in front of a window. *Transforming Maternity*.

2.3.5. Case Studies Involving Delivery in Forensics

Forensic virginity, pregnancy, and childbirth cases don't just reduce to technical tests—they also expose underlying societal cleavages. In most regions where cultural stigmas persist and educational access lags behind, these problems spill over into larger social issues. Zimbabwe, for example, has a Victim-Friendly System that helps professionals navigate the complicated reality of assisting child sexual abuse survivors (Chikadzi et al., 2018). CARE Kenya research typically presents the same picture by indicating that sexual and gender-based violence is very much present, frequently placing unmarried girls aged 9 to 15 at additional risk (Guyo et al., 2009). If you look closely, really, these forensic assessments are intertwined with normative daily standards and legal requirements. Overall, these cases suggest that effective assistance to survivors requires a combination of coordinated support and a willingness to confront long-standing, systemic issues.

2.3.6. Psychological Impact of Delivery on Victims and Families

Delivery tends to leave lasting impressions that extend far beyond bodily pain—it disrupts mental well-being and even familial bonds in ways both surprising and untold. Survivors of rape, for example, may experience a tidal wave of feelings during childbirth and even beyond; the trauma of their original abuse will usually linger and make matters worse.

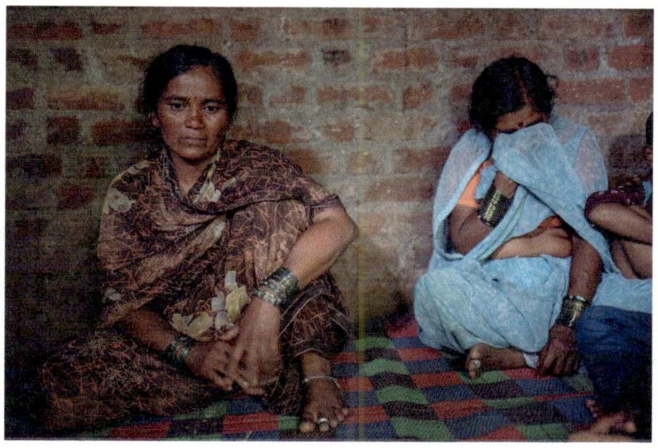

Figure 2.13. Survivors of sexual violence can feel an overwhelming surge of emotions throughout childbirth and even afterward; the trauma from their initial abuse tends to linger and complicate things further.

Source: The Fuller Project. (2024). *Women Sitting on a Mat Inside a Brick-Walled Room in India.* https://fullerproject.org/wp-content/uploads/2024/11/SMK8369-1600x1066.jpg.

In many communities where gender roles are uneven and cultural norms hold tight, the added weight of social stigma can really intensify feelings of anxiety, depression, and even push some toward post-traumatic stress disorder. Support systems are not always up to par either; for example, Zimbabwe's so-called Victim-Friendly System struggles with limited resources and patchy infrastructure (Chikadzi et al., 2018). Research from Kenya also goes in the same direction—most victims are just not aware of legal supports or services that they can access, which only adds to their feelings of isolation and distress (Guyo et al., 2009). Overall, it appears pretty obvious that these issues need to be addressed if we are going to see any significant improvement in mental health for survivors and their families (Figure 2.13).

2.3.7. Ethical Considerations in Delivery-related Forensic Investigations

Forensic investigations related to delivery are full of complexities requiring a straightforward ethical approach—particularly when issues regarding virginity and pregnancy are involved. Medical personnel, police officers, and other people present must prioritize people's dignity and rights, ensuring that whatever they do does not contribute to the already inflicted trauma. You can actually view this ethical requirement in multi-sector systems, such as the Victim-Friendly System, which often faces challenges including resource shortages and weak infrastructure (Chikadzi et al., 2018). For the majority of situations, numerous studies have indicated that an overarching, comprehensive strategy for preventing rape is essential in countering such ethical issues from multiple fronts (Hailegeorgis, 2019). Finally, building an ethical culture is not merely about ticking institutional boxes—it is a vital support for achieving genuine justice and compassionate care in delivery-centered forensic practice.

2.3.8. Challenges in Forensic Analysis of Delivery Evidence

Forensic analysis of delivery evidence is not as straightforward as it appears—it is entwined with problems that tend to obscure the real picture of virginity and pregnancy cases (Figure 2.14). The reality that there is no uniform set of rules across various fields, to some extent, prevents investigators from compiling credible evidence. When you combine insights from medicine, law, and psychology, things inevitably become even more complicated; experts committed to their own profession often bring along ingrained biases, further complicating the process and making it unstable. Additionally, resource constraints—such as a lack of equipment or personnel—tend to exacerbate complications. In most conversations regarding child sexual abuse cases, for instance, it is evident that financial and infrastructure limitations significantly hinder the quality of forensic work (Chikadzi et al., 2018). These issues not only hinder the successful analysis of delivery evidence but can also continue to keep old gender assumptions in circulation in the legal system, shifting how accusations are conceptualized and addressed (Allen et al., 2018).

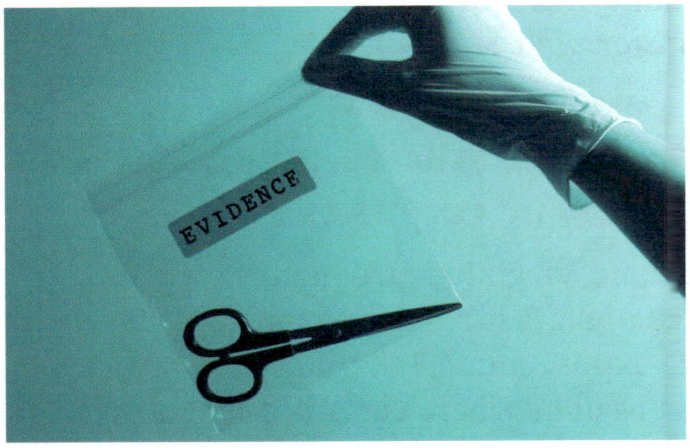

Figure 2.14. Forensic work on delivering evidence is not as simple as it seems—it is tangled up in issues that often cloud the accurate picture of cases involving virginity and pregnancy.

Source: BBC. (n.d.). *Scissors Placed in an Evidence Bag Held by a Gloved Hand.*

2.3.9. Future Trends in the Study of Delivery in Forensics

Societal changes in perceptions about gender and reproductive rights have led to fresh thinking when it comes to analyzing delivery cases. Forensic work used to be almost all about biology; now, the psychological and social complications of pregnancy and giving birth are beginning to get attention – they bring additional layers to the scenario. Cultural practice research – consider, for instance, some of the work on Korekore women – reveals that local understandings often influence reproductive health decisions in ways we had not previously considered. These projects, which occasionally suggest fascinating intersections between bodily considerations, feelings, and social environments (Rural Support Programs Network, 2019), assist us in refiguring forensic procedures to be more capable of supporting sexual violence survivors. In general terms, examining how women navigate complex social pressures appears to provide insight into creating more compassionate and effective practices, illuminating the messy problems that people tend to encounter (Mudzimu et al., 2021).

Test Your Knowledge

1. Name any two clinical signs indicative of recent childbirth.
2. How does a forensic expert confirm recent vaginal delivery during an examination?

2.4. Interconnections Between Virginity, Pregnancy, and Delivery

Learning Outcome

1. Know the relationship between virginity and pregnancy
2. Explain the impact of cultural beliefs on perceptions of virginity and pregnancy
3. Learn the forensic implications of virginity on pregnancy outcomes
4. Describe the role of delivery in the context of virginity and pregnancy
5. Explain case studies highlighting interconnections
6. Discuss the psychological consequences of the interconnections
7. Focus on ethical considerations in addressing these interconnections
8. Describe the legal ramifications of the interconnections in forensic cases
9. Know future research opportunities in the interconnection

Virginity, pregnancy, and childbirth become all tangled together in ways that society and history actually form the forensic aspect of SRH. Virginity tends to come up as a sort of cultural marker that can influence the way that evidence about pregnancy and childbirth is interpreted. It's not merely a social designation—it also becomes entangled with notions of purity that can complicate things for investigators, at times in unexpected ways. Medical professionals, in most situations, must thread these undercurrents, particularly when handling situations of sexual assault where these myths run deep. In The Body of Evidence, one can see that the slow development of forensic medicine typically comes to show just how deeply beliefs in society contort the interpretation of body signals related to virginity and pregnancy. Also, new developments in personalized health technologies remind us that merging holistic, culturally oriented practices into healthcare can actually enhance patient experience and care management.

2.4.1. The Relationship Between Virginity and Pregnancy

Virginity and pregnancy become entangled with old cultural conceptions that intertwine a woman's sexual history with her fertility (Figure 2.15). In most communities, virginity is a heavy moral and social burden, and unwed mothers who become pregnant are usually judged. It is a widespread assumption—one that has been repeated down the ages—that loss of virginity inevitably results in pregnancy, which unfortunately draws a strict line between those who are viewed as virtuous and those described as promiscuous. This type of clear-cut split makes it more difficult when investigating forensic cases, particularly those of sexual assault, where the victim too often finds herself having to establish more than appears reasonable. Historical examples, as also pointed out by Ferraro's work, illustrate how public opinion has influenced outcomes in the law for ages. Even now, forensic nursing collides with the same old notions, which emphasize the urgent need for more effective and well-balanced training in forensic practice to dispel such biases and actually stand up for the victims (Coelho et al., 2016; Ferraro et al., 2022).

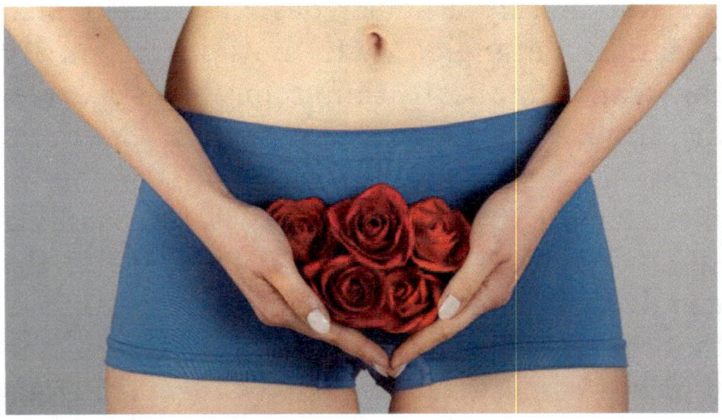

Figure 2.15. Virginity and pregnancy get tangled up in old cultural ideas that mix a woman's sexual past with her ability to bear children.

Source: Health Shots. (2020). *Conceptual Image Related to Virginity*.

2.4.2. The Impact of Cultural Beliefs on Perceptions of Virginity and Pregnancy

Societal perceptions of virginity and pregnancy emerge from entrenched cultural beliefs that contort into complicated issues of women's health. Virginity becomes entangled in honor codes and morality ideals in most communities; this combination, in the vast majority, evokes a persistent stigma surrounding premarital sex. And yes, that stigma only worsens preexisting issues – consider pregnant teenagers who frequently find themselves ostracized from their own communities. When discussing women's health, it becomes apparent that sexual and reproductive issues are not merely prevalent but also suggest broader ethical dilemmas rooted in tradition (De Bürger et al., 2023). In addition to this, gender imbalances and a disturbing level of violence further complicate the situation, particularly in areas where young girls experience high levels of sexual and gender-based abuse (Guyo et al., 2019). Overall, these interconnected factors limit women's access to the necessary healthcare they require, impacting both individual well-being and overall community health.

2.4.3. Forensic Implications of Virginity on Pregnancy Outcomes

Cultural and legal definitions of virginity influence how pregnancy test results are considered in forensic situations—particularly where sexual assault or rape is the concern (Figure 2.16). Virginity becomes imbued with traditional notions of purity and good moral character in most cultures, and that can instantly make survivors get blamed. Frequently, too frequently, a victim's account is brought into doubt merely due to her sexual history, with judicial prejudices making holes in a woman's word. Even when the laws have been revised to typically safeguard the survivors, such deep-seated prejudices remain, resulting in not investigating sufficiently and fewer convictions by and large, which in fact hurts the victims. As Allen et al. (2018) show, the stigma for sexual violence simply will not desist, thus complicating pregnancy information further to disentangle in forensic practice. Concurrently, there exists some intertwining between what society views about virginity and the few support services provided, the blend that interferes directly with the psych and medical treatment survivors receive post-trauma, as Chikadzi et al. (2018) explain.

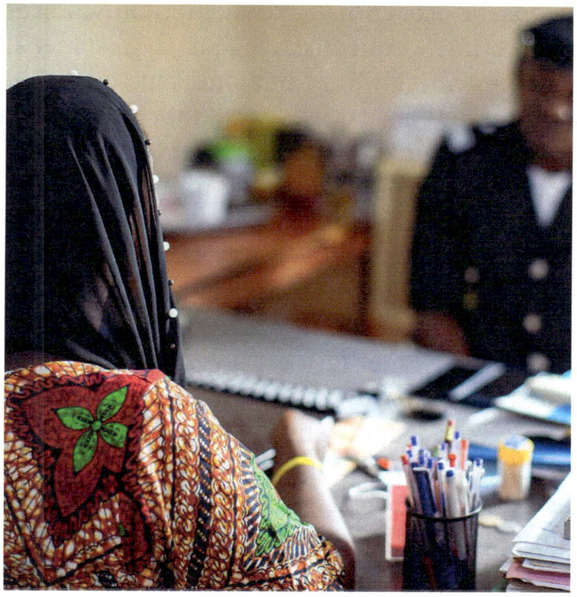

Figure 2.16. Virginity ideas in both culture and law shape how pregnancy outcomes are looked at in forensic cases—especially when sexual assault or rape is involved.

Source: UNFPA. (n.d.). *A Woman Speaking to a Uniformed Officer Across a Desk.*

2.4.4. The Role of Delivery in the Context of Virginity and Pregnancy

Virginity and pregnancy combine in novel ways during giving birth—particularly when viewed through a forensic frame. Giving birth flaunts SRH's messiness, dragging everyday concepts and old cultural narratives into focus. Current studies of Egyptian youth indicate that, in general, providing honest, direct sexual health guidance can actually influence how young people approach pregnancy and motherhood (Abdel-Tawab et al., 2013). Going back, records inform us that previous legal systems tended to judge women according to their sex history, particularly when a birth was considered out of wedlock, adding additional social pressures along the way (Ferraro et al., 2022). Briefly, delivery is not merely the act of giving birth; it is an instant when society's perceptions regarding purity and parenthood collide with a crash, impacting individual lives as well as the community.

2.4.5. Case Studies Highlighting Interconnections

Societal conventions, medical protocols, and legal arrangements all blend to paint a complicated image of virginity, pregnancy, and childbirth in forensic contexts. It is fascinating—case studies tend to highlight that physicians' descriptions of sexual consent will tend to ripple their way through legislative shifts surrounding sexual crimes, illustrating how medicine and law will most often find themselves in some back-and-forth negotiation (Bates et al., 2015). In most instances, if you consider the complexities of human sexuality in regions such as Tehuantepec, you find a mix of practices that not only define how motherhood is felt but also how intimate violence is interpreted, connecting everyday life with its surroundings in unexpected ways (Rodriguez et al., 2011). Age, class, and gender certainly play their roles—occasionally in overlapping, messy ways—shaping forensic evidence, defying any suggestion that these subjects exist separately in neat, distinct ways. When all these elements are combined, they enhance our perspective on forensic work, making discourse around virginity and childbirth into a braided fabric of social threads that continue to recycle themselves.

2.4.6. Psychological Implications of the Interconnections

Virginity, pregnancy, and birth combine a lot of social and psychological pressures, all of which are entwined with the ways that cultures construct sexual morals and womanhood. Everywhere, shame associated with sex before marriage really gets to activate deep-seated emotional problems—such as depression and anxiety—particularly for women who find themselves unexpectedly pregnant outside of marriage.

It becomes even more complicated when normal social or legal assistance is simply not available or falls short in any case. As an example, certain studies indicate that individuals who assist victims of child sexual abuse experience many setbacks, primarily because resources are limited (Chikadzi et al., 2018). And in settings where sexual or gender-based violence is widespread, the absence of explicit legal protection leaves women vulnerable and isolated (Guyo et al., 2009). All of this, by and large, indicates a genuine need for support mechanisms that can address both the emotional highs and lows, as well as the legal hurdles, simultaneously (Figure 2.17).

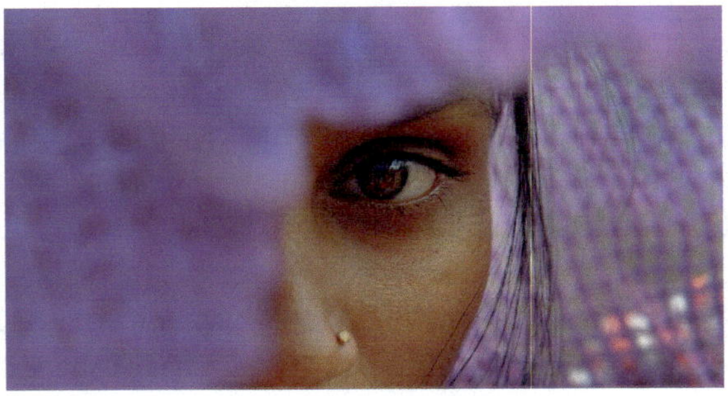

Figure 2.17. Those who help survivors of child sexual abuse face a lot of setbacks, mainly because resources are in short supply.

Source: Human Rights Watch. (2017). *Everyone Blames Me: Barriers to Justice and Support Services for Sexual Assault Survivors in India.*

2.4.7. Ethical Considerations in Addressing These Interconnections

Social concepts of virginity, the complications of pregnancy problems, and the actual on-the-ground challenges of giving birth in forensic situations all combine in ways that require a closer ethical examination. It is not a tidy puzzle—women and children tend to suffer most from these intertwined issues, so this is an obvious public health concern that we cannot sweep under the rug. Adopt research from Ethiopia on preventing rape; such studies indicate that victims require care that is not merely a short-term solution, but one that addresses both current assistance and more profound, deeper-level interventions (Hailegeorgis, 2019). There has been a growing opinion that we cannot count on interventions that come into play after issues arise—what we actually need are robust primary measures to address the social problems at their root. Meanwhile, if you examine how mental health professionals are educated to serve families with children who have been sexually abused, there is clearly a lack of specialized expertise and preparedness; this strongly indicates an immediate need for improved teaching materials. By and large, supporting these training programs could lead to more empathetic and informed responses. Ultimately, bridging such ethical and pragmatic gaps remains critical to managing sensitive cases (Arredeondo et al., 2019).

2.4.8. Legal Ramifications of the Interconnections in Forensic Cases

Forensic cases tend to conceal a web of interrelationships that ultimately change legal conclusions in unexpected ways. Issues such as virginity, pregnancy, and even childbirth suddenly show dimensions—based on common medical facts and larger social narratives—that render legal choices well beyond being black and white. Frequently, observing those themes blend helps clarify what evidence actually matters in court, though it all appears slightly grisly. Take Rodriguez et al. (2011), for instance, which reminds us that human sexuality, in all its twists and turns of complicatedness, does not lend itself to easy legal compartments. You can also observe it in how Irish deaf women explain their experiences; their accounts reveal how society's perceptions of vulnerability can actually warp legal arguments (Meehan et al., 2019). It is as if these legal repercussions transcend mere procedural checklists, reflecting underlying power struggles and long-standing cultural narratives that, in the vast majority of instances, cry out for a closer, more detailed examination. Overall, this combination of factors suggests that we require a broader, more cautious framework for legal systems addressing such delicate and intricate issues.

2.4.9. Future Research Opportunities in the Interconnections

Forensic research recently has been tearing apart the legal designations associated with virginity, pregnancy, and childbirth—even as many questions remain in the air. The legal and medical communities are not precisely operating in silos, as we observe how the concept of consent has changed over time, in general, due to changes in sexual offense legislation (Figure 2.18). Look, when you delve into medicos' concepts of sexual offence and consent, you immediately see that to comprehend these connections is to examine age, class, and gender—the very things that have long influenced the way society understands (Bates et al., 2015). Meanwhile, incorporating local perspectives can actually enhance our understanding of pregnancy and birth practices for health, providing a more comprehensive picture that draws on diverse cultural perceptions. Such an approach not only enlivens scholarly argumentation but is also in accord with contemporary efforts at decolonizing studies, particularly in the sciences of health (Anokwuru et al., 2025).

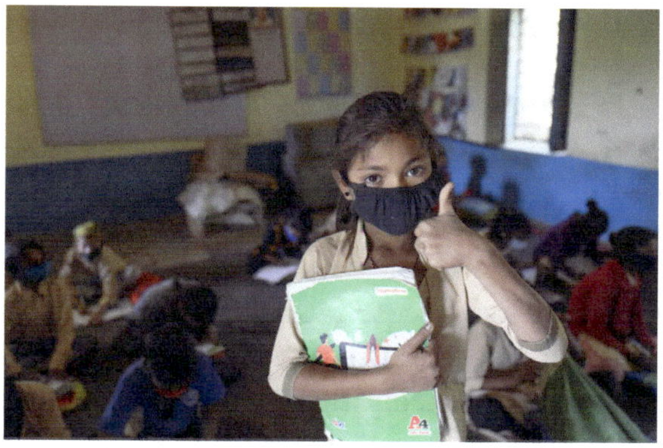

Figure 2.18. The legal and medical worlds are not exactly working in silos, as we see how the definition of consent has evolved over time, generally speaking, thanks to shifts in sexual offense laws.

Source: UNICEF. (n.d.). *Girl in Classroom Wearing a Mask and Giving a Thumbs Up During COVID-19 Pandemic*. https://www.unicef.org/india/sites/unicef.org.india/files/styles/media_large_image/public/UN0595340.jpg.webp?itok=ZtZwWfdd.

Test Your Knowledge

1. Write a note on medico-legal issues related to alleged pregnancy denial.
2. What is the relevance of pregnancy test results in the context of statutory rape allegations?

SUMMARY

Cultural expectations and forensic exams blend in ways that lead us to challenge outdated notions about virginity, pregnancy, and giving birth. If you pay close attention to how forensic procedures operate, you see those pesky, even sloppy stereotypes taint the legal response to sexual violence. Despite the establishment of new legislation—rape shield provisions—designed to safeguard victims, there remain many who still hold on to the notion that women fabricate accusations, one that continues to surface and compels us to reassess our legal approaches (Allen et al., 2018). Also, suppose you consider practices such as virginity testing as viewed by young people. In that case, it is apparent that traditions of the past are set against modern forensic methodologies, where education must extend across both cultural and legal landscapes (Mhlongo et al., 2009). Ultimately, only a wide-ranging, adaptable approach can truly guarantee victims are treated fairly in our forensic systems.

Forensic examination of virginity, pregnancy, and childbirth illustrates how knotted these issues actually are. Studies inform us that practitioners assisting child sexual abuse survivors encounter systemic barriers. Too often, they don't have sufficient training and adequate resources within what is referred to as the Victim-Friendly System (Chikadzi et al., 2018). In most instances, locations like Kenya's North Eastern Province are the witness to high sexual and gender-based violence rates, necessitating a more concerted effort by all the stakeholders (Guyo et al., 2009). Economic issues, cultural taboos, and an ambiguous understanding of legal rights all appear to converge, influencing the lives of women and girls, primarily in the context of sexual health and reproductive rights. When you put it all together, it is clear—albeit not without some flaws—that wide-ranging, well-rounded approaches are necessary to mitigate the aftermath of sexual violence, ultimately improving both survivor care and the overall quality of forensic examinations in these sensitive environments.

KEY TERMS FROM THIS CHAPTER

- Childbirth
- Delivery
- Midwives
- Obstetricians
- Personal healing
- Pregnancy
- Survivors
- Trauma
- Uterus
- Virginity

CRITICAL THINKING QUESTIONS

1. **Which of the following is TRUE regarding the hymen in forensic examination?**
   a. Its presence confirms virginity
   b. Its rupture always indicates sexual intercourse
   c. It can be torn due to non-sexual activities
   d. It cannot be visualized during examination
2. **Which hormone is tested for in pregnancy detection kits used in forensic settings?**
   a. Progesterone
   b. Estrogen
   c. Human Chorionic Gonadotropin (hCG)
   d. Oxytocin
3. **Which of the following is NOT a reliable indicator of virginity?**
   a. Intact hymen
   b. Absence of vaginal laxity
   c. Absence of previous pregnancies
   d. Presence of torn hymen
4. **A positive hCG test in a sexual offence case may support which of the following?**
   a. Virginity
   b. Recent delivery
   c. Pregnancy due to alleged intercourse
   d. Menstrual irregularity
5. **Lochia is a clinical sign associated with which condition?**
   a. Pregnancy
   b. Sexual assault
   c. Recent delivery
   d. Menopause

Short Answer Questions

1. What is the hymen, and is its presence or absence a reliable indicator of virginity?
2. Define virginity from a forensic and medico-legal perspective.
3. Can a woman who has delivered a child still have an intact hymen? Explain briefly.
4. What is the medico-legal significance of determining pregnancy in forensic cases?
5. Name two physical signs suggestive of recent delivery in a female.
6. What tests can confirm early pregnancy in a forensic setting?
7. Why is forensic confirmation of pregnancy important in cases of alleged sexual assault?

Answers to Critical Thinking Questions

1. (c); 2. (c); 3. (a); 4. (c); 5. (c)

REFERENCES

1. Abdel-Tawab, N. G., El Nawawi, N., & Saher, S., (2013). *Breaking the Silence: Learning About Youth Sexual and Reproductive Health in Egypt.* https://core.ac.uk/download/229800133.pdf (accessed on 9th May 2025).
2. Ajagunna, F. O., Ogunwale, A. O., & Oshiname, F. O. (2020). *A Review of the Conceptual Issues, Social Epidemiology, Prevention and Control Efforts Relating to Rape in Nigeria.* https://core.ac.uk/download/478293496.pdf (accessed on 9th May 2025).
3. Allen, A., (2018). *Rape Messaging.* https://core.ac.uk/download/216959128.pdf (accessed on 9th May 2025).
4. Anokwuru, R. A., Du Plessis, M. A. R., Lukhele, S., Magoro, M., et al. (2025). *Working with Indigenous Knowledge.* https://core.ac.uk/download/637920143.pdf (accessed on 9th May 2025).
5. Arredeondo, H. M. A. (2019). *Development & Evaluation of an Introductory Webinar Training for Mental Health Professionals Working with Families of Sexually Abused Children: A Strengths-Based Sociocultural Approach.* https://core.ac.uk/download/288854500.pdf (accessed on 9th May 2025).
6. Asadi, L., Noroozi, M., Salimi, H., Jambarsang, S., & Mardani, F., (2024). A qualitative study on the health system-related needs in women survivors of rape. *BMC Health Services Research, 24.* https://doi.org/10.1186/s12913-024-10852-0.
7. Asadi, L., Noroozi, M., Salimi, H., Mardani, F., & Jambarsang, S., (2023). A qualitative exploration of the psychological needs of women survivors of rape in Iran. *BMC Psychology, 11.* https://doi.org/10.1186/s40359-023-01332-x.
8. Ayday, E., Clayton, E. W., Fellay, J., Gunter, C., et al. (2015). *Privacy in the Genomic Era.* https://core.ac.uk/download/148015081.pdf (accessed on 9th May 2025).
9. Bates, V. L. (2015). *'Not an Exact Science': Medical Approaches to Age and Sexual Offences in England, 1850–1914.* https://core.ac.uk/download/12826778.pdf (accessed on 9th May 2025).
10. Butler, S. M. (2019). *"More Than Mothers: Juries of Matrons and Pleas of the Belly in Medieval England."* https://core.ac.uk/download/534863065.pdf (accessed on 9th May 2025).
11. Chatterji, A. P., Fletcher, L. E., Kaur, M., & Altholz, R., (2015). *Access to Justice for Women: India's Response to Sexual Violence in Conflict and Social Upheaval.* https://core.ac.uk/download/75783197.pdf (accessed on 9th May 2025).
12. Chikadzi, V., Kaseke, E., & Muridzo, N., (2018). *Challenges Faced by Professionals Working in Child Sexual Abuse Multi-Sectorial Forums: A Case of the Victim-Friendly System in Zimbabwe.* https://core.ac.uk/download/268542125.pdf (accessed on 9th May 2025).
13. Coelho, M., Cunha, M., & Libório, R., (2016). *Knowledge Questionnaire Over Forensics Nursing Practices.* https://core.ac.uk/download/70646655.pdf (accessed on 9th May 2025).
14. De Vido, S., (2020). *The Anamnesis.* Manchester University Press eBooks. https://doi.org/10.7765/9781526124982.00006 (accessed on 9th May 2025).
15. De Vido, S., (2020). *Violence Against Women's Health in International Law.* https://doi.org/10.7765/9781526124982.

16. Değer, B., (2023). *Reproductive HEALTH and Ethical Problems in Women's Health.* https://core.ac.uk/download/560378408.pdf (accessed on 9th May 2025).
17. Dixon-Goodall, R. E. (2017). *Infanticide, a Mother's Crime: Expert Evidence and Infanticide Cases, 1688–1955.* https://core.ac.uk/download/556181248.pdf (accessed on 9th May 2025).
18. Farina, P., Leye, E., Ortensi, L., Pecorella, M., et al. (2017). *The Impact of the Law in the Prevention of FGM: Legal Analysis.* https://core.ac.uk/download/153397215.pdf (accessed on 9th May 2025).
19. Ferraro, J. M. (2022). *Nefarious Crimes, Contested Justice.* https://core.ac.uk/download/534897504.pdf (accessed on 9th May 2025).
20. Gitanjali, D., (2011). *A Study on Victims of Sexual Offences.* https://core.ac.uk/download/235663920.pdf (accessed on 9th May 2025).
21. Guyo, J., & Mwangi, G. K. (2009). *An Assessment of Sexual and Gender-Based Violence in Wajir District, North Eastern Kenya.* https://core.ac.uk/download/327313290.pdf (accessed on 9th May 2025).
22. Güzel, H., (2020). B*ecoming-Virgin: Re-virginization Practices in Turkey.* https://core.ac.uk/download/328719675.pdf (accessed on 9th May 2025).
23. Hadi, M., (2016). *An Analysis of Policy and Social Factors Impacting the Uptake of Sexual and Reproductive Health Services in Kabul, Afghanistan.* https://core.ac.uk/download/76946271.pdf (accessed on 9th May 2025).
24. Hailegeorgis, D. S. (2019). *Situation Analysis of Perceptions on Comprehensiveness of Rape Prevention Interventions by Implementing Agencies in Addis Ababa* https://core.ac.uk/download/328838839.pdf (accessed on 9th May 2025).
25. Kilic, S., & Karasin, S. S. (2022). *A Pregnant Adolescence with an Intact Hymen.* https://core.ac.uk/download/612900656.pdf (accessed on 9th May 2025).
26. Lonza, N., (2002). *"Two Souls Lost": Infanticide in the Republic of Dubrovnik (1667–1808).* https://core.ac.uk/download/14391765.pdf (accessed on 9th May 2025).
27. Macher, L., & Raoult, M., (2021). *Surgical Interventions for Women with Female Genital Mutilation/Cutting: (A) How Successful are the Most Common Types of Surgical Interventions for FGM/C Available in Industrialized Countries; and (B) Which Factors Influence Whether the Results are Considered Satisfactory by the Women Receiving Them?* https://core.ac.uk/download/489484199.pdf (accessed on 9th May 2025).
28. Meehan, G. P. (2019). *Flourishing at the Margins: An Exploration of Deaf and Hard-of-Hearing Women's Stories of Their Intimate Lives in Ireland.* https://core.ac.uk/download/297033269.pdf (accessed on 9th May 2025).
29. Mhlongo, S. P. (2009). *Reasons for Undergoing Virginity Testing: A Study of Young People in Rural KwaZulu-Natal, South Africa.* https://core.ac.uk/download/196543934.pdf (accessed on 9th May 2025).
30. Mudzimu, E., (2021). *Religious and Cultural Encounters: Sexual and Reproductive Health and Rights Among the Korekore Women in Zimbabwe.* https://core.ac.uk/download/519038581.pdf (accessed on 9th May 2025).

31. Oja, L., (2022). *Who is the 'Woman' in Human Rights Law: Narratives of Women's Bodies and Sexuality in Reproduction Jurisprudence.* https://core.ac.uk/download/534151240.pdf (accessed on 9th May 2025).

32. Pint, D., Chung, Y., & Heneghan, M. A. (2025). Portal hypertension in pregnancy. *Current Opinion in Gastroenterology.* https://www.semanticscholar.org/paper/83439e33c51c34e15913e507b0d05abe2b9581cb (accessed on 9th May 2025).

33. Rodriguez, V., (2011). *Behind the Scene: The Enactments of Human Sexuality in Tehuantepec, Mexico.* https://core.ac.uk/download/pdf/29237234.pdf (accessed on 9th May 2025).

34. Rural Support Programs Network. (2019). *Building Partnerships for Scaling Access to Justice for Survivors of Sexual Violence in Pakistan.* https://core.ac.uk/download/542480767.pdf (accessed on 9th May 2025).

35. Sheedy, K., Wilson, T., Groesch, K., Diaz-Sylvester, P., Delfino, K., Unal, E. R., & Nelson, E., (2024). Assessment of marijuana use during pregnancy and its effects on neonatal outcomes. *North American Proceedings in Gynecology & Obstetrics.* https://www.semanticscholar.org/paper/5e7b0450309fb41bbc374c43fd8547f7d70aafd8 (accessed on 9th May 2025).

36. State University, Columbus. (2014). *Abstracts 2014: Highlights of Student Research and Creative Endeavors.* https://core.ac.uk/download/147510471.pdf (accessed on 9th May 2025).

37. Violi-Satkoske, V., (2008). *Emergency Contraception, Catholic Hospitals, and Rape.* https://core.ac.uk/download/234047995.pdf (accessed on 9th May 2025).

FORENSIC PSYCHIATRY

3

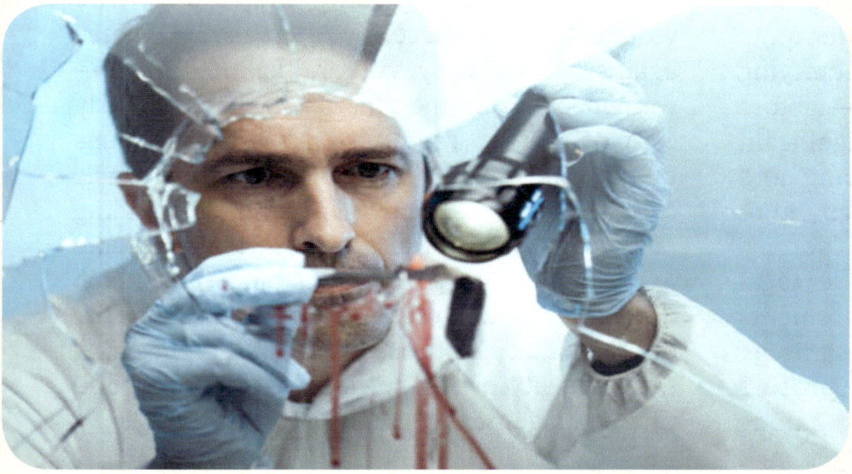

Introduction

Recently, the confluence of mental health and the legal system has truly been on people's minds, leading us to reassess forensic psychiatry. Forensic psychiatry, essentially, attempts to sort out the interplay between mental disorders and legal rules—commingling clinical assessments and legal responsibility issues. Most often, when the World Health Organization gave ICD-11 its stamp of approval, it sparked a range of debates regarding the classification of mental disorders (Stein et al., 2020). This change prompted specialists to reassess entrenched diagnostic criteria and consider how these modifications could be applied in both daily practice and research. Apart from that, since mental illnesses can be highly complicated and intertwined with social and economic issues (Hirdes et al., 2020), wider evaluations become nearly inevitable. Overall, by considering things from these various perspectives, forensic psychiatry appears to emerge as a central discipline that can lead the way towards more successful interventions and improved legal results.

LEARNING OBJECTIVES

After studying this chapter, you will be able to:

1. Understand the role of forensic psychiatrists
2. Know legal implications of forensic psychiatry
3. Explain assessment techniques in forensic psychiatry
4. Discuss treatment and rehabilitation in forensic psychiatry

Definition of Forensic Psychiatry

Forensic psychiatry intersects law and mental health in a complex manner—it rests precisely where legal principles intersect with everyday psychological wisdom (Figure 3.1). It involves the evaluation and treatment of individuals who are in legal trouble, paying particular attention to mental problems that may cause criminal activity or influence whether an individual is fit to stand trial. Specialists here marry their therapeutic experience with a practical working knowledge of the law to assess defendants, quite frequently throwing insight into the underlying reasons behind offenders' behaviors—factors which, often enough, end up playing a significant role in decisions regarding sentencing and rehabilitation. Aware of these nuances, more often than not, assists in treatment planning, which attempts to address both the legal criteria and actual psychological requirements of those being treated. This dual strategy not only promotes an equitable trial process but also enhances overall well-being among those navigating the criminal justice system, a factor increasingly recognized in contemporary discussions of successful mental health care (Shalaby et al., 2020; Young et al., 2020).

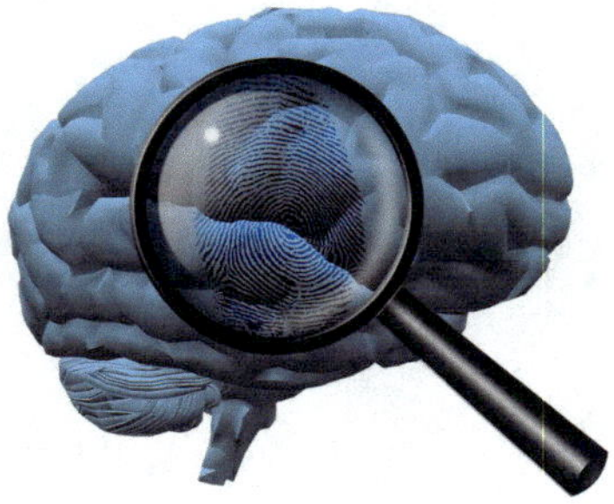

Figure 3.1. Forensic psychiatry.

Source: News-Medical. (n.d.). *Fingerprint Under Magnifying Glass over a Brain Illustration*. https://d1g9yur4m4naub.cloudfront.net/images/Article_Images/ImageForArticle_709_16432978853601663.jpg.

Historical Background of the Field

Forensic psychiatry has developed alongside our changing concepts of mental illness and the law. In the 19th century, judges began to realize that a disturbed mind occasionally qualified as a ground for mitigation of criminal guilt, and before anyone could say the word, psychiatrists had themselves entered courtrooms as definitive expert witnesses. This transformation moved beyond legal rulings; it also subtly shifted public opinions regarding individuals who violate the law. Recently, increased violence against particularly vulnerable individuals—women, children, and others—has made it fairly evident that we require more targeted means of diagnosing and treating problems in forensic contexts (Reza et al., 2013). As our understanding of personality disorders intensified, it became apparent, in the majority of instances, that such difficulties tend to present themselves alongside other mental health issues, again emphasizing the necessity of comprehensive care and good case management (Houghton et al., 2016).

Importance of Forensic Psychiatry in the Legal System

Forensic psychiatry and the law blend in ways that call for real-world skills at unravelling mental health matters—it is not abstract discussion (Figure 3.2). These experts are often summoned in situations where a defendant's mental state is put on trial, particularly in cases involving claims of insanity or diminished responsibility. Judges are increasingly relying on technologies such as neuroimaging—those head scans that attempt to provide hard data about what really goes on in someone's brain—to inform verdicts and even sentencing. Nevertheless, even technologically advanced approaches are not magic; there are times when subtle biases can creep into the way images are interpreted, which obviously demands real-world, well-delineated rules (particularly when synthesizing descriptive diagnoses with anatomical findings [Ferracuti et al., 2018]). In most instances, such a demand for clear rules is as evident as ever. Recent breakthroughs in neuroscience, in broad terms, even suggest the potential for forecasting antisocial behavior—a development that may nudge the way assessments of recidivism risk are addressed (Anderson et al., 2016). Generally, though, technology comes with the reminder that thoughtful human judgment remains the norm.

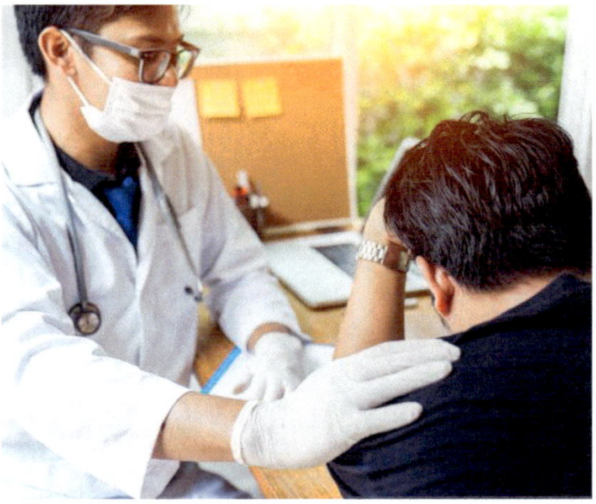

Figure 3.2. Forensic psychiatry and the legal system mix in ways that demand real-world expertise in unpicking mental health issues—it is not just theoretical talk.

Source: American Academy of Forensic Sciences. (n.d.). *Doctor Comforting a Distressed Patient During a Consultation*. https://www.aafs.org/sites/default/files/styles/hero/public/media/images/adobestock_212720158.jpeg?itok=nHmRAe00.

Overview of the Roles of Forensic Psychiatrists

Forensic psychiatrists don't do much more than treat patients in a standard office. They combine mental health expertise with legal expertise, often intervening to investigate a defendant's mental state - and in doing so, can significantly impact the outcome of a criminal case. They are, in most instances, also responsible for caring for psychiatric offenders; consider Italy's Law 81/2014, for instance, which introduced new forms of care for such individuals. However, when facilities fall below standard, it turns out to increase risks for patients as well as the people attempting to care for them (Bellomo et al., 2024). In fact, the pressure of balancing these serious responsibilities at times causes psychiatrists to experience burnout, with over half of them citing the pressure, revealing just how delicate it is to maintain ethical responsibilities alongside taking care of oneself (Wilkie et al., 2024). Overall, the position is both vital and ever-evolving in the dynamic realm of law.

Distinction Between Forensic Psychiatry and General Psychiatry

Forensic and general psychiatry—two overlapping but actually quite distinct sides of mental health practice—both are important, although they each take their own paths. General psychiatry is kept busy diagnosing and treating individuals with cognitive impairments to help improve their day-to-day existence; forensic psychiatry, in the meantime, focuses on individuals entangled in legal problems, frequently grappling with issues regarding competence and accountability. As a general rule, the two specialties require different approaches; consider forensic patients, for instance—they tend to be subject to additional scrutiny of their conduct in legal situations, which isn't typically something you see within everyday psychiatric practice. The negative stigmatizing labels applied to mentally disordered offenders can, in most instances, cloud care by developing negative attitudes within health professionals. Glancing back at the history of how psychiatric care has developed—take Italy's transition in patient management—it becomes evident that altering policies can not only redefine care methods but also transform the way society perceives mental illness.

Current Trends in Forensic Psychiatry

Neuroimaging in forensic psychiatry has actually transformed the way we judge mental states in legal contexts. Increasingly, such tools are utilized to collect factual information that can support or undermine insanity pleas by defendants, often sharpening judicial decisions. There is also a delicate aspect to it—structural neuroimaging at times allows faint cognitive biases to creep in, possibly distorting the way evidence is perceived. To keep such issues at bay, principles emphasizing transparent, descriptive diagnoses and uncomplicated anatomical correlations are crucial (Ferracuti et al., 2018). New research even suggests that neuroimaging could be well-suited to forecasting repeat offending, steering risk assessment in the criminal justice system (Anderson et al., 2016). Overall, this rapidly changing environment requires forensic psychiatrists to tread the intersection of neuroscience and law carefully—balancing new-age techniques with ethical safeguards and always keeping in mind that human behavior is complicated to nail down.

Ethical Considerations in Forensic Psychiatry

Practicing forensic psychiatry involves coping with a range of challenges that require a genuine understanding of ethics—particularly when external factors continue to disrupt the landscape (Figure 3.3). More recently, with escalating global tensions across everything from geopolitics to climatic turmoil, psychiatric assessments tend increasingly to rely on techniques that are both sensitive to cultural idiosyncrasy and underpinned by social justice and human rights. Forensic psychiatrists, for instance, must remain vigilant about how sweeping social concerns may influence patient outcomes and even restrict patients' access to adequate treatment. In general, adherence to established professional standards is crucial in job-required psychological assessments, as failure to do so can have far-reaching consequences for both the individual and society as a whole (American Psychological Association, 2018). Overall, combining advocacy with interdisciplinary collaboration proves essential, enabling forensic psychiatrists to construct more equitable systems that cater to their patients' diverse needs in an ever-evolving world (Bhugra et al., 2024).

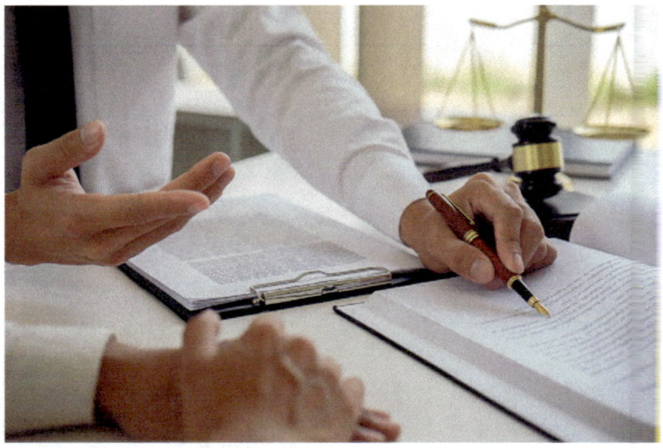

Figure 3.3. Working in forensic psychiatry means dealing with a maze of challenges that call for a real grasp of ethics—especially when outside forces keep shaking things up.

Source: Principium Psychiatry. (2024). *Legal Consultation with Documents, Gavel, and Scales of Justice.* https://www.principiumpsychiatry.com/wp-content/uploads/2024/04/GettyImages-1130660900-scaled.jpg.webp.

Challenges Faced by Forensic Psychiatrists

Technology and forensic psychiatry often blend in unusual ways, introducing significant challenges—particularly in the areas of trust and interpreting digital evidence. Forensic psychiatrists are now venturing into various online information sources, including social media gossip and communication records, and are grappling with concerns such as privacy, maintaining data integrity, and even identifying bias in legal battles. There is pressure on these professionals to delve deeply into the technical details because, honestly, any slight miscalculation could swing the balance in their case analyses and court rulings. And then came COVID-19, which put a wrench in all plans, causing many to quickly transition to telemedicine and remote assessments, thereby disrupting the typical rhythm between patient encounters and examinations (Xu et al., 2024). Overall, professionals are in a dilemma of welcoming cutting-edge technology and ensuring that the essence of forensic assessment remains authentic (Rodchenko et al., 2025).

3.1. The Role of Forensic Psychiatrists

Learning Outcome

1. Learn assessment of mental competency
2. Explain the evaluation of criminal responsibility
3. Discuss risk assessment for future violence
4. Focus on expert testimony in cour
5. Give treatment recommendations for offenders
6. Know collaboration with legal professionals
7. Conduct psychological evaluations
8 Describe research contributions to the field
9. Focus on training and qualifications Required

The forensic psychiatrists actually step in when the mental illness and criminality cross paths—it is not so clean-cut as it sounds. They analyze and treat individuals whose mental struggle gets entwined in legal matters, usually operating under mental illness laws that sound harder than they actually are. Patients, particularly those with intellectual disabilities and challenging behaviors, tend to spend far too long in the hospital primarily because of the risk that they pose to themselves and others (Alexander et al., 2015). These workers are often in the midst of balancing ethical dilemmas, attempting to provide care for their clients while maintaining community safety, under less-than-ideal situations in the majority of cases. Implementing approaches such as Restorative Justice can, all things considered, provide a type of sophisticated moral compass—tempering responsibility with actual therapeutic assistance (Andrews et al., 2015). Ultimately, closing the gap between treatment and legal accountability, forensic psychiatrists assist us in viewing criminal conduct through a mental health prism, making the entire picture slightly more distinct—even though it is still a messy, dynamic process.

3.1.1. Assessment of Mental Competency

Determining whether a person can endure the demands of a trial is not an easy task—It requires a curious mix of legal acumen and gut-level psychological intuition (Figure 3.4). Today's federal standards, codified in 18 U.S.C. § 4241, typically focus on defendants who display apparent, noticeable symptoms of mental illness or defect, tending to miss those whose problems arise from more subtle brain or emotional glitches (Collins et al., 2018).

This narrow focus has many experts worried that it simply does not capture the numerous ways mental challenges arise in modern courtrooms. And then there is the age-old free will controversy, complicating things further by influencing how we determine responsibility for criminal behavior. For the most part, new neuroscience is challenging traditional conceptions of free will, raising more questions about the actual influence on mental competency assessments (Biondi et al., 2017). Overall, these different concerns suggest the need for a rethink of our standards and assessment procedures in a hurry so that the process actually mirrors each defendant's capability to participate actively in their trial.

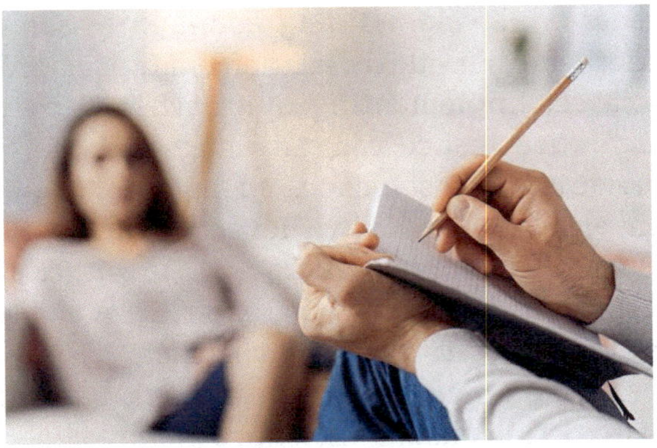

Figure 3.4. Figuring out if someone can handle the rigors of a trial is not simple—it calls for a curious blend of legal know-how and gut-level psychological sense.

Source: PatientPop. (n.d.). *Psychologist Taking Notes During a Therapy Session*. https://sa1s3optim.patientpop.com/assets/docs/83530.jpg.

3.1.2. Evaluation of Criminal Responsibility

Free will and responsibility have long been intertwined, and this combination gives rise to some challenging questions in forensic psychiatry. We used to believe that free will was the basis for assigning blame, but recent research on the brain—broadly speaking—leaves us skeptical about whether this concept actually works in legal contexts. Consider legal insanity cases, for example, in these, determining a defendant's state of mind and intent becomes even more paramount for judges and jurors. Employing models that test for decision-making—such as that four-part method—tends to provide us with a more profound, if imperfect, sense of culpability by combining neuro evidence with mental health assessments (Biondi et al., 2017). Structural neuroimaging has also begun to appear as a means to provide concrete evidence of a defendant's state of mind, directing legal rulings toward more objective ground (Ferracuti et al., 2018). Nevertheless, it is not easy to interpret these scans—biases tend to cloud things, so having strict guidelines is crucial to ensure they are applied correctly in court.

3.1.3. Risk Assessment for Future Violence

Risk assessment of potential future violence is delicate and not something you can pin down with a one-size-fits-all approach, even in forensic psychiatry (Figure 3.5). Experts, who—let's be honest—typically struggle to anticipate violent behavior, now have a new angle with technology such as A.I. neuroprediction that, in most instances, suggests the possibility of finding some neurocognitive markers. These indicators could potentially enhance how we measure risk, particularly in considering patients with psychosis, who, after all, constitute a large chunk of forensic mental health populations (Bijlsma et al., 2020). Applying objective, quantifiable indicators is not only intended to increase public safety but also to introduce an element of consistency and protection to clinical approaches (Kumari et al., 2024). Yet, for all its promise, there is a need to take a step back and ponder—albeit with some hesitancy—the ethical issues and possible downsides of these novel methods, ensuring that any use in forensic settings truly prioritizes both public security and patient care.

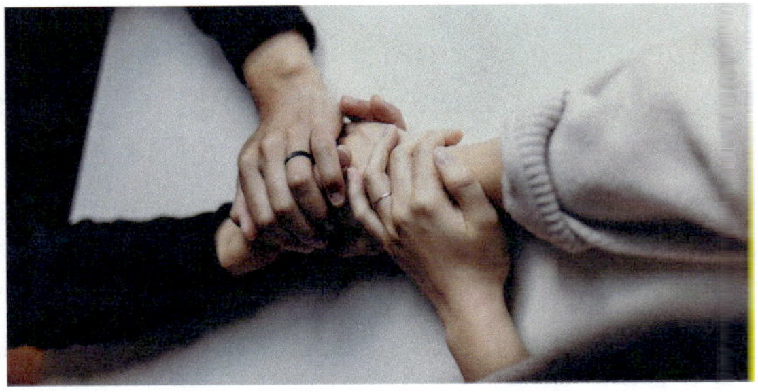

Figure 3.5. Risk assessment for future violence is tricky and not something you can nail down with a one-size-fits-all method, even in forensic psychiatry.

Source: FutureLearn. (2024). *Mental Health Intervention Blog Header.*

3.1.4. Expert Testimony in Court

Expert testimony truly comes into its own when mental health intersects with legal issues—particularly in forensic psychiatry (Figure 3.6). Specialists frequently collaborate with a group of assorted experts when performing evaluations, which serves to uncover how thoroughly crimes, particularly those that involve a sexual component, can disrupt an individual's psychological well-being.

There have been several recent studies (Fokina et al., 2024) that reveal that the mentioned psychological trauma is capable of developing into severe mental issues, thus affecting a victim's health and well-being more than initially anticipated. This clearly demonstrates why having experts in court who are knowledgeable is usually essential. In most instances, courts' consideration of an expert's opinion—even awarding higher marks if the witness is well-credentialed (Cohn et al., 2023)—can tip the decisional balance. Overall, ensuring the expert judgments are trustworthy continues to be essential in arriving at conclusions that are, well, just sufficient.

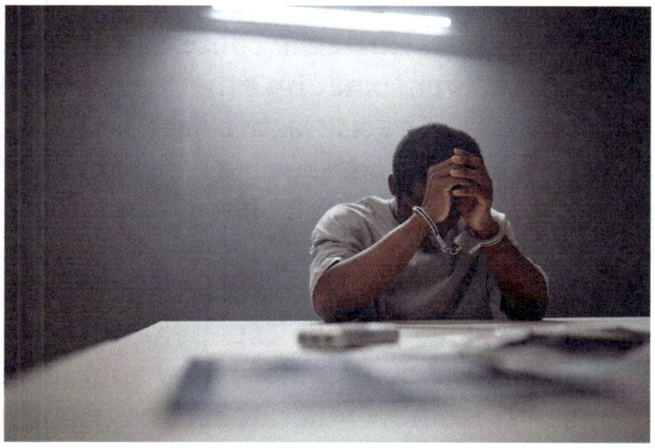

Figure 3.6. Expert testimony plays a crucial role when mental health intersects with legal matters—especially in forensic psychiatry.

Source: Expert Court Reports. (2024). *Mental Health Expert Witness.*

3.1.5. Treatment Recommendations for Offenders

Forensic psychiatry treatment of offenders is not a simple affair—it consists of interventions that combine mental health treatment with reactions to criminality in a rather intractable mixture. Studies indicate that information such as an individual's psychiatric diagnosis and the type of offense they have perpetrated tends to determine outcomes in treatment in ways that are not necessarily intuitive (Weber et al., 2024). You frequently find that those with Cluster B personality disorders or drug offenders are more likely to encounter more roadblocks with court-mandated psychiatric interventions, indicating these populations require refinement of their treatment approaches to their circumstances (Weber et al., 2024). It also happens that how healthcare professionals perceive things makes a difference; forensic psychiatric nurses who are empathic and interested in their patients actually can, at times, form stronger therapeutic relationships, and then the outcome seems to be enhanced. Overall, when coupled with good, practical training for providers, personalized treatment plans improve the overall quality of care, typically reducing recidivism and contributing to a safer society.

3.1.6. Collaboration with Legal Professionals

Forensic psychiatrists team up with legal experts—a combination that becomes critical for securing successful outcomes (Figure 3.7). This collaboration extends beyond merely untangling the psychology of legal cases; it delves deeper into each item of evidence on the table. Today, digital evidence such as social media and online conversations increasingly feature in courtrooms (Rodchenko et al., 2025). In general terms, as AI increasingly sneaks into legal work, it opens up new doors while raising ethical challenges that everyone needs to face. Legal scholars and forensic professionals often find themselves negotiating models that explain risk assessment in terms that inform actual decisions. Ultimately, those circuitous collaborations drive our justice system toward a more equitable configuration, reflecting the complex messiness of human activity and our ongoing need for balanced legal understanding.

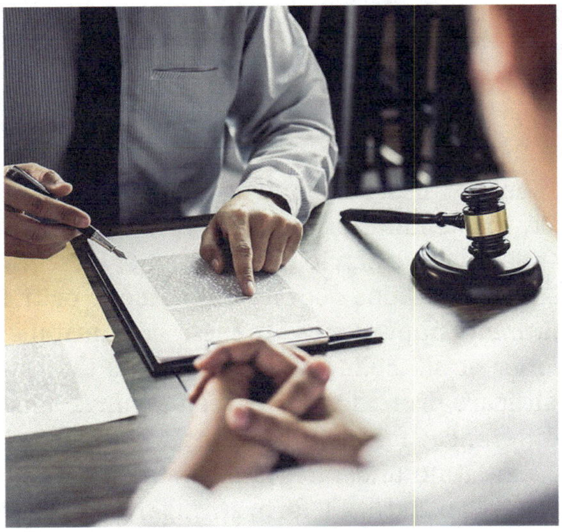

Figure 3.7. Forensic psychiatrists join forces with legal professionals—a union that proves vital for nailing successful outcomes.

Source: Wixstatic. (n.d.). *Forensic Psychiatrists Join Forces with Legal Professionals—A Union That Proves Vital for Nailing Successful Outcomes.* https://static.wixstatic.com/media/b3a4967ff3214a43b9ca98e1b3b8777b.jpg/v1/fill/w_640,h_600,al_c,q_85,usm_0.66_1.00_0.01,enc_avif,quality_auto/b3a4967ff3214a43b9ca98e1b3b8777b.jpg.

3.1.7. Conducting Psychological Evaluations

Today's forensic psychiatry must contend with a whole new array of technology-fueled challenges in psychological assessments. Digital evidence is in the spotlight—its impact is impossible to ignore, and obtaining a clear understanding of its significance is key to sound decision-making. Experts nowadays are not merely examining traditional practices; they are also deconstructing web dialogues and social media sound bites, which, lo and behold, can influence court verdicts in surprising ways. Privacy concerns and issues regarding data integrity have become a routine part of maintaining data integrity (Rodchenko et al., 2025), and these problems repeatedly arise in actual cases. Then there's generative AI (GenAI), which introduces a further permutation into the equation by typically providing novel perspectives that can enhance diagnostic accuracy and assist in shaping treatment strategies (Tortora, 2024). As things continue to change, ongoing training and new guidelines are essentially a requirement to conduct assessments that are both accurate and ethically consistent, aiding in informing judicial decisions with a greater understanding and sophistication.

3.1.8. Research Contributions to the Field

The path of forensic psychiatry has been influenced by a blend of study activities that guide clinicians and theorists in care provision (Figure 3.8). Most now rely on a biopsychosocial model to disentangle the complex problems of mental illness in legal contexts—in most instances, however, some argue that this paradigm winds up too imprecise and eclectic (Stein et al., 2022). Innovations such as neuroimaging and new statistical tools have provided us with new tools for looking inside the thought and affective processes involved in forensic assessment. Meanwhile, the penetration of digital means and community-based approaches has transformed how practitioners engage with clients; this development offers a more holistic perspective on mental health treatment (Beć et al., 2020). Taken as a whole, these advances shed, if imperfectly, some of the discipline's problems and also suggest small, incremental steps toward improvement. For the most part, such research illuminates difficult questions while also encouraging us to continue probing and refining our practices—a good reminder that curiosity is the most important aspect in this constantly evolving field.

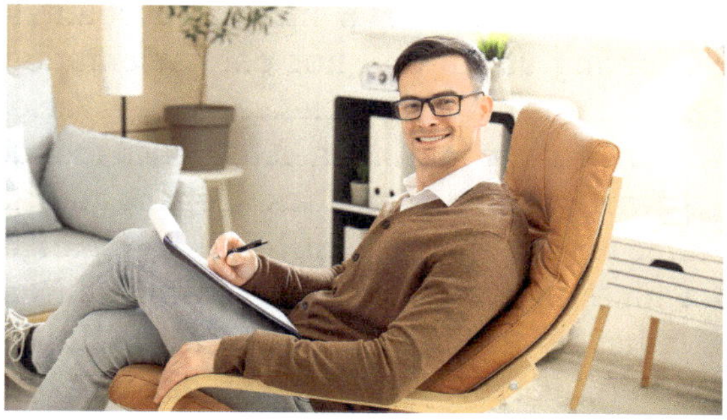

Figure 3.8. Forensic psychiatry's journey has been shaped by a mix of research efforts that inform how clinicians and theorists approach care.

Source: Squarespace. (n.d.). *Blog Post Images*. https://images.squarespace-cdn.com/content/v1/61de209dad96a72dd56bfb92/ef427075-07a3-4c97-9fd8-d0578fee7e3a/blog+post+images%2816%29.png.

3.1.9. Training and Qualifications Required

Being a forensic psychiatrist involves embarking on quite a demanding training path that demands not only general but also specialist qualifications. Most trainees begin by completing a medical degree and then embark on a psychiatry residency—a process that, in the majority of instances, lasts for several years. The Royal College of Psychiatrists, for example, frequently emphasizes that additional higher-level training is required; they cite courses such as the training the trainer (TTT) course, intended to hone teaching skills and develop the consultants of the future. Most trainees identify this type of education as central to fulfilling their curriculum requirements. However, there are still some reservations regarding the efficacy of existing training modules (Murugan et al., 2024). Meanwhile, forensic psychiatry is also changing—today, it is increasingly aligned with cutting-edge technology, so trainees must come to terms with the ethical implications of using artificial intelligence in practice, particularly when predictive evaluations are linked to behavior and environmental conditions (Starke et al., 2023).

Test Your Knowledge

1. Define the role of a forensic psychiatrist and explain how it differs from that of a general (clinical) psychiatrist.
2. What ethical challenges might a forensic psychiatrist face in their work? Provide examples.

3.2. Legal Implications of Forensic Psychiatry

Learning Outcome

1. Understand the insanity defense
2. Explain the role of mental illness in sentencing
3. Know the impact of forensic evaluations on legal outcomes
4. Discuss confidentiality and privilege in forensic settings
5. Focus on the intersection of mental health and criminal law
6. Learn case law influencing forensic psychiatry
7. Describe ethical dilemmas in legal contexts
8. Know the role of forensic psychiatry in civil cases
9. Explain legislative changes affecting forensic practices

Forensic psychiatry today becomes entangled with legal systems in complicated ways. Emerging technology and advanced methods of measuring psychology have, in most instances, opened up possibilities such as A.I. neuroprediction—a potential game changer in risk assessments and even in how violent behavior is identified in court. However, there are snags here; legal and ethical issues that must be examined closely. Researchers, in general, are busy considering the pros and cons to ensure ethical boundaries are not transgressed (Bijlsma et al., 2020).

To add to that, habitual slips in judgment by forensic psychologists refer to pitfalls that might influence legal decisions—a scenario that eminently necessitates improved training and more stringent standards (Castelnuovo et al., 2015). Overall, these considerations underscore the need for a more refined approach to blending forensic psychiatry and legal rules, generating continued debate among professionals, legal scholars, and ethicists.

3.2.1. Understanding the Insanity Defense

Mental illness is a complicated puzzle when it comes to holding legal insanity accountable – it's forcing us to look not only at emotional considerations but brain science as well. Various approaches to the insanity defense, each founded on its own legal measuring stick, keep the question of blame alive. New research, however, highlights brain hints in disorders such as schizophrenia and indicates that when a person's mind isn't functioning correctly, his or her decisions and behaviors are disrupted (Moriarty et al., 2016). Conversations regarding free will introduce a new complication; if mental illness actually gets in the way of a person making choices, as some recent research on the brain appears to suggest, then what we typically use as accountability may require a rethink (Biondi et al., 2017). Ultimately, integrating neuroscience with law requires us to delve into what was truly happening in a person's mind at the time of a crime – and that helps ensure justice is not compromised by the complexity of how mental health influences behavior (Figure 3.9).

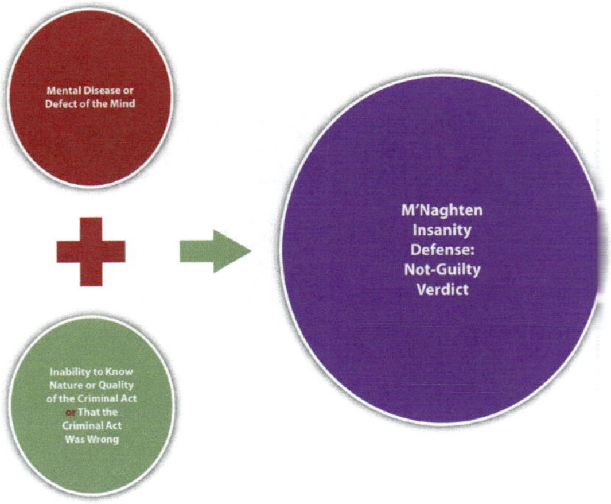

Figure 3.9. The insanity defense.

Source: Saylor Academy. (n.d.). Image. In *Criminal Law*. https://saylordotorg.github.io/text_criminal-law/section_10/a69eb2220e5771e433d240a3bfdec1d3.jpg

3.2.2. The Role of Mental Illness in Sentencing

Criminal justice isn't always cut-and-dry—mental illness tends to get confused with sentencing in ways that raise some serious ethical and legal concerns. More and more, courts observe that a defendant's mental condition can influence the degree to which they actually appear responsible, and this, in many situations, results in sentencing that is more personalized than simply one-size-fits-all. Occasionally, mental illness obscures a person's understanding of what they actually did, so it becomes difficult to assign full moral responsibility. Forensic psychiatry enters the picture here by default; specialists in this branch of study untangle the knotted particulars of one's mindset, and their opinion may influence judges in determining what penalty would best suit. Bigger than checking boxes, however, is the trend toward rehabilitating criminals rather than just issuing penalties, suggesting a more compassionate face of justice. It typically softens entrenched biases and stereotypes in mental health cases as well, keeping the process as equitable as possible. And with continuous learning on mental health for lawyers, if not at one time in totality, at least incrementally, then the stigma melts away, leading the way towards knowledge-informed as well as justice-oriented sentencing.

3.2.3. Impact of Forensic Evaluations on Legal Outcomes

Forensic tests play a significant role in determining the direction of criminal cases (Figure 3.10). They combine psychological testing with brain imaging to demonstrate what a defendant was contemplating at the moment—usually, they are employed to determine accountability. Structural neuroimaging, increasingly applied these days, provides judges a glimpse of a defendant's mental capacity at the time; that added information can truly swing the balance in court. The effectiveness of such tests, in the majority of instances, rests on adhering to standards that help reduce cognitive biases in interpreting evidence—if not, misinterpretation and ill judgment can easily ensue (American Psychological Association, 2018; Ferracuti et al., 2018). Ultimately, whereas forensic testing may vow greater legal fairness, its real effects rely on how meticulously they are utilized and interpreted.

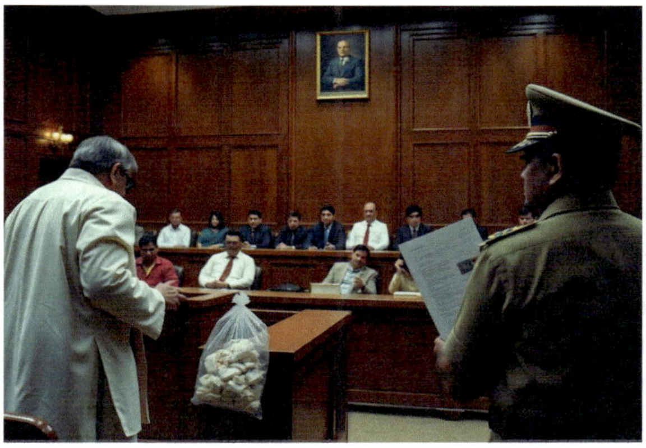

Figure 3.10. Forensic evaluations carry a lot of weight in shaping how criminal cases turn out.

Source: Sulthan, A. K. A. (2025). Drug abuse and criminal law in India – Understanding legal consequences and enforcement. *Spicy Law Firm.*

3.2.4. Confidentiality and Privilege in Forensic Settings

Forensic activity is not as straightforward as it may appear. Legal privilege and confidentiality become entangled in ways that can make everything seem uncertain. Forensic psychiatrists, for example, frequently have two jobs to do simultaneously—they attempt to treat their patients while responding to legal calls, and that does not always go smoothly. Confidentiality, of course, generates trust, which is very important when a person is handling illnesses such as schizophrenia (Besse et al., 2024). There are times, however, when rules or the threat of damage compels one to move; information is leaked out, and patients are left to feel somewhat betrayed. Studies indicate that even the manner in which forensic psychiatric nurses engage with individuals can alter the treatment atmosphere; therefore, some additional, rigorous training could assist in avoiding these ethical tightropes more effectively.

3.2.5. The Intersection of Mental Health and Criminal Law

Dealing with criminal cases becomes complicated when mental health problems enter the equation—our criteria for trial competency are badly in need of an update (Figure 3.11). All things considered, federal statutes such as 18 U.S.C. § 4241 find a defendant incompetent only if a "mental disease or defect" can be identified, usually without regard to other psychological or neurological disorders that may impair a person's capacity to stand trial (Collins et al., 2018).

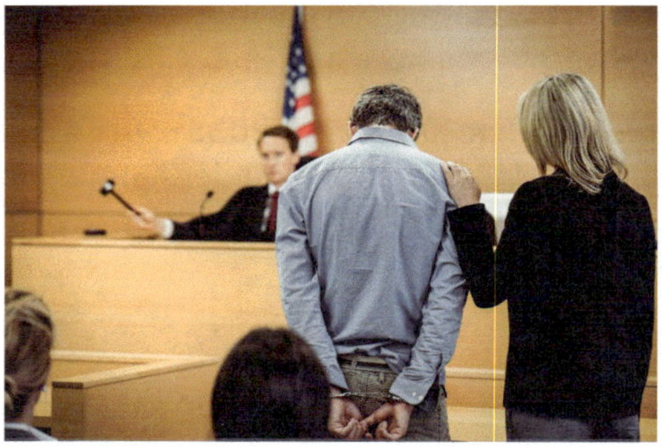

Figure 3.11. Handling criminal cases gets tricky when mental health issues mix in—our standards for trial competence seem long overdue for a refresh.

Source: Adobe Stock. (n.d.). *Person in a Lab Conducting Forensic Analysis* https://b2257157.smushcdn.com/2257157/wp-content/uploads/2020/04/AdobeStock_76100700-2048x1365-1.jpg?lossy=1&strip=1&webp=1.

This narrow focus has the effect of creating disproportionate judicial outcomes and casts a shadow over the legal process, revealing defects in both the laws themselves and their application by judges. It should also be observed that most criminal defendants struggle with mental illnesses, a fact that highlights a lack in legal training; with the majority of instances, the exploration of how mental health impacts criminal responsibility fails to receive the necessary attention it deserves (Redding, 2025). Addressing them could not only lead the way to more equitable trials but also shed further light on how mental health integrates into criminal activity—an understanding key to advancing the way our justice system functions.

3.2.6. Case Law Influencing Forensic Psychiatry

Jurisprudence and psychiatry are beginning to blend in unexpected patterns. Case law continues to evolve, and it now brings neuroimaging into the fray—a turn that has caused courts to reconsider the cognitive aspects of criminal behavior. Judges, by and large, are reassessing the significance to assign to brain scan evidence, and this is provoking actual debate. Structural scans are supposed to provide us with an objective view of a person's mental condition (including elements of mens rea). Still, their application tends to become entangled in cognitive biases that can distort the results (Ferracuti et al., 2018).

Recently, considerable discussion has centered on the use of brain scans to predict antisocial behavior, highlighting the validity of such evaluations (Anderson et al., 2016). As neuroscience gets intertwined into legal proceedings, it is coming into view that definite guidelines are semi-necessary if these technologies are to operate reasonably well in forensic assessments, and finally, they could actually reform how both legal determinations and psychiatric assessments are made.

3.2.7. Ethical Dilemmas in Legal Contexts

Forensic psychiatry has been advancing rapidly, and blending new technology with sound thinking has produced some genuine puzzles that don't have a simple solution. One such excellent case in point is the rise of AI applied to risk assessment—a development that comes freighted with ethical concerns, particularly if these "black box" models preserve their workings as a secret, which can seriously tamper with transparency and accountability in court proceedings. Opponents argue that a lack of understanding of how these AI systems make decisions can lead to unjust outcomes, particularly in critical areas such as criminal jurisprudence. Telepsychiatry, meanwhile, is opening up new possibilities by increasing access to mental health care. Still, it also raises controversies around patient confidentiality, adequate informed consent, and adherence to long-standing medical ethics. For the most part, legislation falls behind technological advances, creating loopholes that could jeopardize patient rights and security (Chatzi, 2024). In total, these concerns necessitate an interdisciplinary discussion and more informed regulatory action to effectively address the numerous complexities and challenges in current forensic psychiatry.

3.2.8. The Role of Forensic Psychiatry in Civil Cases

When psychology and law combine, it can become very complicated—particularly in civil matters, where forensic psychiatry often takes over (Figure 3.12). Experts screen an individual's mental state during disputes involving the law, providing input that courts use to make decisions about matters such as liability, competency, and damages. More recent research (Callan et al., 2018) has indicated that as psychiatric treatment varies, especially with marginalized populations, it can influence legal decisions, so getting risk assessment right becomes terribly significant. Newer neuroscientific approaches have, in the vast majority of cases, improved outcomes prediction, somewhat closing the science-practice divide (Anderson et al., 2016). Overall, applying forensic psychiatry to civil matters not only assists in serving justice but also ensures that mental health issues are not overlooked, seeking more equitable treatment for all parties concerned.

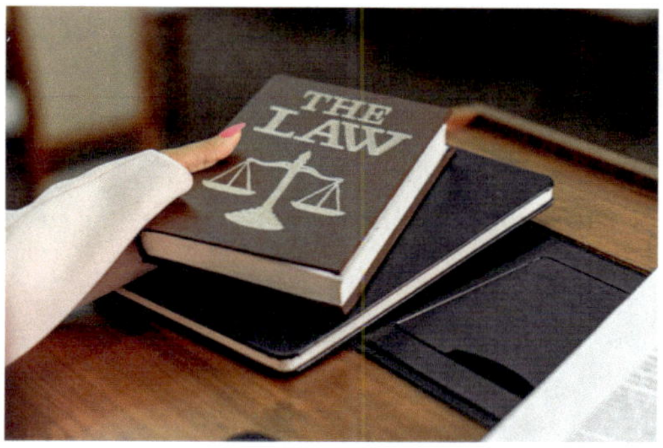

Figure 3.12. When law and psychology intersect, things can become quite complex—especially in civil cases, where forensic psychiatry usually intervenes.

Source: FCPsych Experts. (2024). *A Woman Holding a Book About Law.* https://www.fcpsychexperts.com/wp-content/uploads/2024/12/1.A-woman-holding-a-book-about-law-1-2-1.png.

3.2.9. Legislative Changes Affecting Forensic Practices

Legal rules have been changing considerably in recent times, and forensic psychiatry bears the brunt in ways that are not always easy to interpret. Patients ' rights are becoming more emphasized, and more effort is made towards decisions that are based on sound evidence rather than gut feeling. Consider the new therapeutic leave regulations in mental health facilities, for instance—these reforms imply that discharges in today's era require a more systematic and organized methodology. Studies, the majority of the time, indicate that while supervised leave at times has obvious advantages, its more extensive implementation is still inhibited by the absence of compelling evidence; thus, many decisions wind up depending on intuitive assessments instead of hard facts (Barlow et al., 2018). Discussion across the intersection of law and psychology also suggests that a firmer, more vibrant educational system could spark genuine innovation in forensic care, propelling the practice toward a more comprehensive and informed approach (Barlow et al., 2018). Overall, these developments in the legal arena remind us that forensic psychiatry will always require ongoing study and adjustments to its policies to remain current.

Test Your Knowledge

1. What is the legal significance of a forensic psychiatric evaluation?
2. In what situations can a forensic psychiatrist breach confidentiality?
3. What is the role of a forensic psychiatrist in civil cases?

3.3. Assessment Techniques in Forensic Psychiatry

Learning Outcome

1. Understand clinical interviews and their importance
2. Learn psychological testing methods
3. Identify risk assessment tools and their validity
4. Discuss the use of collateral information in assessments
5. Focus on cultural considerations in evaluations
6. Identify challenges in assessing malingering
7. Describe the role of neuroimaging in forensic assessments
8. Analyze standardized assessment instruments
9. Know the limitations of current assessment techniques

Forensic psychiatry isn't a tidy discipline—sorting out various psychological characteristics actually counts when clinicians must make good decisions. Research indicates that, in the majority of instances, experienced experts are likely to rely on their instincts rather than strict tools when verifying aspects such as moral judgment and conscience (Tiemersma et al., 2022). This type of intuitive inclination can at times confuse treatment decisions and risk management outcomes. Even other studies indicate that forensic professionals, rather than employing open and productive interviewing methods, often adhere to closed or leading questions, which ultimately scratch the surface of essential facts (Leach et al., 2022). Overall, these considerations suggest that additional, hands-on training and broad-based assessment measures might not only enhance the accuracy of sound evaluations but also provide a more profound insight into the psychological aspects of forensic practice.

3.3.1. Clinical Interviews and their Importance

Clinical interviews are an essential part of forensic psychiatry—they are not merely standard discussions but an important means of penetrating a defendant's mind (Figure 3.13). Clinicians tend to combine formal techniques with natural conversation to construct a picture of a person's present state, their history, and any possible red flags. Consider, for instance, the case of young "Paul" (Scognamiglio et al., 2024). He has suffered some quite extreme childhood trauma, and in his interview, subtle clues such as dissociation and mood swings tend to surface, often in unexpected ways. Recently, methods such as videoconferencing are being incorporated into these tests; these instruments can produce more engaging sessions—and, in some cases, even reduce distractions (Christensen et al., 2024). Overall, these interviews are not just about arranging treatment plans. They actually influence the way risks are assessed and can result in more successful rehabilitation approaches in a forensic context.

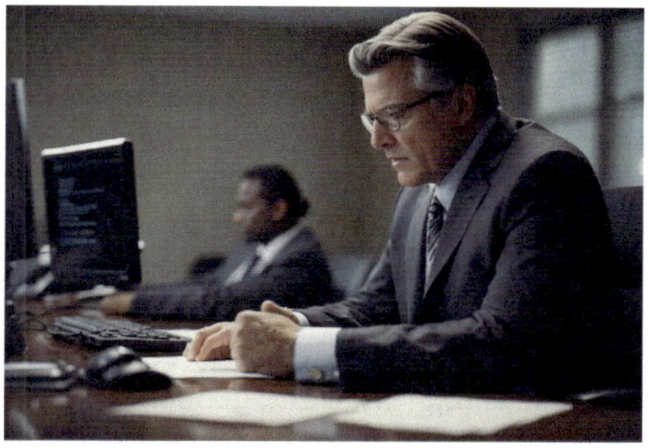

Figure 3.13. Clinical interviews play a massive role in forensic psychiatry—they are not just routine talks but a key way to get inside a defendant's mind.

Source: MVS Psychology. (2024). *Screenshot of Psychological Service or Consultation Interface.* https://www.mvspsychology.com.au/wp-content/uploads/2024/04/Screenshot-2024-04-18-at-12.11.47-AM.jpg.webp.

3.3.2. Psychological Testing Methods

Psychological testing assumes a low-key but vital role in forensic psychiatry, particularly when attempting to decipher the mental status of individuals mired in legal proceedings. Experts in many instances employ a blend of strategies—traditional testing, thorough neuropsychological assessments, and even a few loose ends, qualitative approaches—to accumulate fragments of information that are significant in court. For instance, one neuropsychological testing study in general tended to indicate that these tests are able to isolate cognitive issues in organic mental disorders from those found in other psychiatric conditions by highlighting aspects such as auditory-speech memory and some neurodynamic characteristics (Pilechev et al., 2024). Judges increasingly rely on expert opinions, and recent Hungarian research even suggests what may constitute the ideal forensic expert (Baran et al., 2024). In the end, these testing approaches not only aid in more precise diagnoses but also strengthen the overall credibility of psychiatric examinations in courtrooms.

3.3.3. Risk Assessment Tools and Their Validity

Forensic psychiatry has been moving towards the application of structured risk assessment, and as a consequence, this development naturally raises questions concerning the extent to which these instruments are truly effective (Figure 3.14). In a typical situation, there are more than 400 various instruments developed worldwide, each used in a different manner – either in a chaotic acute psychiatric ward or a specialized forensic environment. Recent research typically indicates that if you examine the overall scores from those instruments, they will beat those more open-ended judgments at predicting things such as violent or sexual crime, after adjusting for some potential study bias. Yet, this trend does appear to highlight a rather evident need for additional improvement. Technicians and researchers are committed to the notion that we should enhance the specificity and accuracy of these measures, particularly given the diverse combination of populations and settings they represent (Viljoen et al., 2024). Furthermore, when considering differential performance across scales such as the HCR-20 and START, it highlights the ongoing and persistent need for periodic reviews and adjustments to maintain the effectiveness of these methods in risk management within forensic psychiatry (Rosca et al., 2025).

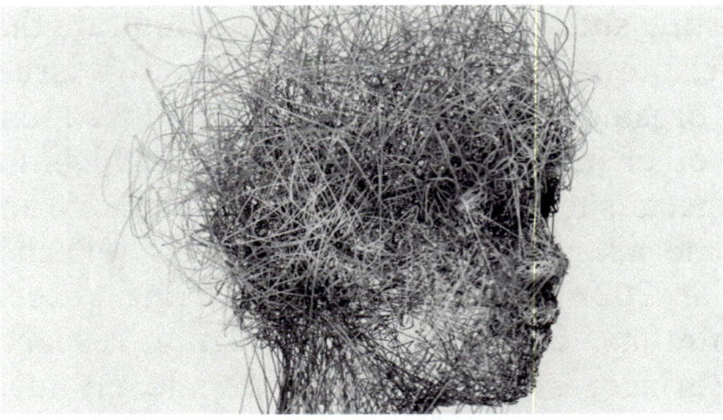

Figure 3.14. Forensic psychiatry has been shifting its focus toward using structured risk assessments, and naturally, this shift invites questions about how well these tools actually work.

Source: Psypack. (2025). *Adverse Childhood Experiences (ACEs).*

3.3.4. Use of Collateral Information in Assessments

Forensic assessments typically require blending various forms of information to create a full, solid picture. When legal cases are at stake, firsthand accounts often lack essential details, and additional background—such as previous medical records, prior encounters with the law, and even social environments—fills in the gaps to reveal details that would otherwise go unnoticed. In the majority, advancements in electronic evidence collection highlight the critical importance of having trustworthy data for informed decisions. Neuropsychological examinations also break down the way individuals think and demonstrate how such processes can influence legal matters (Pilechev et al., 2024). Ultimately, attentively integrating this additional information not only enhances confidence in forensic psychiatry reports but also highlights the particular expertise required to analyze complex psychological exams (Rodchenko et al., 2025).

3.3.5. Cultural Considerations in Evaluations

Trauma and cultural identity intertwine in ways that actually determine how forensic psychiatric assessments conclude. It happens that getting a real sense of someone's cultural background – particularly for asylum seekers – is just the absolute key to understanding their mental state. Examiners who have received good training in cultural sensitivity can often establish a safe space where people feel comfortable enough to discuss past, painful experiences. Consider, for instance, torture or chronic violence histories; these types of traumatic stressors tend to blend with cultural factors that transform the way in which people recount their histories. Such intricacy requires not merely empathy, but also collaboration with interpreters who already possess familiarity with local cultural and situational nuances in each case (Franks et al., 2024). Furthermore, with contemporary issues such as migration and geopolitical unrest, forensic psychiatrists will, in most cases, need to adjust their approach, ensuring that respect for diversity is always paramount in both clinical and legal evaluations (Smith et al., 2024).

3.3.6. Challenges in Assessing Malingering

Evaluating malingering is a complex process (Figure 3.15). Evaluators will frequently struggle with a muddle of cues emanating from psychological, neurocognitive, and somatic processes – cues that can be quickly exaggerated. In most instances, failure to consider response bias can result in misinterpretation with significant legal implications (Granacher et al., 2015). Disorders such as schizophrenia spectrum disorder merely compound the complexity, particularly when criminal responsibility is being separated (Chille et al., 2023). Most experts rely on a combination of performance testing and symptom validity testing alongside collaboration with specialists from other disciplines. This multi-disciplinary approach, although imperfect, is imperative in identifying true instances of malingering and in avoiding legal pitfalls resulting from unstable psychiatric assessments.

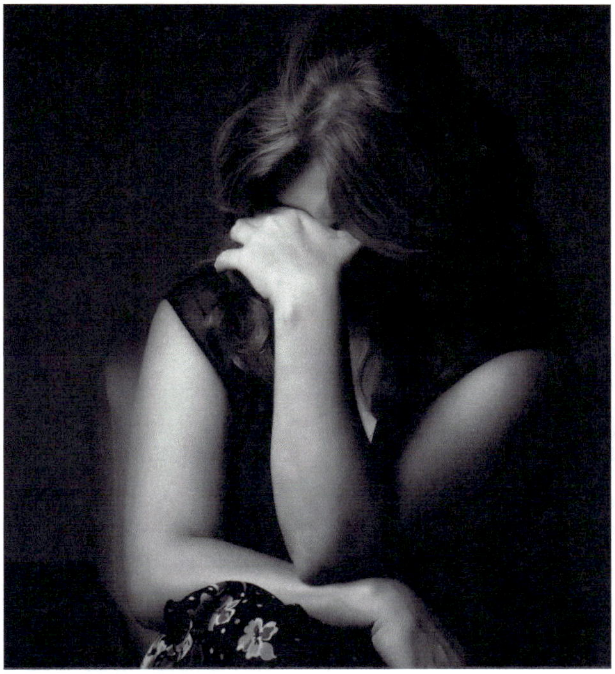

Figure 3.15. Assessing malingering is not a simple task.

Source: Your Local Psychiatrist NYC. (2023). *Amerigroup as a Health Insurance Provider.* https://yourlocalpsychiatrist.nyc/wp-content/uploads/2023/09/Amerigroup-as-a-Health-Insurance-Provider-1.webp.

3.3.7. The Role of Neuroimaging in Forensic Assessments

Neuroimaging has truly revolutionized forensic evaluations; its relentless improvement offers new methods for examining the structure and activity of the brain, which ultimately allows professionals to uncover the hidden sources of behavior. Brain scans enable forensic psychiatrists to glimpse someone's mental life in the context of legal proceedings—a perspective that is useful and enlightening. You can detect such problems as traumatic brain injury or indicators of neurodegeneration, and research (Onar et al., 2025) even suggests that such issues are frequently overlooked in forensic practice, something that might alter our assessment of criminal responsibility, in most instances. With courts increasingly considering electronic data, neuroimaging provides a dose of hard facts that may support or challenge conventional psychological assessments (Rodchenko et al., 2025). Overall, this technology is more than a diagnostic aid; it has become a means to make forensic psychiatry fairer and more precise.

3.3.8. Standardized Assessment Instruments

Standardized assessment instruments emerge in forensic psychiatry, reflecting the discipline's effort to establish robust diagnostic structures, despite the relative clumsiness of psychological assessments

(Figure 3.16). Forensic psychiatrists rely on clinical scales that translate one-of-a-kind case information into straightforward numbers, which serve to pump up both reliability and overall soundness, in general terms.

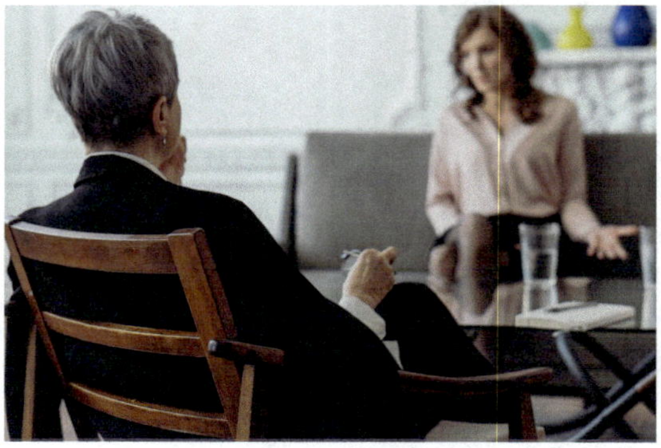

Figure 3.16. Standardized assessment tools emerge in forensic psychiatry, reflecting the field's effort to establish robust diagnostic frameworks despite the inherent complexity of psychological evaluations.

Source: Research.com. (n.d.). *Forensic Psychology Careers.* https://research.com/resized/uploads/Forensic_Psychology_Careers_bc7e837eea.jpg?format=large.

This is particularly important in legal contexts, where a personal story may have very concrete implications. One method—translational cross-validation—attempts to strike a balance between clinical decisions in daily practice and biological assessment, thereby honing diagnostic precision (Najar et al., 2024). Additionally, these measures appear to enhance practitioners' self-confidence, providing them with a broader understanding of combined strategies for psychiatric treatment (Villagomez et al., 2024). Overall, such tools not only facilitate a more stable approach but also foster a team ethos that really enables professionals to deal with complex mental health issues.

3.3.9. Limitations of Current Assessment Techniques

Forensic psychiatry is confronted with actual challenges in evaluating mental health, primarily because such conditions are profound and multi-layered. Most times, existing methods fail to capture all the complexities of psychological disorders. Consider, for instance, conventional devices that place a great deal of reliance on personal interviews and subjective perceptions—such dependency can foster inconsistencies, even biases, in identifying issues. Novel methods that boast cutting-edge technology hold promise but continue to encounter problems such as restricted access, specialized machinery, and additional training needs. Telehealth, applied during remote forensic assessments, has some advantages but also raises questions about whether these sessions accurately measure an individual's state of mind; such questions necessitate acareful weighing of related disadvantages (Fujisawa et al., 2023; Lee et al., 2025). Overall, addressing these issues is essential if forensic psychiatric evaluations are to be more valid and reliable.

Test Your Knowledge

1. What is the purpose of a forensic psychiatric evaluation?
2. Name two structured tools used for violence risk assessment.

3.4. Treatment and Rehabilitation in Forensic Psychiatry

Learning Outcome

1. Understand an overview of treatment modalities
2. Know the importance of individualized treatment plans
3. Explain the role of psychotherapy in rehabilitation
4. Describe medication management for offenders
5. Identify challenges in treating incarcerated individuals
6. Focus on community-based treatment options
7 Learn about recidivism and its implications for treatment
7 Discuss ethical considerations in treatment
8. Know success stories and case studies

Treatment and rehabilitation of the mentally ill offenders is not as straightforward as one may believe; it requires an actual plunge into every individual's story. In most situations, phenomenological observations depict that older offenders facing mental issues tend to favor the prison setting rather than conventional psychiatric institutions. It appears that, surprisingly, prisons are able to provide more informal social encounters and some extra liberty—factors that serve to enhance individual confidence and introduce a sense of connection to life outside (Broekaert et al., 2015). These results somewhat encourage us to develop rehabilitation approaches that support emotional well-being while also monitoring risks. The debate regarding therapeutic leave in secure environments also highlights the fact that clinical care and risk management tend to converge, urging us to move toward a more holistic approach (Barlow et al., 2018). In general, as ideas and practices evolve, continued research remains pivotal in the formulation of interventions that respect offender dignity while prioritizing public safety.

3.4.1. Overview of Treatment Modalities

Mental illnesses and the criminal justice system inevitably intersect in ways that require a range of treatments attuned to the specific challenges presented by forensic patients (Figure 3.17). Forensic psychiatry combines talk therapy with medication in most cases—therapies that essentially attack the root mental problems, which occasionally result in criminal behavior. Good care doesn't merely reduce symptoms; it also seeks to enhance an individual's capacity for recovery and reintroduction into day-to-day existence. Most people feel, across the majority of instances, that incorporating mental health lessons into the curriculum at law schools is needed, given the fact that so many professionals have to deal with troubled individuals yet lack a substantial foundation in understanding these issues (Redding, 2025). The concept of "balanced care" is gaining traction, proposing that services be provided in forms that reflect patients' actual environments—aiding them in transitioning more easily through various stages of care. All things being equal, such blended and adaptive strategies are essential both to improved treatment outcomes and to making our communities safer.

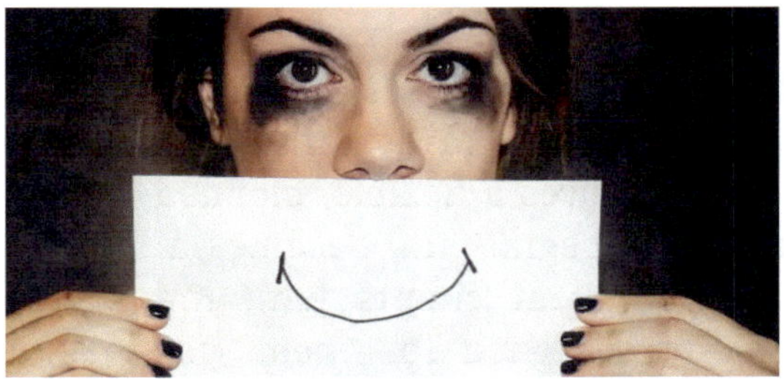

Figure 3.17. Mental health issues and the criminal justice system often collide in ways that call for a variety of treatments tuned to the unique challenges faced by forensic patients.

Source: Kelley, E. (2024). Eliminating discriminatory practices against the mentally ill in the criminal justice system. *Elizabeth Kelley Law.*

3.4.2. Importance of Individualized Treatment Plans

Forensic psychiatry is filled with complexity that challenges us to develop care plans as distinctive as the patients they treat. Treatment here involves not only repairing mental illness but also confronting everyday elements such as family affiliation and community ties. Research finds that astonishingly high levels of patients within such environments become separated from regular contact with families - just about 30% of them do maintain contact - and such lapses can, in most instances, blow a gasket in rehabilitation and reintegration activities (Fojcik et al., 2025). Regular family participation often prevents progress, as discharge support typically follows. In general terms, the emergence of generative AI is starting to turn the tide; by mining through enormous pools of data, it provides new means of refining both diagnosis and rehabilitation techniques (Tortora, 2024). Ultimately, by recognizing each individual's unique idiosyncrasies and implementing interventions tailored to the individual, forensic psychiatry can perhaps have a smoother and more efficient path to recovery.

3.4.3. Role of Psychotherapy in Rehabilitation

Rehabilitating individuals in forensic contexts is a challenging and demanding business—it actually requires a flexible, blended approach. Therapy, to begin with, becomes a real thing. When you treat clients with interventions explicitly designed for them, you begin to understand why they behave the way they do, and you also brush against the emotions and underlying psychological forces that drive their behavior. In general, Evidence-Based Practice (EBP) emphasizes treating every individual as an individual; however, in most correctional settings, this notion is often set aside by the prevalent Risk–Need–Responsivity model, which prioritizes evaluating risks over building genuine relationships (Gannon et al., 2014). Blending psychotherapy with psychiatry can provide practitioners with an opportunity to develop a greater, more authentic relationship with clients—a form of encouraging environment that fosters healing and self-improvement. The formal training that psychiatrists receive further enables them to tackle such challenges—leaving them, in many cases, better positioned to enhance rehabilitation outcomes in such environments (Jasti et al., 2005). All in all, adding psychotherapy into the rehab mix not only helps lower repeat offenses but also boosts the overall mental well-being of offenders (Figure 3.18).

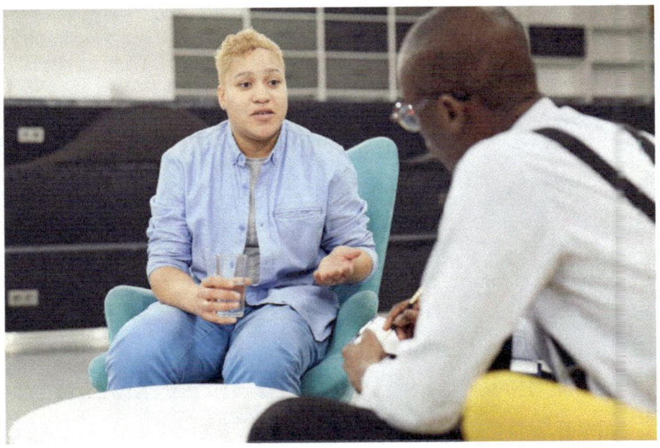

Figure 3.18. Role of psychotherapy in rehabilitation.

Source: Maryville University. (2021). *Bachelor of Arts in Psychology.* https://online.maryville.edu/wp-content/uploads/sites/97/2021/12/mvubafpsy.jpg.

3.4.4. Medication Management for Offenders

Medically managing offenders actually begins with being aware of what is happening in their heads and the situations about their treatments. Offenders in forensic contexts, for instance, tend to present signs of complex mental health struggles—consider Cluster B personality disorders—which, as Weber et al. (2024) indicate, can really get around in their ability to complete court-ordered treatments and keep up with their medication regimens. In Italy, once Law 81/2014 took effect, things in community care became a bit more complicated; issues related to resources began arising; additional concerns for both the patients and individuals on the front lines (Bellomo et al., 2024). As a rule, combining systemized med routines with structured therapy plans is no longer a nice-to-have—it is a necessity. It addresses short-term psychiatric requirements and, for the most part, sets the stage for improved rehab outcomes and decreases the likelihood of future encounters with the police.

3.4.5. Challenges in Treating Incarcerated Individuals

Forensic psychiatry is not as simple as it may appear to be—knowing the knotted realities surrounding imprisonment is essential.

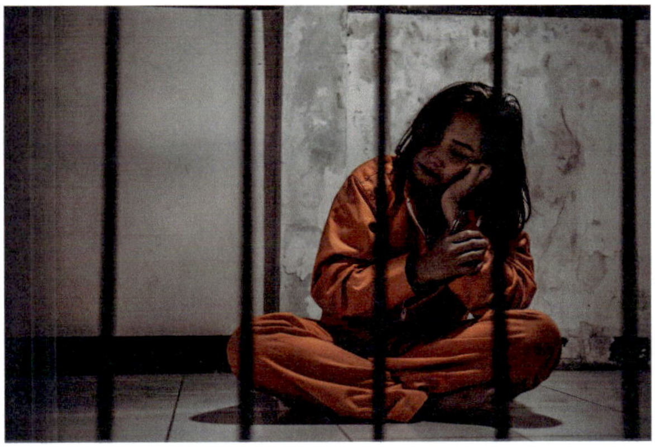

Figure 3.19. Challenges in treating incarcerated individuals.

Source: Rutgers University. (2021). *Women_ Prison.* https://www.rutgers.edu/sites/default/files/2021-09/Women_Prison.jpg.

In most prisons, patients struggle with untreated mental illnesses as well as the double stigma of having both their condition and their criminal history. Several studies suggest that many primary care physicians aren't receiving sufficient training in psychiatry (Jayasankar et al., 2022), and this lack of expertise only serves to widen the gaps in treatment. Since the onset of COVID-19, the transition to remote therapies has introduced another messy element; some people have actually become more invested in tele-therapy, but not meeting face-to-face appears to interfere with building the type of trust that is so important, particularly for those working with antisocial behaviors (Yakeley, 2021). Overall, an integration of traditional treatment and innovative methods would be necessary to enhance mental health outcomes among these vulnerable groups (Figure 3.19).

3.4.6. Community-Based Treatment Options

Current shifts in mental health treatment indicate that we desperately require good, community-based treatment alternatives. As institutional care declines, many who suffer from severe mental illness find their way into prisons—places now compelled to function as the primary providers of mental health treatment. This trend, in most cases, creates cycles of violence and frequent recidivism, highlighting apparent failures of our current approaches. Addressing these problems is not as simple as it may appear; it requires a multi-faceted solution that relies on local services and produces genuinely supportive settings for vulnerable people. Increases in awareness and decreases in barriers to care may quite possibly reduce harm's effects, as we notice them in institutional settings, that is, mentally troubled, economic, and spikes of violent crime (Rushforth et al., 2015; Dezsö et al., 2019). Altogether, our investment in solutions that are focused on the community is a critical step if we aim to achieve improved forensic psychiatry for better health and justice.

3.4.7. Recidivism and Its Implications for Treatment

Recidivism is an ugly issue that forces us to blend disciplines in ways that are not necessarily by the book – combining brain science with innovative technology flips forensic psychiatry on its head. The old ways, for instance, have all too often failed when it comes to actually predicting criminal behavior, and now there is a suggestion that A.I. neuroprediction could be onto something by indicating faint neurocognitive markers associated with reoffending. In most instances, existing analyses even encourage us to examine these methods more closely (Bijlsma et al., 2020). Such predictions do more than refine risk calculations; they also direct us towards interventions that may decrease the likelihood of recidivism. Of course, all such progress brings its own moral conundrums—namely, how it may affect treatment and legal rights. Nevertheless, recent research shows that neuroimaging, quirkiness notwithstanding, can actually forecast recidivism, revealing the complex tango between brain activity and criminal behavior (Anderson et al., 2016). Overall, integrating neuroscience into treatment plans could be the change agent that strengthens rehabilitation in forensic contexts.

3.4.8. Ethical Considerations in Treatment

Treatment in forensic psychiatry is not a neat affair—it is knotted up in problems that actually force us to re-examine our ethical underpinnings. New technology, particularly generative AI, is now an integral part of day-to-day clinical practice and, by and large, it heralds a combination of exciting progress with unforeseen ethical challenges. Despite the ability of AI to refine risk assessments and enhance rehabilitation strategies, its application continues to raise concerns regarding patient autonomy, informed consent, and data protection (Tortora, 2024). In the meantime, urgent geopolitical and environmental concerns add further complexity, highlighting how external pressures can influence both treatment efficacy and our ethical obligations (Smith et al., 2024). In most instances, forensic psychiatrists are left to practice in an environment where social justice and cultural sensitivity have to blend with ethical principles that prioritize patient care, even if the road ahead is messy and unpredictable (Figure 3.20).

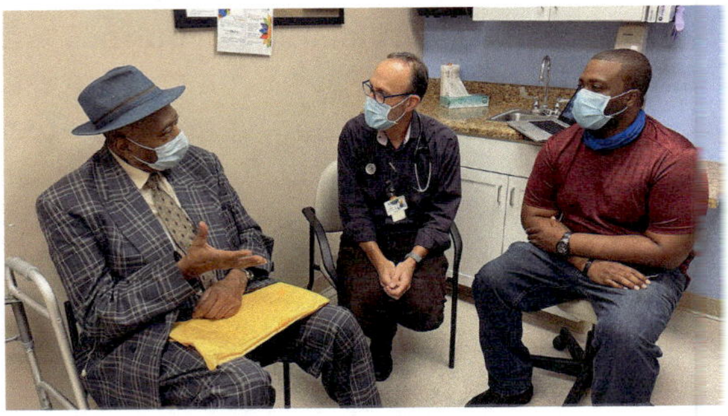

Figure 3.20. Ethical considerations.

Source: Association of American Medical Colleges (AAMC). (n.d.). *Ashkin Green Clinic, Chapel Hill.* https://www.aamc.org/sites/default/files/aamcnews-ashkin-green-clinic-chapel-hill.jpg.

3.4.9. Success Stories and Case Studies

Peer support services, commonly referred to as PSSs, have been quietly working to transform mental health care and generate some truly uplifting stories. Individuals who have struggled with mental health issues themselves seem to group in a manner that provides each other a true boost (Shalaby et al., 2020)—exchanging experiences that instill hope, self-esteem, and an actual desire to continue treatment. More often than not, these mundane transactions function as a bridge, mitigating the harsh chasm between the agony of mental illness and the promise of reasonable care, which in turn can significantly enhance life for individuals in forensic settings. It should also be noted that a comprehension of the way an organisation functions has its own role; i.e., health organisations are putting greater emphasis on better cybersecurity (i.e., the types of protection for sensitive patient information) as theyseek to incorporate wedded holistic psychiatric techniques in their methodology

(Jalali et al., 2018). In most instances, these developing forensic psychiatric practices do more than address mental illness issues—they promote the safety of our most vulnerable citizenry.

Test Your Knowledge

1. What are the primary goals of treatment in forensic psychiatry?
2. How does treatment in forensic settings differ from treatment in general psychiatry?
3. How is risk management integrated into forensic psychiatric treatment?

SUMMARY

Forensic psychiatry is not a cut-and-dry situation – it combines law with the complexities of the human mind, and staying on top of both can get quite complicated. Recently, with the COVID 19 outbreak, things changed almost overnight; video calls stepped in to keep patient check-ups and evaluations going, even though staff opinions were mixed, with some wondering if these methods truly did justice to a complete, professional observation (Christensen et al., 2024). We find that examining victims versus accused added another level of understanding to the mental health trends common in this area. Typically, victims bring with them a unique set of issues, usually associated with past traumas, and the accused often present with additional issues such as psychosis, addiction, and other similar concomitant problems (Şair et al., 2022). When you combine it all, the blend of psychiatry and legal examination continues to compel us to continually revise our practices—trying to safeguard individual rights while still maintaining the depth necessary for sound mental health evaluations.

Forensic psychiatry relies on understanding how mental health concerns intersect with legal matters—this intersection truly sits at the heart of the discipline. Consider schizophrenia spectrum disorder, for instance; it reaches more than 50 million individuals across the globe and is usually a priority in criminal responsibility matters due to its ability to change behavior and thinking drastically (Chille et al., 2023). This illness is not straightforward by any means—it makes us excavate its symptoms, struggle with challenging diagnostic obstacles, and try to determine how it crosses over with the world of law. And then there is the entire forensic evaluation process, which is less concerned with pinpointing the precise diagnosis but also has a way of identifying legal side biases (de Robb et al., 2022). By and large, risk assessment instruments—whether they rely on cold, complex data or on the nuances of professional judgment—have a significant role in determining recidivism patterns and influencing more individualized interventions in forensic contexts. Together, these observations reveal a complicated, occasionally volatile pas de deux between psychiatric understanding and legal framework in the relentless pursuit of equitable justice and successful treatment.

KEY TERMS FROM THIS CHAPTER

- Courtrooms
- Expert testimony
- Intellectual disabilities
- Legal insanity
- Mental health
- Neuroprediction
- Patients
- Criminal behavior
- Healthcare professionals
- Jurors
- Legal responsibility
- Moral guide
- Online chats
- Psychology

CRITICAL THINKING QUESTIONS

1. **What is the primary role of a forensic psychiatrist?**
   a. To provide long-term therapy to psychiatric patients
   b. To determine the criminal responsibility and competency of individuals in legal settings
   c. To prescribe medications only in correctional facilities
   d. To perform only psychological testing
2. **Which of the following is a commonly used tool to assess risk of violence?**
   a. MMPI-2
   b. Rorschach Inkblot Test
   c. HCR-20
   d. TAT (Thematic Apperception Test)
3. **What does malingering refer to?**
   a. A genuine mental illness that is hard to treat
   b. A psychotic state brought on by drug use
   c. The intentional faking of symptoms for secondary gain
   d. A personality disorder marked by deceitfulness
4. **Which of the following is not typically assessed during a competency to stand trial evaluation?**
   a. Ability to understand courtroom procedures
   b. Ability to consult with a lawyer
   c. Intelligence quotient (IQ)
   d. Understanding of charges and potential penalties
5. **The legal term "insanity" is best described as:**
   a. A diagnosis listed in the DSM-5
   b. A legal concept referring to criminal responsibility
   c. A synonym for schizophrenia
   d. A condition that always leads to hospitalization

Short Answer Questions

1. What is forensic psychiatry, and how does it differ from general psychiatry?
2. What are the key ethical principles guiding forensic psychiatry?
3. What role does a forensic psychiatrist play in civil commitment hearings?
4. How does forensic psychiatry interact with the legal system?
5. What is the difference between criminal responsibility and legal insanity?
6. Describe the process of conducting a forensic psychiatric evaluation.

Answers to Critical Thinking Questions

1. (b); 2. (c); 3. (c); 4. (c); 5. (b)

REFERENCES

1. Alexander, R., Chester, V., Devapriam, J., McCarthy, J., et al. (2015). "Why can't they be in the community?" A policy and practice analysis of transforming care for offenders with intellectual disability. *Advances in Mental Health and Intellectual Disabilities.* https://core.ac.uk/download/41990943.pdf (accessed on 9th May 2025).
2. American Psychological Association, & Melchert, T. P. (2018). *Professional Practice Guidelines for Occupationally Mandated Psychological Evaluations.* https://core.ac.uk/download/231843503.pdf (accessed on 9th May 2025).
3. Anderson, N. E., Gaudet, L. M., Kerkmans, J. P., Kiehl, K. A., et al. (2016). *Can Neuroscience Help Predict Future Antisocial Behavior?* https://core.ac.uk/download/144231730.pdf (accessed on 9th May 2025).
4. Andrews, D. A., Appelbaum, P. S., Arrigo, B. A., Engelhardt, H. T., Glaser, B., Gutheil, T. G., Johnstone, G., et al. (2015). *Restorative Justice-Informed Moral Acquaintance: Resolving the Dual Role Problem in Correctional and Forensic Practice.* https://core.ac.uk/download/30712423.pdf (accessed on 9th May 2025).
5. Baran, B., Szabó, F. Á., Lisincki, A., Vida, L., Czobor, P., Jekkel, É., & Szuromi, B., (2024). The preferences of Hungarian judges with regard to forensic psychiatry and forensic psychology experts. *European Psychiatry, 67,* S580. https://www.semanticscholar.org/paper/295fe62bb68b709f8e01fb6705fb98647471e32e (accessed on 9th May 2025).
6. Barlow, E. M., & Dickens, G. L. (2018). *Systematic Review of Therapeutic Leave in Inpatient Mental Health Services.* https://core.ac.uk/download/228178293.pdf (accessed on 9th May 2025).
7. Barlow, E. M., & Dickens, G. L. (2018). *Therapeutic Leave from Secure Mental Health Inpatient Services: A Review.* https://core.ac.uk/download/228178535.pdf (accessed on 9th May 2025).
8. Beć, K. B., Grabska, J., & Huck, C. W. (2020). Near-infrared spectroscopy in bio-applications. *Molecules, 25,* 2948. https://doi.org/10.3390/molecules25122948.
9. Bellomo, A., Cecere, A., Mandarelli, G., Gaggiano, C., Giallanella, D., Meglio, M., Iorio, U., et al. (2024). Psychiatrists on forensic psychiatry after the law 81/2014 in Italy: Findings from a national pilot survey. *International Review of Psychiatry, 36*(7), 777–783. https://www.semanticscholar.org/paper/96665d7c4e35395f45941e22401ef568317572f6 (accessed on 9th May 2025).
10. Besse, M., Gather, J., Schiffer, B., & Zilles-Wegner, D., (2024). Electroconvulsive therapy in forensic psychiatry: A systematic review. *The Journal of ECT.* https://www.semanticscholar.org/paper/259c35a38553610e19cec456a0ce82124335557f (accessed on 9th May 2025).
11. Bhugra, D., Moura, H. F., Liebrenz, M., Ogunwale, A., et al. (2024). *Mental Health and Justice Beyond Borders: Global Crises, Sociopolitical Determinants, and Contemporary Practices in Forensic Psychiatry.* https://core.ac.uk/download/618391722.pdf (accessed on 9th May 2025).
12. Bijlsma, J., Ferracuti, S., Meynen, G., Tortora, M., et al. (2020). *Neuroprediction and A.I. in Forensic Psychiatry and Criminal Justice: A Neurolaw Perspective.* https://core.ac.uk/download/323191898.pdf (accessed on 9th May 2025).
13. Biondi, M., Ferracuti, S., Mandarelli, G., Meynen, G., et al. (2017). *Free Will, Neuroscience, and Choice: Towards a Decisional Capacity Model for Insanity Defense Evaluations.* https://core.ac.uk/download/98339734.pdf (accessed on 9th May 2025).

14. Broekaert, E., De Smet, S., Ryan, D., Van Hecke, N., et al. (2015). *Treatment and Control: A Qualitative Study of Older Mentally Ill Offenders' Perceptions on their Detention and Care Trajectory.* https://core.ac.uk/download/55807198.pdf (accessed on 9th May 2025).

15. Callan, A. F., Ineichen, B., Lawlor, C., Morgan, C., Morgan, C., Morgan, C., et al. (2018). *Ethnic Inequalities and Pathways to Care in Psychosis in England: A Systematic Review and Meta-Analysis.* https://core.ac.uk/download/287581294.pdf (accessed on 9th May 2025).

16. Carabellese, F. F., & Parente, L., (2025). *The Italian General Psychiatry and Forensic Psychiatry Treatment Model: A Unique Story.* CNS Spectrums. https://www.semanticscholar.org/paper/718ce10a7bb8e45f162d6684a4bd3f691d8da16c (accessed on 9th May 2025).

17. Castelnuovo, G., Faccio, E., Iudici, A., Salvini, A., et al. (2015). *The Clinical Assessment in the Legal Field: An Empirical Study of Bias and Limitations in Forensic Expertise.* https://core.ac.uk/download/80156168.pdf (accessed on 9th May 2025).

18. Chatzi, M., (2024). The ethical and legal dilemmas of telepsychiatry. *Bioethica.* https://www.semanticscholar.org/paper/7ed24b3a98f3edd5ea6ff655f447f836a2cb3f45 (accessed on 9th May 2025).

19. Chille, T. A. (2023). *The Relationship Between Schizophrenia Spectrum Disorder and Criminal Responsibility.* https://core.ac.uk/download/572738070.pdf (accessed on 9th May 2025).

20. Christensen, L. F., Sørensen, L., & Johansen, K. K. (2024). Staff experiences with videoconferences during the COVID-19 pandemic in forensic psychiatry outpatients. *Nordic Journal of Psychiatry, 78*, 370–375. https://www.semanticscholar.org/paper/ebab13c55a452bf2bf30ea017cfcd9ffa3b601c8 (accessed on 9th May 2025).

21. Cohn, J., & Karlin, J., (2023). Forensic practitioner testimony and jury instructions involving insanity defense. *The Journal of the American Academy of Psychiatry and the Law, 51*, 442–444. https://www.semanticscholar.org/paper/615c73a2b016c2434e08b589d72e22617c65a721 (accessed on 9th May 2025).

22. Collins, D., (2018). *Re-Evaluating Competence to Stand Trial.* https://core.ac.uk/download/213021567.pdf (accessed on 9th May 2025).

23. De Vries Robbé, M., & Van Der Wolf, M., (2022). *Contemplations and Discussions on the Quality of Forensic Assessment in Sentencing: Puzzling Pieces for Decision Makers.* https://core.ac.uk/download/562123422.pdf (accessed on 9th May 2025).

24. Dezsö, D., Gauger, U., Kogan, I., Konrad, N., et al. (2019). *Violent Behavior During Psychiatric Inpatient Treatment in a German Prison Hospital.* https://core.ac.uk/download/286097310.pdf (accessed on 9th May 2025).

25. Ferracuti, S., Miolla, A., Sartori, G., Scarpazza, C., et al. (2018). *The Charm of Structural Neuroimaging in Insanity Evaluations: Guidelines to Avoid Misinterpretation of the Findings.* https://core.ac.uk/download/188827245.pdf (accessed on 9th May 2025).

26. Fojcik, J., Górski, M., & Krzystanek, M., (2025). Marginalization of family life among patients in forensic psychiatry units. *Psychiatria i Psychologia Kliniczna.* https://www.semanticscholar.org/paper/d7194014636d8a5426b60a4bae4b6f701d8fe218 (accessed on 9th May 2025).

27. Fokina, E. V., Barinov, E. H., Barinov, A. E., Fokin, A. S., & Cherkalina, E. N. (2024). Peculiarities of commissions of forensic medical examinations in criminal cases related to crimes against sexual inviolability. *Russian Journal of Forensic Medicine.* https://www.semanticscholar.org/

paper/fdd918d883b0ac3c895f32b679dbe6e0b40a4cc0 (accessed on 9th May 2025).

28. Franks, A., Ali, D. A., & Adi, A., (2024). Clinical and legal considerations when optimizing trauma narratives in immigration law evaluations. *The Journal of the American Academy of Psychiatry and the Law*. https://www.semanticscholar.org/paper/9025a10fc53d77ca71f9821936e64a3a9f1735eb (accessed on 9th May 2025).

29. Fujisawa, R., Konichi, R., & Miziara, I., (2023). Teleforensics in Brazil: Literature review and analysis from the point of view of forensic medicine. *Perspectivas em Medicina Legal e Perícias Médicas*. https://www.semanticscholar.org/paper/a59428f8679a5e4d31c7f7b1d9ed3a8a5a019c28 (accessed on 9th May 2025).

30. Gannon, T. A., & Ward, T., (2014). *Where Has all the Psychology Gone? A Critical Review Of Evidence-Based Psychological Practice in Correctional Settings*. https://core.ac.uk/download/30703980.pdf (accessed on 9th May 2025).

31. Granacher, R. P., & Wygant, D. B. (2015). *Assessment of Validity and Response Bias in Neuropsychiatric Evaluations*. https://core.ac.uk/download/232633889.pdf (accessed on 9th May 2025).

32. Hirdes, J. P., Van, E. C., Ferris, J., Franco, M., Fries, B. E., Heikkilä, J., Hirdes, A., et al. (2020). The interRAI suite of mental health assessment instruments: An integrated system for the continuum of care. *Frontiers in Psychiatry, 10*. https://doi.org/10.3389/fpsyt.2019.00926 (accessed on 9th May 2025).

33. Houghton, K., & Jones, E., (2016). *To Formulate or not to Formulate? A Case Study*. https://core.ac.uk/download/80694193.pdf (accessed on 9th May 2025).

34. Jalali, M. S., & Kaiser, J., (2018). Cybersecurity in hospitals: A systematic, organizational perspective. *Journal of Medical Internet Research, 20*, e10059. https://doi.org/10.2196/10059.

35. Jasti, M., & Kakkilaya, S., (2005). *Psychiatric Training in the United Kingdom*. https://core.ac.uk/download/pdf/86232.pdf (accessed on 9th May 2025).

36. Jayasankar, P., Nirisha, P., Manjunatha, N., Kumar, C., Gajera, G. V., Malathesh, B., Pandey, P., et al. (2022). Are the collaborative video consultations module in diploma in primary care psychiatry helpful? *Indian Journal of Psychiatry, 64*, S516–S520. https://www.semanticscholar.org/paper/d8b4d1a7e2a484c8dc62822f15e238ca4f585459 (accessed on 9th May 2025).

37. Kumari, V., & Sen, P., (2024). *Editorial: Objective and Measurable Predictors of Violence Risk and Outcome Among Forensic Patients with Psychosis*. https://core.ac.uk/download/599582831.pdf (accessed on 9th May 2025).

38. Leach, C., Brown, F., Pryor, L., Powell, M. B., & Harden, S., (2022). Eliciting an offence narrative: What types of questions do forensic mental health practitioners ask? *Psychiatry, Psychology and Law, 30*, 536–552. https://www.semanticscholar.org/paper/edad44db0603b93a602569941aaac5bd69779b65 (accessed on 9th May 2025).

39. Lee, I. H., & Ma, L., (2025). Integrating machine learning, optical sensors, and robotics for advanced food quality assessment and food processing. *Food Innovation and Advances*. https://www.semanticscholar.org/paper/a14d433c3119c2f2b8550567458fef57c2b2d12a (accessed on 9th May 2025).

40. Moriarty, J. C. (2016). *Seeing Voices: Potential Neuroscience Contributions to a Reconstruction of Legal Insanity*. https://core.ac.uk/download/144231734.pdf (accessed on 9th May 2025).

41. Murugan, M., Sangoi, B., & Nainar, F., (2024). Evaluating the Training the Trainer course for psychiatry higher trainees in the West Midlands. *BJPsych Open, 10*, S114–S115. https://www.semanticscholar.org/paper/85e5e7502fc808530d2585b41c5b01f78a769590 (accessed on 9th May 2025).

42. Najar, D., Dichev, J., & Stoyanov, D., (2024). Towards new methodology for cross-validation of clinical evaluation scales and functional MRI in psychiatry. *Journal of Clinical Medicine, 13.* https://www.semanticscholar.org/paper/6e6f1824d8cf17f233ce1a6d221ab01f79cd67f1 (accessed on 9th May 2025).

43. Onar, G., Azizoğlu, S. İ., Büyükakça, E., & Oncu, F., (2025). Assessing the role of mega cisterna magna in criminal responsibility: Implications for neurocognitive disorders in forensic evaluations. *BMC Psychiatry, 25.* https://www.semanticscholar.org/paper/d4387710134ea9a9c09b75bb3f47603ccb5f169e (accessed on 9th May 2025).

44. Pilechev, D., Mikadze, Y., Vandysh-Bubko, V., & Adamovich, T., (2024). Neuropsychological assessment and verification of cognitive impairments in forensic psychiatry patients. *Psychology and Law.* https://www.semanticscholar.org/paper/132cbec218f13b748fc6083f9d529f67e5fa75f6 (accessed on 9th May 2025).

45. Redding, R., (2025). *Why it is Essential to Teach About Mental Health Issues in Criminal Law (and a Primer on How to Do it).* https://core.ac.uk/download/pdf/7158772.pdf (accessed on 9th May 2025).

46. Reza, A., Fanniff, A. M., Smith, A. M. A., Van Wijk, A. P. H., Grabell, A. S., Gray, A. S., Harrell, A. V., et al. (2013). *Sexual Abuse—Current Medico-Legal, Forensic and Psychiatric Aspects.* https://core.ac.uk/download/53286244.pdf (accessed on 9th May 2025).

47. Rodchenko, L., Ilnytskyi, M., Velhan, O., Tolmachov, O., Shevchuk, R., & Kovalenko, V., (2025). Judicial decisions in the era of information technology: Review of electronic evidence and its role in forensic psychiatry expertise. *Journal of Lifestyle and SDGs Review.* https://www.semanticscholar.org/paper/bbdf98f41c89a208df6849fec333a9e9aa6d383b (accessed on 9th May 2025).

48. Rosca, M. A., La Charité-Harbec, O., Allard, J. M., Borduas, P. S., & Hudon, A., (2025). Violence risk assessment tools used in forensic and acute psychiatry in North America: A scoping review. *Psychiatry International.* https://www.semanticscholar.org/paper/6165587b5b71f3d1ea123d8000b6def2e52b6229 (accessed on 9th May 2025).

49. Rushforth, J., (2015). *Guilty by Reason of Insanity: Unforeseen Consequences of California's Deinstitutionalization Policy.* https://core.ac.uk/download/70414608.pdf (accessed on 9th May 2025).

50. Şair, Y., Doğan, B., & Dirlik, M., (2022). The clinical features of victims and offenders admitted to the forensic psychiatry outpatient clinic: A single-center retrospective analysis. *Meandros Medical and Dental Journal.* https://www.semanticscholar.org/paper/f59493af0e3fd21c90b17af7deb9dd4057d546da (accessed on 9th May 2025).

51. Scognamiglio, C., Sorge, A., Borrelli, G., Perrella, R., & Saita, E., (2024). Exploring the connection between childhood trauma, dissociation, and borderline personality disorder in forensic psychiatry: A comprehensive case study. *Frontiers in Psychology, 15.* https://www.semanticscholar.org/paper/b15cbcd06cfbea4698ae9fe9a36a00c00be7a9a3 (accessed on 9th May 2025).

52. Shalaby, R., & Agyapong, V. I. O. (2020). Peer support in mental health: Literature review. *JMIR Mental Health, 7*, e15572. https://doi.org/10.2196/15572.

53. Smith, A., Ogunwale, A., Moura, H., Bhugra, D., Ventriglio, A., & Liebrenz, M., (2024). Mental health and justice beyond borders: Global crises, sociopolitical determinants, and contemporary practices in forensic psychiatry. *International Review of Psychiatry, 36*(7), 784–793. https://www.semanticscholar.org/paper/a9d133b2e17ba615bc81e4dda5b3b4e3933bb6ae (accessed on 9th May 2025).

54. Starke, G., D'Imperio, A., & Ienca, M., (2023). Out of their minds? Externalist challenges for using AI in forensic psychiatry. *Frontiers in Psychiatry, 14*. https://www.semanticscholar.org/paper/05333fac7fe2fc91a03970331ce476e8d10e513e (accessed on 9th May 2025).

55. Stein, D. J., Szatmári, P., Gäebel, W., Berk, M., Vieta, E., Maj, M., de Vries, Y. A., et al. (2020). Mental, behavioral and neurodevelopmental disorders in the ICD-11: An international perspective on key changes and controversies. *BMC Medicine, 18*. https://doi.org/10.1186/s12916-020-1495-2 (accessed on 9th May 2025).

56. Tiemersma, J., Noom, M., Stoffelsen, R., Popma, A., & Schalkwijk, F. S. (2022). Conceptualization and conscience assessment in adolescence in forensic mental healthcare: Experts' perspectives. *The Journal of Forensic Psychiatry & Psychology, 33*, 673–691. https://www.semanticscholar.org/paper/5dfc5ef54bb80801a998a291ebc4248c0733a41c (accessed on 9th May 2025).

57. Tortora, L., (2024). Beyond discrimination: Generative AI applications and ethical challenges in forensic psychiatry. *Frontiers in Psychiatry, 15*. https://www.semanticscholar.org/paper/ed9ac39ff084fedf916380ab19b472bb683c580c (accessed on 9th May 2025).

58. Viljoen, J. L., Goossens, I., Monjazeb, S., Cochrane, D. M., Vargen, L. M., Jonnson, M. R., Blanchard, A. J. E., et al. (2024). Are risk assessment tools more accurate than unstructured judgments in predicting violent, any, and sexual offending? A meta-analysis of direct comparison studies. *Behavioral Sciences & the Law, 43*, 75–113. https://www.semanticscholar.org/paper/99b9a6cd575b4995ca23f155ae85339d40b6eeba (accessed on 9th May 2025).

59. Villagomez, A., Dunne, R., Brooks, A. J., Chen, M. K., Ricker, M., Kang, S., & Ranjbar, N., (2024). Evaluation of integrative medicine in residency-psychiatry curriculum. *Academic Psychiatry, 48*, 587–592. https://www.semanticscholar.org/paper/1570b55fc9e9cb57d34d6338eb2ab841b1f37ec8 (accessed on 9th May 2025).

60. Weber, K., Morier, S., Menu, C., Bertschy, P., Herrmann, F. R., & Giannakopoulos, P., (2024). Court-ordered forensic psychiatry treatment in prison: Determinants of outcome and risk mitigation. *Frontiers in Psychiatry, 15*. https://www.semanticscholar.org/paper/ee8e83eb7aaa444ac3d7a8ed5d284e7025279416 (accessed on 9th May 2025).

61. Wilkie, T., Jones, R. M., Ramshaw, L. A. L., Glancy, G., Groat, L., & Chatterjee, S., (2024). Contributors to physician burnout and well-being in forensic psychiatrists in Canada. *The Journal of the American Academy of Psychiatry and the Law, 52*, 41–50. https://www.semanticscholar.org/paper/c0fcf6d30672dc648ddbf4f14985cbc32262dc77 (accessed on 9th May 2025).

62. Xu, Y., Parkin, J. A., & Cunningham, N., (2024). The impact of COVID-19 on clinical forensic medicine and forensic psychiatry: A literature review. *Medicine, Science and the Law*. https://www.semanticscholar.org/paper/7268fe235f38b57a0c1a0200cc0388b8014cac54 (accessed on 9th May 2025).

GENERAL TOXICOLOGY

4

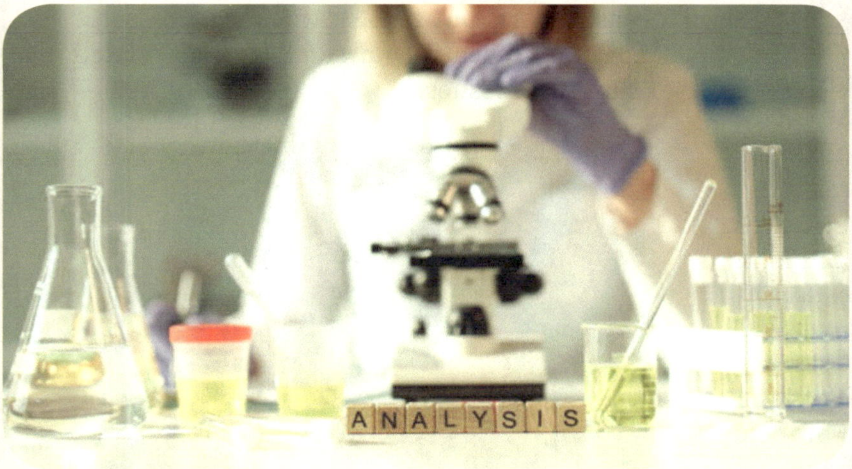

LEARNING OBJECTIVES

After studying this chapter, you will be able to:

1. Explain types of toxic substances
2. Describe methods of toxicological analysis
3. Learn case studies in forensic toxicology

Introduction

Combining toxicology and forensic work plays a huge role in solving tricky cases of chemical exposure and poisoning. These days, environmental and synthetic chemicals seem to be everywhere, and understanding their impact on our bodies is crucial for both public health and legal cases. Basic toxicology provides investigators with the knowledge to identify harmful substances, assess how these chemicals affect our health, and even link exposures to adverse outcomes. Lately, there has been a buzz about breakthroughs – think improved testing methods and the rise of molecularly imprinted polymers (MIPs) (Lowdon et al., 2020) – which demonstrate that our forensic tools are continually evolving. Additionally, there is a growing push to examine emerging contaminants, such as per- and polyfluoroalkyl substances (PFAS), which further underscores the importance of a comprehensive, multidimensional approach to toxicology for both environmental care and forensic practice (Guelfo et al., 2021). All in all, this mixed strategy not only builds a stronger case but also really backs the ongoing search for justice in toxic exposure scenarios.

Definition of Toxicology

There is a messy, almost tangled connection between forensic science and toxicology that shows how chemicals can seriously mess with our health and behavior, particularly when things get criminal. Toxicology is really just the study of how bad chemicals hurt us – it brings to light dangers from things like everyday environmental toxins or the drugs we encounter, often offering clues that help figure out where harm might come from. Sometimes, taking a close look at bodily fluids and tissues for these unwanted substances reveals hidden evidence that might otherwise slip by unnoticed; this kind of detailed work is crucial. In many instances, such analysis not only helps nail down the cause of death but also ties specific substances to criminal acts, a role that turns out to be pretty key in chasing down justice. Forensic toxicologists, aside from merely identifying and measuring toxins, also have the challenging task of interpreting what these findings mean in legal terms (as noted in current research on forensic prevention methodologies (Batiuk et al., 2024) and advances in digital criminalistics (Tiapkin et al., 2023)). This dual role underscores just how critical their work really is.

Importance of Toxicology in Forensics

Toxicology often takes center stage in forensics, acting as a sort of silent detective in figuring out why someone died and who might be to blame (Figure 4.1). It is not just about identifying illegal drugs or prescribed medications – the analysis digs in to measure substances. It offers clues that investigators lean on even when things are not crystal clear. Forensic toxicologists, wedded to techniques such as mass spectrometry (MS) and gas chromatography (GC), sometimes uncover evidence that might otherwise slip by unnoticed, and this can turn an autopsy report into something far more revealing than it initially appears. In many sudden death cases, pinpointing substances can hint at recurring patterns of misuse or even accidental overdoses, as some recent studies bringing necropsy data and sudden cardiac deaths to light (Tseng et al., 2018; Lechien et al., 2020) suggest. Overall, integrating these toxicological insights with other investigative methods not only advances forensic work but also, in most cases, helps shape public health and safety efforts related to substance issues.

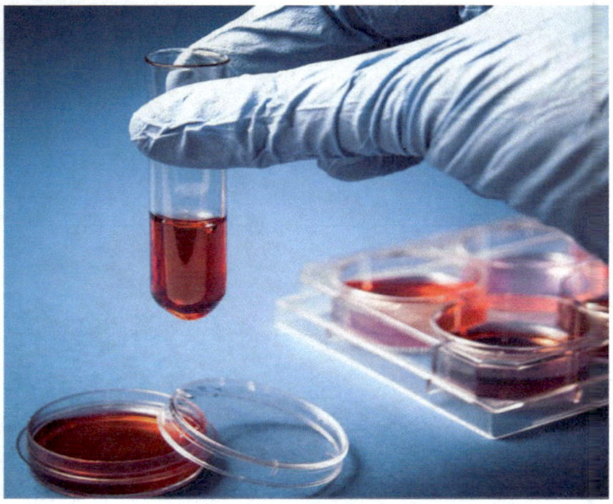

Figure 4.1. Importance of toxicology in forensics.

Source: Fondelco Institute. (n.d.). *Toxicology*. https://www.fondelco.in/institute/assets/images/Toxicology2.jpg.

Historical Context of Toxicology in Criminal Investigations

The journey of forensic toxicology winds through a mix of historical moments that have reshaped crime investigations. In the 1800s, public interest in sensational trials not only exposed flaws in the justice system but also underscored a need for a more scientific approach in legal settings. Consider the 1827 case of William Sheen—his wrongful conviction plainly revealed what happens when toxic tests are not up to snuff.

By the 1900s, new tactics emerged; for example, tapping into different biological samples, such as hair and sweat, opened unexpected doors for tracking drug exposure, thereby sharpening investigative work (de Campos et al., 2021). In most cases, this blend of shifting public expectations and steady scientific progress has transformed toxicology into a key player in the drive for fairness in criminal cases.

Overview of Toxic Substances Commonly Encountered

Toxic substances matter a lot in forensic science—it really all boils down to knowing how different kinds of these compounds affect human health and legal cases. You get heavy metals, organic solvents, assorted drugs, and each one kind of messes with analysis in its own peculiar way. Take heavy metals like lead or arsenic, for example; they are quite sneaky, often accumulating in the body without any obvious symptoms initially. Then there is something like benzene, an organic solvent that often appears in cases of sudden poisoning, so quick identification is usually essential. Lately, new psychoactive substances have started showing up, and honestly, they sometimes manage to dodge the typical tests. In most cases, forensic toxicologists lean on broad screening and detailed analysis techniques to figure out what went wrong after unnatural deaths or suspected drug incidents (Issa et al., 2019; Almeida et al. 2025).

Role of Toxicologists in the Legal System

Criminal investigations can become messy—a tangled web where toxicologists unexpectedly find themselves in the spotlight as crucial players in the legal arena. These specialists study toxins and their effects on living bodies; they provide insights into poisoning cases and other situations where harmful substances impact a victim's health. They do not stop at simply identifying a dangerous chemical—rather, they investigate how these substances interact with human biology, a detail that often proves crucial in determining the cause of an injury or even a death (Boriwala et al., 2024). Relying on methods like chromatography and MS, toxicologists analyze evidence with great care, ensuring forensic work rests on solid, scientific ground (Ashok et al., 2013). This layered method not only sets the stage for determining liability but also helps law enforcement trace suspects and unravel hidden motives. In most cases, blending toxicological expertise into legal processes really strengthens our pursuit of justice in cases marked by complexity, ambiguity, and the occasional unexpected twist (Figure 4.2).

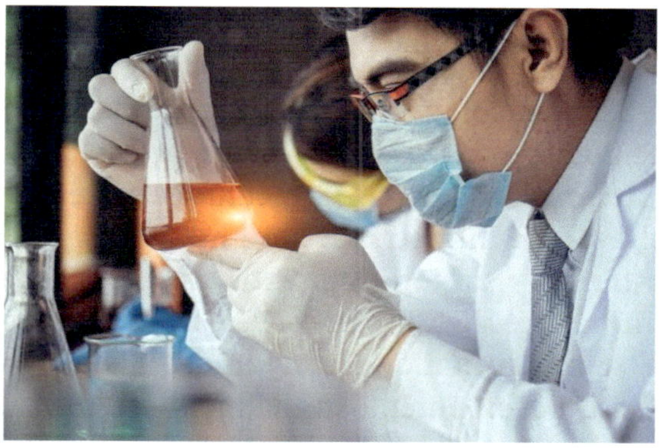

Figure 4.2. Role of toxicologists in the legal system.

Source: Tulane University School of Public Health and Tropical Medicine. (2021). *What Does a Toxicologist Do?* https://publichealth.tulane.edu/wp-content/uploads/sites/3/2021/11/blog-toxicologist.jpg.

Scope of Forensic Toxicology

Forensic science is not just about one strict approach; toxicology, for instance, weaves together legal inquiry with scientific work in surprising ways. Its primary goal is, generally speaking, to test biological samples—be they blood, tissue, or other types of fluids—for drugs, toxins, and other harmful substances that often prove to be crucial evidence in criminal cases. Advanced analytical techniques continue to evolve, allowing methods like MS to detect multiple substances simultaneously, thereby enhancing both the accuracy and speed of these tests (Vincenti et al., 2013). Sometimes, though, the details can feel overwhelming. Additionally, collaboration is crucial—legal professionals and forensic scientists meet in workshops and casual settings to gain a deeper understanding of toxicology's evidentiary role in court. In most cases, this mixed approach not only enhances the trustworthiness of forensic results but also reminds us that toxicology plays a crucial role in the overall pursuit of justice.

Methodologies Used in Forensic Toxicology

Analytical methods have significantly impacted forensic toxicology, transforming it into a field that now operates with greater precision and trustworthiness. You see, techniques like SPME (solid-phase microextraction) have emerged as eco-friendly options for extracting chemicals from biological samples—even from materials like vitreous humor. Lately, there has been a notable development: individuals are utilizing biosorbents, such as cork sheet strips, a move that accelerates extraction while reducing solvent usage.

This clever trick works wonders when analyzing psychoactive medications, which is particularly important in cases involving mental health issues, and it aligns with green chemistry ideals (Ossanes et al., 2023). On another front, pairing liquid chromatography with tandem MS brings some seriously robust quantification for a wide range of analytes, ensuring that postmortem analyses end up with data you can bank on in legal settings (Casparsen, 2024). Altogether, these shifts highlight toxicology's key role in the justice system and continue to push forensic science forward, reminding us that even small tweaks can make a significant difference.

Significance of Accurate Toxicological Analysis

Toxicological analysis holds a critical position in forensic science—it is what often ensures that justice is served and our public remains safe (Figure 4.3). Getting the right read on substances found in biological samples can significantly impact the outcome of criminal probes and legal debates. Sometimes, though, delays occur—often because labs are understaffed or underresourced—which, as noted by the Johannesburg Forensic Pathology Service (Hansmeyer et al., 2016), ultimately slows down the entire justice process. In many cases, these setbacks hint that faster, more reliable screening is needed to ease the load on labs and help the legal system run smoothly. At the same time, the rise of new psychoactive drugs keeps mixing things up in toxicology, meaning experts have to stay nimble to keep up with shifting drug trends (Council A on the Misuse of Drugs, 2011). All in all, nailing the analysis not only boosts law enforcement efforts but also plays a significant role in maintaining community health.

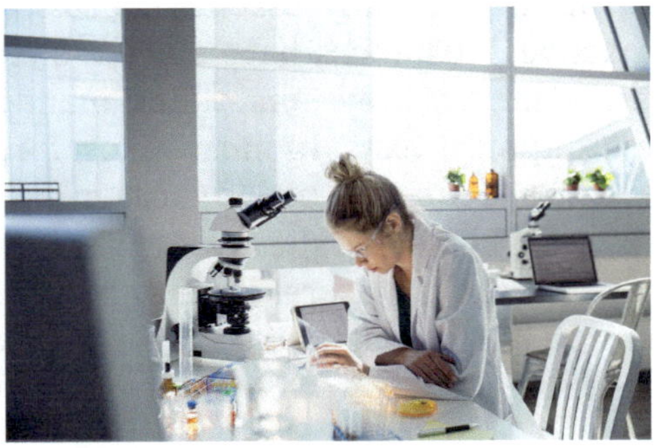

Figure 4.3. Toxicological analysis holds a critical spot in forensic science—it is what often makes sure that justice is served and our public stays safe.

Source: Saylor Academy. (n.d.). *Photograph of a Chemical Engineer Conducting Lab Work with a Microscope.* Saylor Academy. https://images.ctfassets.net/pdf29us7flmy/5sD4RDeft3TewRDWIDFsiF/7e7c5f9a5e8c6a19cc13dc26690e7[illegible]38/chemical-engineer-labwork-microscope.jpg.

4.1. Types of Toxic Substances

Learning Outcome

1. Understand classification of toxic substances
2. Identify commonly encountered drugs in forensic cases
3. Explain environmental toxins and their impact
4. Focus on heavy metals and their forensic relevance
5. Describe biological toxins and their effects
6. Discuss alcohol and its role in forensic toxicology
7. Know synthetic drugs and emerging trends
8. Identify poisonous plants and their identification
9. Know industrial chemicals and their forensic implications

Forensic toxicology often begins with identifying various toxins – they originate from diverse sources and exhibit unexpected effects. Synthetic cannabinoids, for instance, have become a hot topic lately because they pack a lot more punch than you would expect and tend to behave unpredictably. You usually end up splitting cannabinoids into a few groups: there are those our bodies make naturally, ones that come straight from plants, and then these lab-made versions.

The synthetic ones often appear in products marketed as herbal smoking blends or herbal incense, like Spice or K2 (Alves et al., 2020). They are built to latch onto cannabinoid receptors with a lot of force, sometimes producing effects that far surpass natural cannabis. New versions continue to emerge, which means regulators must continually update drug control lists (Zeppenfeld et al., 2022). In most cases, the rise in severe intoxications and even fatalities linked to these substances makes it clear that forensic toxicology needs to ramp up its monitoring and intervention efforts.

4.1.1. Classification of Toxic Substances

Forensic toxicology relies on sorting toxic substances clearly so that analysts stay sharp and legal processes are on point. We tend to group these chemicals by where they come from and how they affect us, with synthetic cannabinoids now popping up a lot in chatter about new drugs. They imitate natural cannabis in many ways, yet carry an extra punch thanks to their unpredictable toxicity and sheer strength. Recent work generally shows that these synthetic variants are sometimes tied to sudden intoxications and even fatalities, a signal that our regulatory playbook might need regular updates (Alves et al., 2020). The scene gets even messier when you factor in the ever-growing list of new psychoactive substances (NPS)—which truly makes detection a bit of a puzzle. One promising approach is metabolomics, which examines the biochemical pathways these substances leave behind and may eventually help identify reliable forensic biomarkers (Steuer et al., 2019) (Figure 4.4).

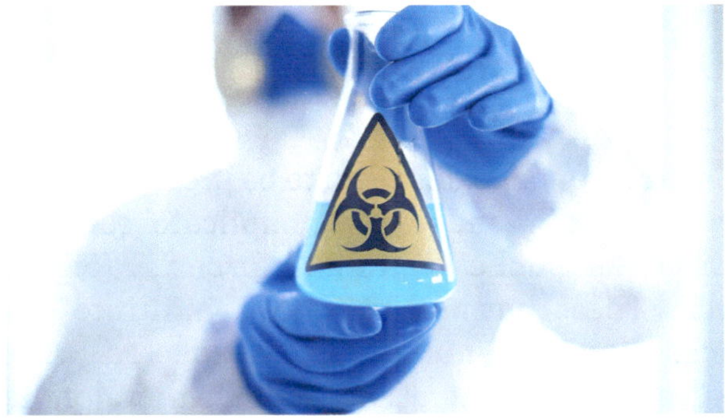

Figure 4.4. Toxic substances.

Source: Eaton Injury Law. (2024). *Equipment Exposure to Toxic Substances Accidents.*

4.1.2. Commonly Encountered Drugs in Forensic Cases

Forensic toxicology today has become increasingly complex, largely because investigators encounter a wide range of substances. Opiates, amphetamines, and benzodiazepines pop up pretty often in these cases – each one tossing up its own set of challenges when it comes to detection and analysis. Take opiates, for example; they are generally tied to overdose incidents, which means labs often have to use strict sampling and detailed analysis methods to pinpoint the exact compounds. Then there is the growing use of synthetic cannabinoids, which only adds to the mess with their unpredictable effects and metabolites that refuse to follow expected patterns, creating hurdles for experts. (Jones et al., 2021; Zeppenfeld et al., 2022). In many cases, recent studies have suggested that building solid, tailored methods for these drugs is crucial for nailing down accuracy and reliability in investigations. Meanwhile, as patterns of drug abuse shift and advancements in analytical technology become more intertwined—almost wedded, you might say—the protocols in forensic toxicology are constantly being reshaped, ultimately boosting our ability to crack even the trickiest cases.

4.1.3. Environmental Toxins and Their Impact

Environmental toxins seem to be present around every corner and often complicate complex issues for public health and forensics (Figure 4.5). These harmful chemicals infiltrate our ecosystems in numerous unexpected ways – from industrial waste and farm runoff to particles settling out of the air. Their effects are not minor; they can trigger long-term illnesses and even sudden bouts of poisoning. For cases where someone has been poisoned or an area has been contaminated, figuring out exactly what these substances are and tracking their origins becomes crucial, often in rather unpredictable ways. Methods like Gas Chromatography-Mass Spectrometry (GC-MS) enable experts to both pinpoint and measure these compounds, thereby enhancing forensic investigations and, in most cases, supporting legal claims (Sinha et al., 2023). Besides that, digging into the origins of toxins sometimes sparks local health projects and even helps shape rules aimed at reducing exposure and risks (Seaman et al., 2001). All in all, the complex relationship between environmental toxins and their effects remains a key, yet challenging, area of study in the field of toxicology.

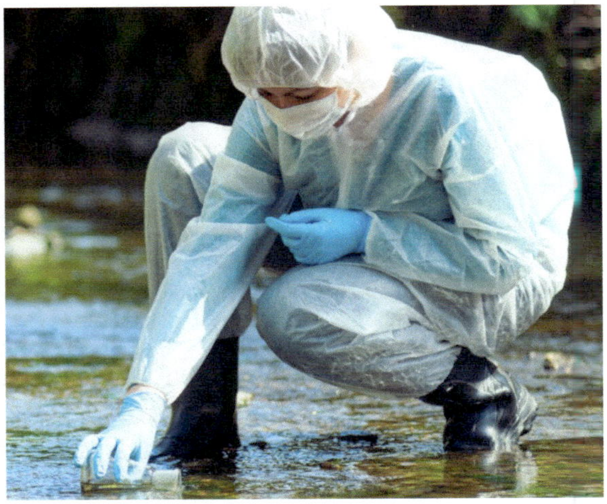

Figure 4.5. Environmental toxins.

Source: Bruker Corporation. (2024). *Environmental Forensics: Water Sample Analysis by a Female Scientist.* https://www.bruker.com/en/applications/detection-and-environmental/forensics/environmental-forensics/_jcr_content/root/sections/section_1467103126/sectionpar/twocolumns/contentpar-2/image.coreimg.82.1280.jpeg/1603648505991/bopt-cml-environmental-env-forensics-water-sample-woman-scientist.jpeg.

4.1.4. Heavy Metals and Their Forensic Relevance

Environmental contamination is not just a buzzword—it is deeply linked to public health, and this complex connection has prompted researchers to explore how heavy metals can reveal what is truly happening. You often find these metals in soil or water, typically indicating human interference, and in many studies, they emerge as key markers. For example, researchers have noted that when metals like copper, cadmium, and lead show up in higher-than-normal amounts, it tends to go hand in hand with real ecological upheaval; think of the coastal stretch by the Styr River, where chemical pollution seems to whisper secrets about exposure and risk (Popovych et al., 2025). Likewise, water analyses at the Verkhnetobolsky and Karatomarsky reservoirs suggest that the way these metals drift and gather can shed a bit of light on environmental misdeeds (Yskak et al., 2024). Generally speaking, grasping these complex relationships not only helps pinpoint the origins of contamination but also adds a new layer to our understanding of toxic profiles, which are crucial for both forensic work and public health policy.

4.1.5. Biological Toxins and Their Effects

Biological toxins and their impact on our health form a fascinating topic in forensic toxicology (Figure 4.6). They come from a mix of sources—plants, animals, or even tiny microorganisms—and these naturally occurring compounds can mess with our body's normal rhythms, sometimes leading to serious health issues. With new analytical methods coming into play, finding and pinning down these toxins has become a high priority; in most cases, forensic science now relies on tools that make the job a bit less lab-intensive. Take ambient ionization mass spectrometry (AIMS), for instance—it has been touted as a breakthrough because it allows experts to quickly analyze samples without extensive preparation (Henderson et al., 2024). The study of cannabinoids, for example, not only sheds light on the benefits they might offer but also on the risks they carry; this research blurs the lines between nature's raw materials and their potential links to conditions like neurodegenerative diseases and cancer (Voicu et al., 2023). All in all, gaining a solid understanding of these connections is crucial to advancing forensic toxicology and, ultimately, making our communities safer.

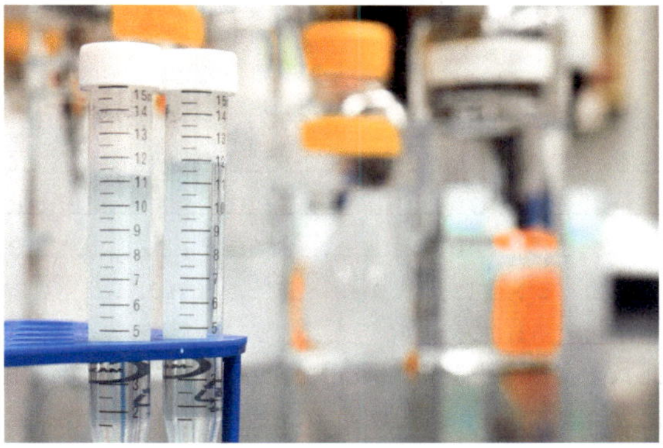

Figure 4.6. Biological toxins.

Source: Forensic Resources. (2019). *Biology Blurred Background.* https://forensicresources.org/wp-content/uploads/2019/05/biology-blur-blurred-background-954585-1024x683.jpg.

4.1.6. Alcohol and Its Role in Forensic Toxicology

Alcohol plays a significant role when trying to figure out how people act and how their bodies respond to substances in forensic cases. It is not just a peripheral detail—since alcohol is arguably one of the most common psychoactive agents out there, it is closely linked with investigations involving accidents, traumatic events, or cases of driving under the influence. Getting an accurate blood alcohol concentration (BAC) reading often helps clear up what happened, which, in most cases, can affect both legal judgments and public health guidelines. Interestingly, recent work in metabolomics has shown that alcohol levels can shift after death, adding extra challenges in nailing down the time of death or exactly how much alcohol might have tipped the scales in a fatal outcome (Evison et al., 2011). All things considered, these issues point to a need for strong, carefully thought-out forensic methods to untangle the subtle yet crucial effects alcohol has on toxicological outcomes (Hoeland et al., 2021).

4.1.7. Synthetic Drugs and Emerging Trends

Forensic toxicology is getting pretty tangled these days—novel psychoactive substances (NPS) keep showing up and ruffling the feathers of labs that must identify and analyze them. Recent reports, which are generally quite alarming, note that U.S. laboratories have recorded over 1,940 instances of seized drugs containing these substances, reflecting a drug market that is shifting faster than expected.

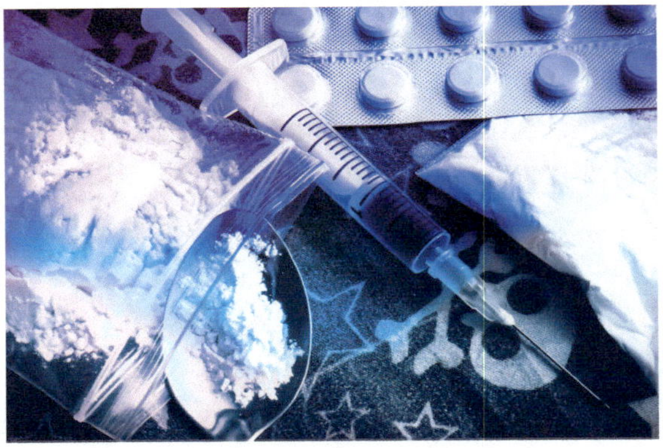

Figure 4.7. Synthetic drugs.

Source: Bruker Corporation. (n.d.). *Forensic Drug Analysis – Drug Abuse.* https://www.bruker.com/en/applications/detection-and-environmental/forensics/forensic-drug-analysis/_jcr_content/root/sections/section_1545192128/sectionpar/twocolumns_212198396/contentpar-2/image.coreimg.82.1280.png/1604083373819/drug-abuse.png.

Novel synthetic opioids (NSO), with fluorofentanyl featuring prominently, seem to be steering a large part of these trends, and that is not something labs can easily ignore. Regional profiles are not uniform either; a mix of synthetic cannabinoids and cathinones appears in various areas, making it more challenging to validate analytical methods (Ellefsen et al., 2024). As opioid misuse steadily rises, researchers have begun to adopt untargeted metabolomics—an approach that, in most cases, could lead to more effective detection strategies—which underscores the pressing need for more robust forensic frameworks in the field (Amante et al., 2021) (Figure 4.7).

4.1.8. Poisonous Plants and Their Identification

Poisonous plants come up a lot in forensic toxicology, especially when investigators are piecing together poisoning cases. It is not just identifying these dangerous greens – one also has to distinguish the symptoms they cause from those of various illnesses, a challenge that forensic medicine has grappled with for ages. In most cases, this began in the late 18th century, when forensic toxicology started paying closer attention to toxins from plants like belladonna and henbane (Coley, 1991)—plants whose effects can resemble serious health issues. Nowadays, clinical toxicology texts still include guidance on these hazardous flora, offering advice on how to recognize and manage emergencies when poisoning occurs (Dunlop, 1957). A solid understanding of the nature of these botanical toxins can greatly assist forensic experts, influencing not only legal outcomes but also everyday public health and safety. Clearly, getting those identifications right is crucial for both preventing and treating poisoning cases.

4.1.9. Industrial Chemicals and Their Forensic Implications

Industrial chemicals are becoming increasingly complex these days, leaving forensic toxicologists scratching their heads as they try to sort through contaminant puzzles (Figure 4.8). PFAS—yes, those per- and polyfluoroalkyl substances that hang around in our environment—have become a big issue, mainly since they are used almost everywhere and their chemistry is anything but simple. In most cases, determining which PFAS compounds are present and tracking their environmental pathways proves to be a challenging task; some studies (Guelfo et al., 2021) even suggest that we require more precise analytical tools and smarter risk management strategies. Then there's road runoff debris—such as particles from worn tires—that is now linked to sudden, lethal effects in aquatic species (Peter et al., 2018). All of this really shows how the jumble of industrial chemicals and forensic science is not just an academic debate; it has real consequences for environmental health and pushes us to rethink regulatory standards. Clearly, keeping up with innovative toxicology research is crucial when chemical challenges continue to evolve.

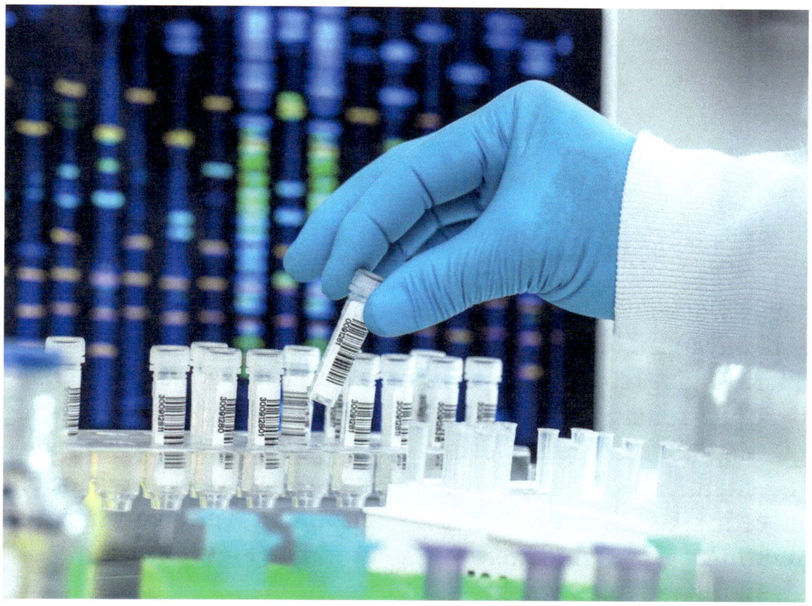

Figure 4.8. Industrial chemicals.

Source: Medindia. (n.d.). *Industrial Chemicals.* https://d1g9yur4m4naub.cloudfront.net/images/Article_Images/ImageForArticle_1409_17367808340863516.jpg.

Test Your Knowledge

1. Classify toxic substances based on their origin.
2. Give two examples of biological toxins.
3. What are the main classes of chemical toxicants?

4.2. Methods of Toxicological Analysis

Learning Outcome

1. Sample collection and preservation
2. Screening techniques in toxicology
3. Confirmatory testing methods
4. Role of chromatography in analysis
5. Mass spectrometry applications
6. Immunoassays in toxicology
7. Interpretation of toxicological results
8. Quality control in toxicological testing
9. Challenges in toxicological analysis

Toxicology and forensic work often intersect in unexpected ways, with advanced testing playing a significant role in resolving complex cases. Labs now employ super-sensitive methods, such as UHPLC–QqQ-MS/MS, that detect even the tiniest traces of chemicals. For example, hydroxyzine (HZ) and cetirizine (CZ) are detected in body fluids, providing crucial information when dealing with drug-related impairments or even fatalities (Ałopaś-Konowałek et al., 2024). Generally speaking, these breakthroughs enable forensic experts to measure these substances accurately, even when they are present at very low levels, which helps gauge their effects on brain function and behavior. In many cases, professionals in the field discuss the versatility of these toxicology methods, whether used in postmortem work or for assessing impairment in criminal cases (Casparsen, 2024). All in all, as analytical techniques continue to evolve, the resulting toxicological data becomes more reliable, and the whole forensic process ends up with a sturdier backbone.

4.2.1. Sample Collection and Preservation

ccurate forensic toxicology relies heavily on maintaining the integrity of samples—it all comes down to how they are collected and then properly preserved. In many instances, the delay between collecting a sample and actually analyzing it can allow the evidence to slowly degrade, potentially leading to misleading outcomes. Some studies, for example, generally show that certain drugs break down pretty fast when left at room temperature; that means you really have to use quick preservation methods—techniques like adding toluene seem to work, though the rates of compound stability can shift with different temperature conditions (Zhen et al., 2017). Now, turning to forensic entomotoxicology (basically, the branch that examines toxins in insects), preserving larvae is absolutely key because poor preservation can compromise their integrity—and, yes, that, in turn, undermines the reliability of toxicological findings (Mbatha et al., 2018). In most cases, adhering to consistent and proper sample collection and storage practices is not only important but also necessary for forensic experts to obtain accurate assessments and, ultimately, valid conclusions from the evidence at hand (Figure 4.9).

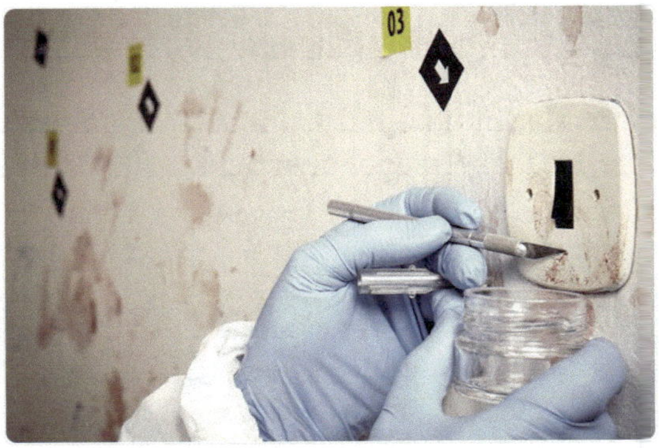

Figure 4.9. Sample collection.

Source: Medindia. (2020). *Forensic Investigator Examining Evidence with Magnifying Glass.*

4.2.2. Screening Techniques in Toxicology

Advanced screening methods play a massive role in forensic toxicology today (Figure

4.10). Liquid chromatography paired with tandem mass spectrometry (LC-MS-MS) is a standout tool—often chosen for its ability to efficiently sort through a wide range of drugs in biological samples, with urine being a common focus. Researchers have generally found that this method can flag nearly 95 substances, demonstrating solid sensitivity and reproducibility, with detection rates typically exceeding 90% in many test cases (dos Santos et al., 2024). At the same time, immunoassay techniques—used by companies such as Randox and Siemens—yield rapid preliminary results that significantly enhance the overall lab workflow. Sure, these methods differ a bit in their exact detection abilities and specificity. Still, they are invaluable as the first checkpoint before confirmatory tests (like GC-MS or HPLC-MS) step in Alwaeel et al. (2022). Taken all together, these overlapping approaches underscore why a varied and layered strategy is so important when addressing substance abuse in forensic investigations.

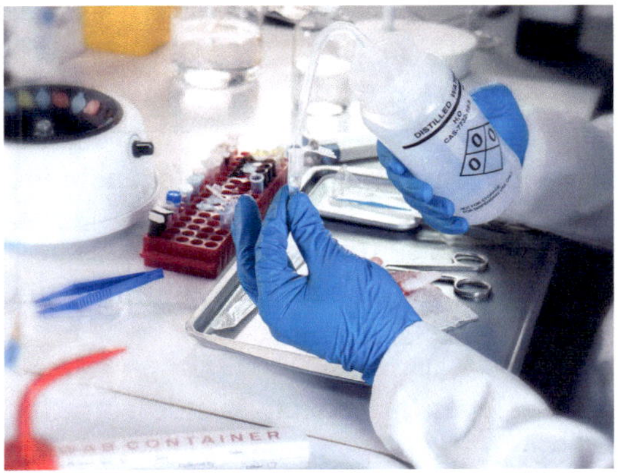

Figure 4.10. Advanced screening methods play a huge role in forensic toxicology today.

Source: SCIEX. (n.d.). *Forensic and Homeland Security Tools.* https://sciex.com/adobe/dynamicmedia/deliver/dm-aid--a7b6819b-9560-4a1c-be72-bc8f122459fc/forensics-homeland-menu-2000x1500.jpg?quality=75&width=1920.

4.2.3. Confirmatory Testing Methods

Forensic toxicology kicks off with the challenge of nailing down what substances are present and exactly how much is there—usually through some pretty strict methods to make sure the outcomes are solid. Confirmatory tests jump in to back up the initial screenings, using techniques like GC-MS and liquid chromatography-tandem mass spectrometry (LC-MS/MS) to give that extra layer of validation. These advanced approaches prove especially essential when dealing with emerging drugs and novel psychoactive substances (NPS) that, in most cases, bring along unique hurdles due to their intricate makeup and the way they shift rapidly in the drug market. All this, in turn, highlights why checking alternative biological matrices can be so valuable—recent literature suggests that these can sometimes offer critical insights into drug exposure over longer detection windows, especially when traditional specimens are not available. In the end, incorporating methods like metabolomics not only enhances the accuracy of confirmatory tests but also helps identify biomarkers of drug use, leading to a more comprehensive understanding of toxicological profiles in forensic investigations (de Campos et al., 2021; Steuer et al., 2019).

4.2.4. Role of Chromatography in Analysis

Forensic toxicology continues to push labs to update their methods to detect a wide range of chemicals. Chromatography is central here—it separates samples and identifies different compounds found in body fluids or tissues. Recent work, for example, has identified new substances, such as bromazolam, detected using techniques like liquid chromatography paired with mass spectrometry (LC-MS), which proved crucial for investigations in Indiana in 2023 (Shanks et al., 2024). In many cases, smaller-scale procedures—think dispersive liquid-liquid microextraction combined with liquid chromatography-tandem MS—have really improved how sensitive and selective analyses can be, allowing experts to pick up on both well-known drugs and emerging ones like ketamine and its variants (Oliveira et al., 2024). All in all, chromatography remains a key tool for unraveling the toxic effects of new compounds in forensic science (Figure 4.11).

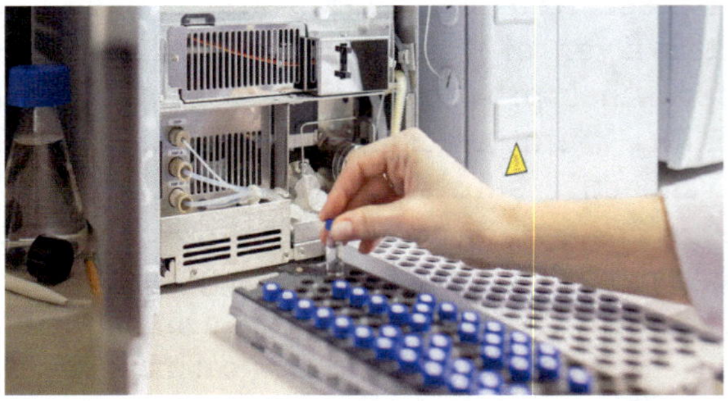

Figure 4.11. Chromatography separates samples and identifies different compounds present in body fluids or tissues.

Source: Nebiolab. (2024). *Speak to our scientist marketing benefit.* https://www.nebiolab.com/wp-content/uploads/2024/11/speak-to-our-scientist-marketing-benefit-bg1.webp.

4.2.5. Mass Spectrometry (MS) Applications

Analytical techniques have undergone a significant upgrade over the years, and forensic toxicology is no exception—in fact, the use of MS has had a profound impact. This tool, essentially a device that measures the weight of molecules, can detect even the tiniest traces of substances; you could say it reveals details that might otherwise go unnoticed.

Researchers now frequently detect challenging toxicants in biological samples, which not only speeds up the process but also makes it more accurate. In most cases, these machines help reveal how contaminants—such as PCBs in environmental samples—enter the environment and interact with living things, sometimes in complex and intricate ways. New methods even incorporate multivariate statistical checks to sort through complex data, further pushing the limits of forensic work (Corl et al., 2015). All said, it is clear that advancements in MS are, generally speaking, indispensable for today's forensic toxicology.

4.2.6. Immunoassays in Toxicology

Immunoassays have significantly transformed toxicology, particularly in forensic work (Figure 4.12). Labs now rely on antibodies that bind to specific chemicals, which means even the tiniest traces do not go unnoticed—vital when samples may be less than pristine.

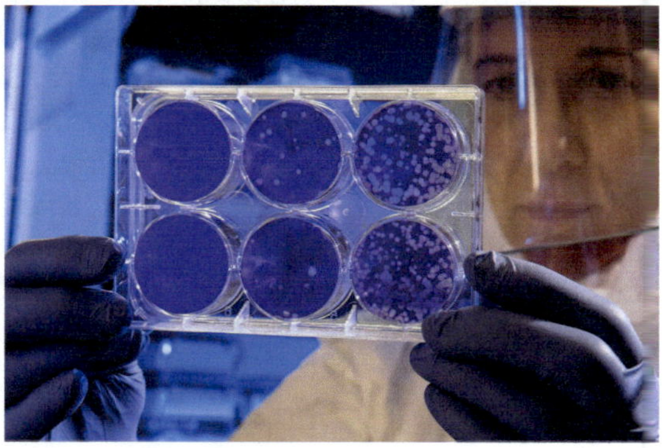

Figure 4.12. Immunoassays in forensic work.

Source: Centers for Disease Control and Prevention. (2019). Scientist examining plaque assay results. *Unsplash*.

This clever approach is not confined to one lane; it is utilized for everything from detecting drugs in biological fluids to identifying environmental toxins. One notable twist involves merging screen-printed electrodes with electroanalysis, a move that is proving to be both affordable and practical, allowing for on-site, real-time testing (Aía-Ferrari et al., 2021). In most cases, the recent push for hydrogen isotope labelling with deuterium and tritium is offering additional insight into how these compounds function in the body. This generally seems to boost both the clarity and dependability of toxicological assessments (Atzrodt et al., 2017).

4.2.7. Interpretation of Toxicological Results

Interpreting toxicology results is not as cut-and-dried as it might seem—it lies squarely at the center of many forensic cases. Instead of following a neat checklist, experts need to juggle a mix of factors; for example, they consider everything from the time since death and the body's physical condition to the practical details of how blood was collected. Sometimes, quirky elements like postmortem redistribution or even a bit too much preservative can throw the numbers off, misleading conclusions about both cause and manner of death. Often, labs rely on tools like High-Performance Liquid Chromatography-MS and GC-MS to pinpoint substances with precision; generally speaking, these methods have helped clarify episodes of acute intoxication or overdose, as seen in studies that illuminated the circumstances leading to death (Dinis-Oliveira, 2024). And when various substances—ranging from drugs such as cocaine to everyday prescription meds—are in play, the need for spot-on, carefully weighed analysis becomes even more apparent (Candia et al., 2022).

4.2.8. Quality Control in Toxicological Testing

Reliability in toxicological testing is crucial in forensics—results can have significant legal implications (Figure 4.13). It is not simply about achieving a result; ensuring that methods are thoroughly checked and that outcomes remain consistent fosters solid scientific trust. You have to look at everyday details, such as how samples are handled, the way lab procedures run, and even the surrounding conditions, because any one of these can hide a potential slip-up. In most cases, studies show that adding newer technologies, such as nanotechnology in these tests, opens up exciting, innovative opportunities while also presenting fresh challenges for risk assessments and worker safety (Adamec et al., 2019). For this reason, forensic labs typically need to implement strict quality control measures that not only enhance accuracy but also address these emerging issues (Capiau et al., 2016). All in all, this mix of careful checks and balances is crucial—if we want toxicology to remain an essential part of the justice system.

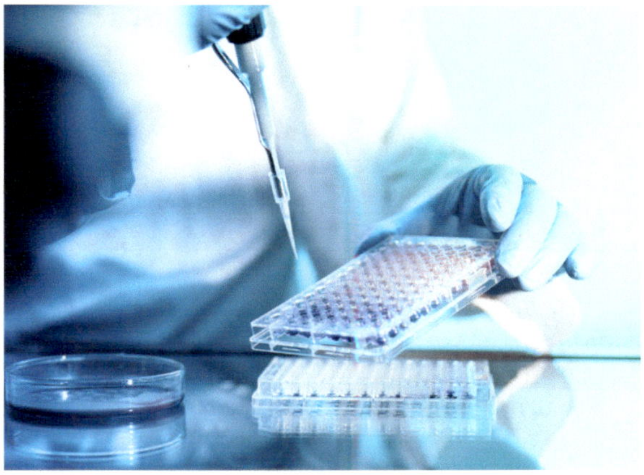

Figure 4.13. Reliability in toxicological testing is a must in forensics.

Source: Alabama Department of Forensic Sciences. (n.d.). *Toxicology Laboratory Equipment.* https://adfs.alabama.gov/Content/ADFSTheme/images/toxicology/toxicology-image-14.jpg.

4.2.9. Challenges in Toxicological Analysis

Forensic science has improved toxicology testing a lot, but plenty of issues still pop up. NPS keep appearing, so labs have to update their testing methods repeatedly; this twist makes it more challenging to establish a standard detection method. Sometimes older screening tools just are not enough, mainly when they deal with unusual mixes like xylazine paired with synthetic opioids, which ramp up overdose risks (OYález et al., 2024). Nanoparticles, for instance, show promise for detecting even tiny traces;

however, their use requires strict guidelines to prevent problems such as oxidative DNA damage (Verma et al., 2024). Illegal drug synthesis adds another messy layer, often leading to errors in toxicology reports. Generally speaking, a blended strategy—improving detection tech while also boosting forensic toxicology training—is key to handling these shifting challenges effectively.

Test Your Knowledge

1. What is the purpose of toxicological analysis?
2. Name two biological samples commonly used in toxicological testing.
3. What is gas chromatography (GC), and how is it used in toxicology?

4.3. Case Studies in Forensic Toxicology

Learning Outcome

1. Discuss landmark cases involving toxicology
2. Perform analysis of drug overdose cases
3. Know poisoning cases and their investigations
4. Explain the role of toxicology in homicide investigations
5. Describe toxicological evidence in DUI cases
6. Understand historical cases that shaped forensic toxicology
7. Explain the use of toxicology in exhumation cases
8. Know the impact of toxicology on wrongful convictions
9. Describe future implications of case studies in toxicology

Forensic investigations lean heavily on toxicology, which gives us key details that can push outcomes in court. Case studies remind us how toxicology often untangles complex situations by revealing substances that are not immediately apparent. Sometimes, looking at drug amounts in bodily samples can sort out the timing in cases like overdoses or impaired driving. New methods in handling evidence and keeping track of its chain—and I mean, really keeping it secure—matter a great deal in ensuring our findings remain solid. In many cases, challenges with lab resources and quality control arise, sparking calls for tighter oversight and clearer guidelines (Garrett et al., 2020). And, you know, maintaining a good chain of custody is critical for maintaining the authenticity of evidence, especially when technology is constantly evolving how we collect this kind of data (Argo et al., 2023).

4.3.1. Landmark Cases Involving Toxicology

Forensics and toxicology have undergone significant changes over time, and a few major cases have significantly advanced their development. Dried blood spots (DBS), for instance, initially began as a tool for newborn screening but have since become a game-changer in the field. This method now pops up in places like drug testing and even when checking for environmental toxins, especially in situations where taking regular blood seems too harsh or feels invasive (Kesel et al., 2012). There's also that mix of social behaviors and legal issues—take, say, cases of sexual assault—where patterns in the evidence point to a clear link between toxicology and our legal system. In most instances, it appears that rapid, accurate testing is crucial for preserving essential evidence (Kumar et al., 2014) (Figure 4.14).

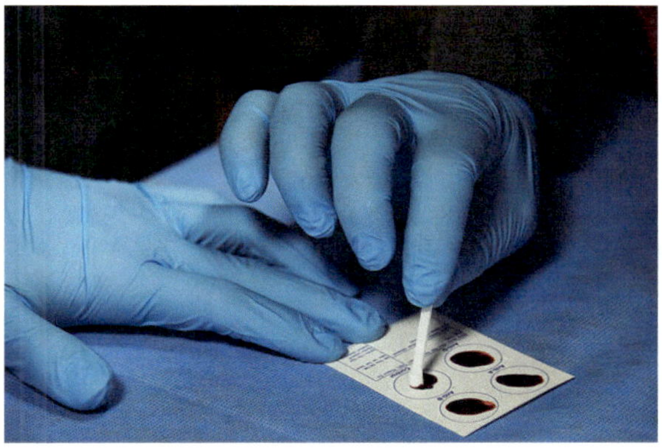

Figure 4.14. Dried blood spots (DBS) in forensics.

Source: Norgen Biotek Corp. (2022). *Dried Blood Spot (DBS) Sample on Filter Paper.*

4.3.2. Analysis of Drug Overdose Cases

Overdose numbers have surged in a way that grabs attention—opioids and stimulants, in particular, seem to be at the core of a deep-rooted public health issue that really needs a closer look. Studies keep hinting at a pattern: young men, often self-employed, show up more frequently than others, with their demographics and drug-use habits repeatedly emerging as key factors. When you examine these cases, it becomes clear, generally speaking, that our current prevention and intervention tactics are falling short of what is needed to alleviate the heavy toll these substances impose on society. In most cases, research suggests that a significant share of overdoses stems from intentional misuse, which only adds more layers to the already complex challenges of treatment and rehabilitation. And it is not just about individual health—the crisis spills over into massive socio-economic costs, from skyrocketing healthcare expenses to lost productivity, piling extra strain on medical systems. All in all, as the opioid epidemic stubbornly persists, confronting its multifaceted nature remains essential for paving the way toward a healthier tomorrow (Dana-Siadat et al., 2014; McLevain et al., 2021).

4.3.3. Poisoning Cases and Their Investigations

Investigating poisoning cases is not exactly straightforward—it is a messy scene in forensic work where figuring out what truly went down often calls for a mix of approaches (Figure 4.15). Poisons can vary a lot; you have the older substances like arsenic and cyanide, along with newer synthetic chemicals that sometimes pretend to be natural illnesses, occasionally (yes, occasionally) leading doctors astray in clinical settings (Soltaninejad, 2023). Generally speaking, when drug mixtures become particularly complex, experts rely on advanced methods, such as tandem mass spectrometry, to detect even the tiniest traces of toxins in samples (Soltaninejad, 2023). In the realm of veterinary forensics, things get equally tangled; for instance, when rodenticides like bromadiolone are involved, investigators often have to use customized protocols to make sense of the scene. Ultimately, both human and animal poisoning cases demand intensive, almost obsessive scrutiny and modern methods—sometimes even investigators wedded traditional techniques with cutting-edge instrumentation—to firmly tie toxins to fatalities, underscoring the intricate, if messy, bond between toxicology and forensic investigation.

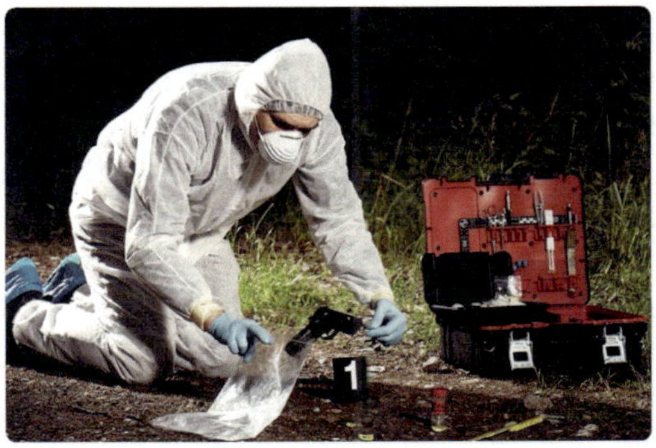

Figure 4.15. Investigating poisoning cases in forensics.

Source: Couperfield. (2015). Crime scene investigation – collecting pistol and cartridges by technician. *Shutterstock*.

4.3.4. Role of Toxicology in Homicide Investigations

Homicide work usually means getting into the details and really digging to sort out what might have driven someone to act. Toxicology jumps in here, checking what substances might have thrown off a victim's state right before death. A study in South Africa showed a strong link between drug use and violent outcomes - hair tests revealed that about 82.2% of cases had signs of long-term substance abuse (Mnisi et al., 2023). This kind of evidence tends to underscore how toxicology helps connect drug habits with violent behavior. Still, there are snags - lab backlogs and quality control issues often pop up (as noted when folks discuss resource allocation (Garrett et al., 2020)) - so tackling these problems becomes pretty key for keeping homicide investigations on track and accurate.

4.3.5. Toxicological Evidence in DUI Cases

Toxicology now plays a key role in solving DUI puzzles. Labs have turned to more brilliant, more hands-on methods when old tests just do not cut it anymore—especially with substances like carfentanil, which often slip through the cracks. One study even pointed out that carfentanil ranked as the second most common drug found in DUI blood samples, usually showing up alongside other opioids and similar mind-altering agents (Tiscione et al., 2018). You can also see tools like paper spray tandem mass spectrometry in action; this method enables labs to quickly measure amphetamines in blood, providing fast and reliable results in a matter of seconds (Teunissen et al., 2017). As these techniques continue to evolve, they are poised to enhance the accuracy of toxicological evidence, which in most cases will impact both legal outcomes and public safety (Figure 4.16).

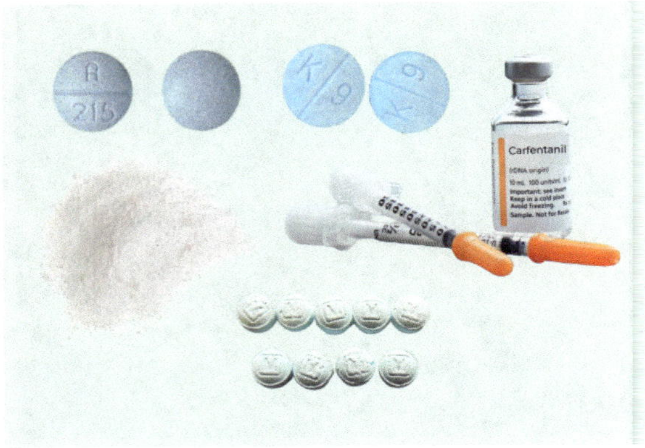

Figure 4.16. Carfentanil ranked as the second most common drug found in DUI blood samples.

Source: Mountainside Treatment Center. (2024). *Carfentanil.*

4.3.6. Historical Cases That Shaped Forensic Toxicology

The journey of forensic toxicology has been driven by a mix of landmark cases that have pushed courts to demand solid scientific proof. Take the Anna Nicole Smith case—an example that showed how vital lab tests can be in pinpointing a death's cause, and it even shed light on how pharmaceuticals can mess with our behavior and health. Cases like this, among others, have prompted experts to reconsider their approaches, often reevaluating how old practices measure toxic substances. With more voices calling for clear and honest answers, the field now relies on sharper techniques that can pinpoint and measure dangerous chemicals more precisely. These upgrades not only support deeper investigations but also broaden our understanding of substance misuse and its ripple effects on society. In the end, it hints that toxicology is not just basic lab work anymore—it is a key part of justice and public health, a view echoed in current chats about physician health programs that now wed modern monitoring tools to boost patient care (Burnier et al., 2019; Polles et al., 2021).

4.3.7. Use of Toxicology in Exhumation Cases

Often in forensic work, toxicology tests open a window into what really happened at the time of death—even if sometimes exhumation gets thrown into the mix. When an initial autopsy does not clear things up or when a hint of foul play surfaces, checking out chemical traces can be a game-changer. Take sodium nitrite, for example; its ingestion usually sets off a chain reaction of worrisome effects, spurring blood issues known as methemoglobinemia that, by starving the body of oxygen, may eventually lead to heart failure. One notable case in which, after a young woman's exhumation, experts uncovered clear signs of sodium nitrite toxicity—details backed up by other forensic clues—and all of that pointed toward suicide (Zerbo et al., 2023). Generally speaking, grasping the role of toxicology in these investigations highlights its value in untangling the messy complications of drug overdoses, as seen in society's tussle with opioid crises and the sometimes life-saving impact of naloxone (Campbell, 2020) (Figure 4.17).

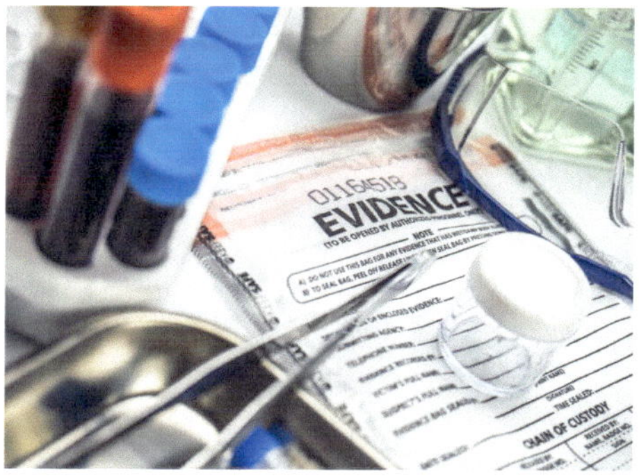

Figure 4.17. When an initial autopsy does not clear things up or when a hint of foul play surfaces, checking out chemical traces can be a game-changer.

Source: Top Lab Direct. (2022). *Vials of blood with evidence bag and other lab equipment.* https://toplabdirect.com/wp-content/uploads/2022/07/Vials-of-blood-with-evidence-bag-and-other-lab-equipment.jpg.

4.3.8. Impact of Toxicology on Wrongful Convictions

Toxicology and wrongful convictions often come together in ways that show our forensic system is not as solid as we would like to think, generally speaking. Sometimes, mistakes in toxicology tests end up misreading the substances found in both victims and suspects, and that shaky evidence can lead to wrongful convictions.

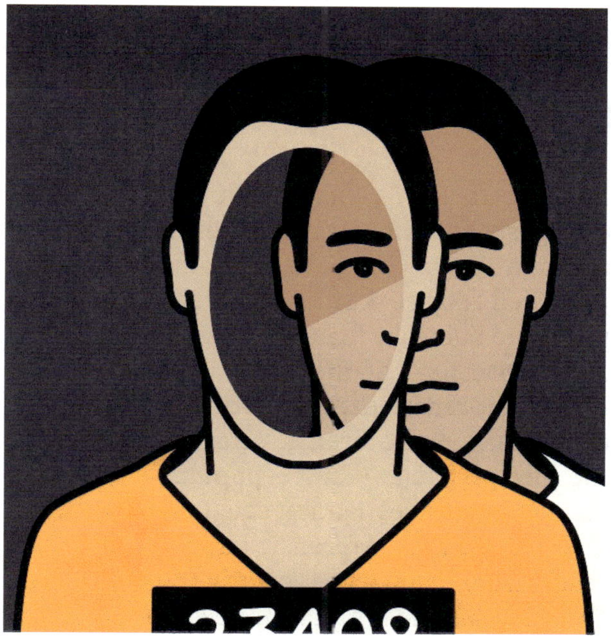

Figure 4.18. Mistakes in toxicology tests end up misreading the substances found in both victims and suspects, and that shaky evidence can lead to wrongful convictions.

Source: The New Yorker. (n.d.). *161024_r28894.* https://media.newyorker.com/photos/59097af2019dfc3494ea35e3/master/pass/161024_r28894.jpg.

A review of data from the National Registry of Exonerations suggests that many of these slip-ups stem more from miscommunication or loose reporting standards than from outright misidentifications by scientists (Morgan, 2023). You may also notice that unconscious biases among examiners tend to complicate the situation even further, making it even more complex (Kukucka et al., 2022). This is not just about isolated errors—the whole picture reveals some deep flaws in how we handle forensic evidence and advocates for reforms to enhance the reliability of toxicological assessments. Without such changes, the risk of convicting the innocent stays worryingly high, which calls for more rigorous oversight and greater accountability in forensic toxicology (Figure 4.18).

4.3.9. Future Implications of Case Studies in Toxicology

Forensic toxicology has undergone significant changes over time—case studies now reveal shifts in how the field is both taught and practiced (Figure 4.19). These reports give us a peek into behavior linked with toxic substances and also bring out the messy, real-world side of what forensic experts actually face. Public excitement about forensic science has been on the rise, especially since popular shows like Crime Scene Investigation caught on; this trend makes it clear that forensic education needs to reach more people, particularly those often left out of STEM. One program, for example, aimed at high school students of color, demonstrates that focused teaching efforts can significantly help build a new generation of forensic professionals prepared to address today's challenges in toxicology (Elrick et al., 2018). Additionally, there is a growing emphasis on collaboration across borders—in fact, international curriculum partnerships highlight the pressing need for comprehensive training that keeps pace with global issues and the everyday realities of forensic work (Anthony et al., 2019).

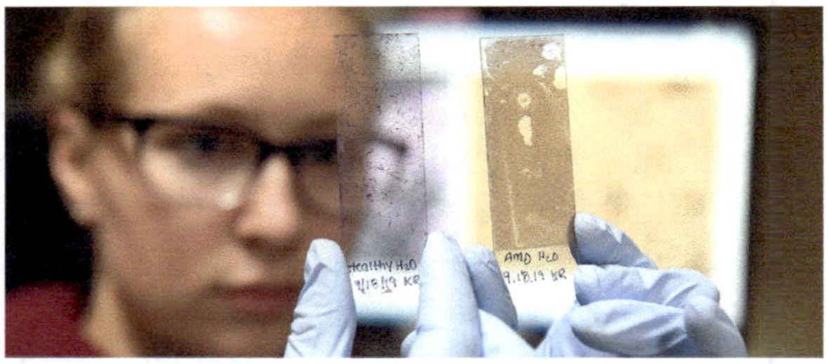

Figure 4.19. Forensic toxicology has undergone significant changes over time—case studies now reveal shifts in how the field is both taught and practiced.

Source: Harrisburg University. (n.d.). *Forensic Science*. https://www.harrisburgu.edu/wp-content/uploads/forensic-science-1600x686.jpg.

Test Your Knowledge

1. What role does toxicological analysis play in determining the cause of death?
2. How can forensic toxicology help distinguish between accidental and intentional poisoning?

SUMMARY

Advances in forensic toxicology are reshaping the way analyses are done, with a blend of new methods that help ensure more reliable results. In several studies, substances such as Zinc Sulfate—often used as an adulterant—have been shown to skew urine drug test outcomes; research even suggests that it messes with the accuracy of immunoassays designed to detect substance abuse (Capiau et al., 2016). It is interesting to note that Ethyl glucuronide (EtG), despite its own set of challenges, appears to offer a promising marker for alcohol consumption, opening up some rather exciting paths for future exploration in toxicology (Cawley et al., 2016). Techniques continue to evolve in unpredictable ways, and this ever-changing mix alongside the complexities of various toxic substances generally calls for ongoing research and adaptation in forensic practices. In many cases, these new approaches and findings—albeit sometimes imperfect—are crucial for deepening our overall understanding. Ultimately, understanding these intertwined factors can help the justice system navigate the complex landscape of substance-related cases more effectively.

Forensic toxicology is loaded with complex challenges and unexpected connections. Real cases continue to demonstrate the importance of recognizing signs of intoxication—whether in hospital settings or during legal investigations (Dinis-Oliveira, 2022). A strong educational base is crucial here, as numerous examples emphasize the importance of understanding what intoxication looks like in practice. New methods in analysis – such as the IAEA-CRP intercomparison exercise – generally enhance both precision and accuracy, ultimately making evidence from all sources, whether biological or not, more trustworthy (Quarta et al., 2022). Mixing fresh teaching ideas with modern lab techniques is not just about routine tests; it builds a broader, more flexible grasp of the field. In most cases, this blend of hands-on practice and in-depth learning is what drives forensic toxicology forward, helping it remain credible, effective, and prepared for future challenges.

KEY TERMS FROM THIS CHAPTER

- Chain reaction
- Custody
- Documentation
- Hair analysis
- Mislabeling
- Psychoactive substances
- Traits
- Contamination
- Data sharing
- Forensic databases
- Misinterpretation
- Poisoning
- Social stigma

CRITICAL THINKING QUESTIONS

1. **Which of the following is a toxin, not a toxicant?**
   a. Lead
   b. Mercury
   c. Snake venom
   d. Carbon monoxide
2. **What is the primary organ responsible for detoxification of chemicals in the body?**
   a. Heart
   b. Liver
   c. Kidney
   d. Lungs
3. **The therapeutic index is defined as:**
   a. The maximum tolerated dose of a drug
   b. The difference between absorption and elimination
   c. The ratio of toxic dose to effective dose
   d. The time taken for a drug to reach peak plasma levels
4. **Which route of toxin exposure is generally the fastest in terms of onset?**
   a. Oral
   b. Inhalation
   c. Dermal
   d. Rectal
5. **Chronic toxicity refers to adverse effects that occur:**
   a. Immediately after a single dose
   b. After repeated exposure over a long time
   c. Only with high doses
   d. Only with toxins injected intravenously

Short Answer Questions

1. What is the definition of toxicology?
2. What is the difference between a toxin and a toxicant?
3. How do dose and exposure duration influence toxicity?
4. Name two routes of exposure to toxic substances.
5. What is the difference between acute and chronic toxicity?
6. How does mass spectrometry (MS) enhance toxicological analysis?

Answers to Critical Thinking Questions

1. (c); 2. (b); 3. (c); 4. (b); 5. (b)

REFERENCES

1. Achsoni, R., Istislam, I., Kumoro, H. S., Widiarto, R., et al. (2020). *Reconstruction of the Position of the Honorary Council of Election Administrators in the Judicial System in Indonesia.* https://core.ac.uk/download/353470262.pdf (accessed on 9th May 2025).
2. Adamec, V., Köbölová, K., Pavlíková, S., Procházková, D., et al. (2019). *Current Approaches of Occupational and Safety Health Management in Work Environments Containing Nanoparticles.* https://core.ac.uk/download/287648860.pdf (accessed on 9th May 2025).
3. Advisory Council on the Misuse of Drugs. (2011). *Consideration of the Novel Psychoactive Substances ('Legal Highs').* https://core.ac.uk/download/1643031.pdf (accessed on 9th May 2025).
4. Ahmad, M. U., Athanasiou, T., Balyasnikova, S., Ehsanullah, M., et al. (2017). *Assessing the Use of Magnetic Resonance Imaging Virtopsy as an Alternative to Autopsy: A Systematic Review and Meta-Analysis.* https://core.ac.uk/download/131167245.pdf (accessed on 9th May 2025).
5. Almeida, A., Brandt, S. D., Christie, R., de Morais, J., et al. (2025). Technical report on N-(1-amino-3,3-dimethyl-1-oxobutan-2-yl)-1-(cyclohexylmethyl)-1H-indazole-3-carboxamide (ADB-CHMINACA): Annex 1 to the risk assessment report on N-(1-amino-3,3-dimethyl-1-oxobutan-2-yl)-1-(cyclohexylmethyl)-1H-indazole-3-carboxamide (ADB-CHMINACA). https://core.ac.uk/download/144574946.pdf (accessed on 9th May 2025).
6. Alves, V. L., Gonçalves, J., Aguiar, J., Teixeira, H. M., & Câmara, J. S. (2020). The synthetic cannabinoids phenomenon: From structure to toxicological properties. A review. *Critical Reviews in Toxicology, 50*, 359–382. https://doi.org/10.1080/10408444.2020.1762539.
7. Alwaeel, M., Gomaa, R., Ansari, N., & Nader, L., (2022). A comparative analysis of three different immunoassay techniques for screening of drugs of abuse in urine and their confirmation using GC-MS & HPLC-MS. *The Egyptian Journal of Forensic Sciences and Applied Toxicology.* https://www.semanticscholar.org/paper/622ac1a70bf975b663866e275dfd1c18171af97e (accessed on 9th May 2025).
8. Amante, E., Alladio, E., Rizzo, R., Di Corcia, D., Negri, P., Visintin, L., Guglielmotto, M., et al. (2021). Untargeted metabolomics in forensic toxicology: A new approach for the detection of fentanyl intake in urine samples. *Molecules, 26.* https://www.semanticscholar.org/paper/70174e749d29d46f6ffec26ab6b1d5a6d23c6aa3 (accessed on 9th May 2025).
9. Anthony, J. M., Magni, P. A., & Zuha, R. M. (2019). Forensic science and student mobility programs in the Indo-Pacific region: Unveiling the potential of an international and intercultural project in forensic science education. *Journal of Applied Learning & Teaching.* https://core.ac.uk/download/335016467.pdf (accessed on 9th May 2025).
10. Argo, A., Cannella, G., Scalzo, G., Puntarello, M., Buscemi, R., Zerbo, S., & D'Anna, T., (2023). The chain of custody in the era of modern forensics: From the classic procedures for gathering evidence to the new challenges related to digital data. *Healthcare.* https://core.ac.uk/download/599096302.pdf (accessed on 9th May 2025).
11. Atzrodt, J., Derdau, V., Kerr, W. J., & Reid, M., (2017). Deuterium- and tritium-labelled compounds: Applications in the life sciences. *Angewandte Chemie International Edition, 57*, 1758–1784. https://doi.org/10.1002/anie.201704146.

12. Barroso, J. M. P., Bernardo, B., Santos, V., São, M. F., et al. (2024). *Innovation and Breakthroughs Across Different Fields.* https://core.ac.uk/download/639216714.pdf (accessed on 9th May 2025).

13. Batiuk, O. V., & Novykova, O. O. (2024). Methodology of forensic prevention of crimes against the foundations of national security. *Kyiv Law Journal.* https://www.semanticscholar.org/paper/347467116ec637de7c92fd9a70bae0382ac0cb7f (accessed on 9th May 2025).

14. Boriwala, A., & Hankare, M., (2024). *Literature Review About Forensic Toxicology and Poisoning.* https://core.ac.uk/download/617189933.pdf (accessed on 9th May 2025).

15. Burnier, M., & Egan, B. M. (2019). Adherence in hypertension. *Circulation Research, 124*, 1124–1140. https://doi.org/10.1161/circresaha.118.313220.

16. Busardò, F. P., & Jones, A. W. (2014). GHB pharmacology and toxicology: Acute intoxication, concentrations in blood and urine in forensic cases and treatment of the withdrawal syndrome. *Current Neuropharmacology, 13*, 47–70. https://doi.org/10.2174/1570159x13666141210215423 (accessed on 9th May 2025).

17. Campbell, N., (2020). *OD: Naloxone and the Politics of Overdose.* The MIT Press eBooks. https://doi.org/10.7551/mitpress/12054.001.0001.

18. Capiau, S., Stove, C., & Velghe, S., (2016). *Opening the Toolbox of Alternative Sampling Strategies in Clinical Routine: A Key Role for (LC-)MS/MS.* https://core.ac.uk/download/84043363.pdf (accessed on 9th May 2025).

19. Cappelletti, S., Piacentino, D., Fineschi, V., Frati, P., D'Errico, S., & Aromatario, M., (2019). Mercuric chloride poisoning: Symptoms, analysis, therapies, and autoptic findings. A review of the literature. *Critical Reviews in Toxicology, 49*, 329–341. https://doi.org/10.1080/10408444.2019.1621262.

20. Caron, C., (2022). *To Certify or Not to Certify? A Proposed Graduate Course and Universal Certification for Forensic Expert Witnesses.* https://core.ac.uk/download/524806204.pdf (accessed on 9th May 2025).

21. Casparsen, C., (2024). The role of toxicology in forensic investigations. *International Journal of Forensic Medicine.* https://www.semanticscholar.org/paper/da3c2ea594c2d9e2608a802503025b50e5cb0849 (accessed on 9th May 2025).

22. Cawley, S. M. (2016). *The Effects of Zinc Sulfate on Ethyl Glucuronide Immunoassay Urine Testing.* https://open.bu.edu/bitstream/2144/16768/1/Cawley_bu_0017N_11829.pdf (accessed on 9th May 2025).

23. Chłopaś-Konowałek, A., Szpot, P., Zawadzki, M., Kukuła-Koch, W., & Dudzińska, E., (2024). Development of two ultra-sensitive UHPLC–QqQ-MS/MS methods for the simultaneous determination of hydroxyzine and its active metabolite (cetirizine) in human blood: Applications to real cases of forensic toxicology. *Archives of Toxicology, 98*, 3987–4012. https://www.semanticscholar.org/paper/5abebc4a71880ae31ad76c7857015698943e8751 (accessed on 9th May 2025).

24. Cinosi, E., Martinotti, G., Simonato, P., Singh, D., Demetrovics, Z., Román-Urrestarazu, A., Bersani, F. S., et al. (2015). Following "the roots" of kratom (*Mitragyna speciosa*): The evolution of an enhancer from a traditional use to increase work and productivity in Southeast Asia to a recreational psychoactive drug in Western countries. *BioMed Research International, 2015*, 1–11. https://doi.org/10.1155/2015/968786.

25. Coley, N., (1991). Alfred Swaine Taylor, MD, (1806–1880): Forensic toxicologist. *Medical History, 35*, 409–427. https://www.semanticscholar.org/paper/29f08be0bfa18cebbce53e1736cf63c89713bf2c (accessed on 9th May 2025).

26. Corl, W. E. (2015). *Polychlorinated Biphenyl Source Identification in Fish Tissue Using a Multivariate Statistical Evaluation of Congeners and Stable Isotope Ratio Mass Spectrometry.* https://www.semanticscholar.org/paper/006313119efd911f70545b291ee8e00d011ba084 (accessed on 9th May 2025).

27. Dana-Siadat, Z., Eizadi-Mood, N., Gheshlaghi, F., Masoumi, M., et al. (2014). Demographic factors, duration and costs of hospitalization, and causes of death in patients intoxicated with opioids and amphetamines. *International Journal of Medical Toxicology and Forensic Medicine.* https://core.ac.uk/download/483635462.pdf (accessed on 9th May 2025).

28. Dashora, A., Joshi, B., Sahu, D., Deepak, M., et al. (2013). *Techniques Used for Biochemical Investigation in Relation to Forensic Analysis.* https://core.ac.uk/download/482242353.pdf (accessed on 9th May 2025).

29. de Campos, E. G., da Costa, B. R. B., dos Santos, F. S., Monedeiro, F., Alves, M. N. R., Santos, W. J. R., & De Martinis, B. S. (2021). Alternative matrices in forensic toxicology: A critical review. *Forensic Toxicology, 40*, 1–18. https://doi.org/10.1007/s11419-021-00596-5.

30. De Kesel, P., Ingels, A. S., Lambert, W., Stove, C., et al. (2012). *Dried Blood Spots in Toxicology: From the Cradle to the Grave?* https://core.ac.uk/download/55802542.pdf (accessed on 9th May 2025).

31. Di Candia, D., Giordano, G., Boracchi, M., & Zoja, R., (2022). Postmortem forensic toxicology cases: A retrospective review from Milan, Italy. *Journal of Forensic Sciences, 67*, 1640–1650. https://www.semanticscholar.org/paper/cd5a304d2f8586048e70c9a9c1dd8d0cf6c8cae1 (accessed on 9th May 2025).

32. Dinis-Oliveira, R., (2022). One image is worth more than a thousand words: Producing an atlas of medical signs for teaching clinical and forensic toxicology. *Forensic Sciences Research, 7*, 815–822. https://www.semanticscholar.org/paper/8f90eec1804d9c9870922162c6d24e0499c8e45e (accessed on 9th May 2025).

33. Dunlop, D., (1957). Diagnosis and treatment of poisoning. *British Medical Journal, 2*, 203. https://www.semanticscholar.org/paper/3d01ffb07bc70be49dafef60b9a28d1858140074 (accessed on 9th May 2025).

34. Ellefsen, K. N., Papsun, D. M., Mata, D. C., Ayala, J. L., Modell, C., Goodson, L. J., & Truver, M. T. (2024). Seized drug reporting of NPS helps to guide regional toxicological practice: A 17 month review between 2022 and 2023. *Journal of Forensic Sciences, 69*, 1392–1399. https://www.semanticscholar.org/paper/3ceba0cd6d09812d4206d48efadd9b9f2a547091 (accessed on 9th May 2025).

35. Elrick, D., Hargrave, C., Hargrave, C., Yu, T., et al. (2018). *Integrating Online Instruction and Hands-on Laboratory Activities for Summer Learning for Students of Color: A Design Case in Forensic Science.* https://core.ac.uk/download/212851070.pdf (accessed on 9th May 2025).

36. Evison, M., (2011). *Written Evidence Submitted by Northumbria University Centre for Forensic Science (FSS 70).* https://core.ac.uk/download/80693790.pdf (accessed on 9th May 2025).

37. Fellmann, F., van El, C., Charron, P., Michaud, K., Howard, H., Boers, S. N., Clarke, A., et al. (2019).

European recommendations integrating genetic testing into multidisciplinary management of sudden cardiac death. *European Journal of Human Genetics, 27*, 1763–1773. https://doi.org/10.1038/s41431-019-0445-y.

38. García-Miranda, F. A., Rowley-Neale, S. J., & Banks, C. E. (2021). Screen-printed electrodes: Transitioning the laboratory into the field. *Talanta Open, 3*, 100032. https://doi.org/10.1016/j.talo.2021.100032.
39. Garrett, B. L. (2020). *The Costs and Benefits of Forensics*. https://core.ac.uk/download/322820151.pdf (accessed on 9th May 2025).
40. Gillies, A., (2015). *Mapping Current and Potential Sources of Routine Data Capture on New Psychoactive Substances in Scotland*. https://core.ac.uk/download/132846012.pdf (accessed on 9th May 2025).
41. González, O. Y., & Silva-Torres, L. A. (2024). Opioid abuse, the escalating crisis, xylazine co-use, and the forensic toxicology challenges. *Forensic Science Today*. https://www.semanticscholar.org/paper/b76f3826e295fe0e9d95a2473427c43e6b74609e (accessed on 9th May 2025).
42. Guelfo, J. L., Korzeniowski, S. H., Mills, M. A., Anderson, J. K., Anderson, R. H., Arblaster, J., Conder, J., et al. (2021). Environmental sources, chemistry, fate, and transport of per- and polyfluoroalkyl substances: State of the science, key knowledge gaps, and recommendations presented at the August 2019 SETAC Focus Topic Meeting. *Environmental Toxicology and Chemistry, 40*, 3234–3260. https://doi.org/10.1002/etc.5182.
43. Hansmeyer, C. G. (2016). *Near-Body Drugs of Abuse Testing in a Post Mortem Medico-Legal Population in South Africa: A Pilot Study*. https://core.ac.uk/download/188770368.pdf (accessed on 9th May 2025).
44. Henderson, A., Heaney, L. M., & Rankin-Turner, S., (2024). Ambient ionization mass spectrometry for drug and toxin analysis: A review of the recent literature. *Drug Testing and Analysis, 16*, 1323–1344. https://doi.org/10.1002/dta.3644.
45. Hoeland, K. M. (2021). *Investigating the Potential of Postmortem Metabolomics in Mammalian Decomposition Studies in Outdoor Settings*. https://core.ac.uk/download/524887815.pdf (accessed on 9th May 2025).
46. Issa, S. Y. (2019). *Forensic Toxicology*. https://core.ac.uk/download/322440626.pdf (accessed on 9th May 2025).
47. Jones, S., McGowan, C. K., Boyle, S., Ke, Y., Chan, C. H. M., & Hwang, H. J. (2021). An overview of sample preparation in forensic toxicology. *Wiley Interdisciplinary Reviews: Forensic Science, 4*. https://doi.org/10.1002/wfs2.1436.
48. Kazantsev, R., & Yatsenko, I., (2022). Forensic veterinary diagnosis of dog's fatal poisoning with anticoagulant rodenticide – bromadiolone. *Naukovij Vìsnik Veterinarnoï Medicini*. https://www.semanticscholar.org/paper/fa152ce9e0ca5cd9315cf4113731c24fd282fe22 (accessed on 9th May 2025).
49. Kintz, P., (2018). Hair analysis in forensic toxicology: An updated review with a special focus on pitfalls. *Current Pharmaceutical Design, 23*. https://doi.org/10.2174/1381612823666170929155628.
50. Kukucka, J., & Dror, I. E. (2022). *Human Factors in Forensic Science: Psychological Causes of Bias and Error*. https://doi.org/10.31234/osf.io/8pqyt.

51. Kumar, S. P., Rana, A. S., Sehgal, A. K., Sharma, R., et al. (2014). *A Study of Sexual Assaults in Northern Range of Himachal Pradesh.* https://core.ac.uk/download/483635474.pdf (accessed on 9th May 2025).

52. Lechien, J. R., Chiesa-Estomba, C. M., Hans, S., Barillari, M. R., Jouffe, L., & Saussez, S., (2020). Loss of smell and taste in 2013 European patients with mild to moderate COVID-19. *Annals of Internal Medicine, 173*, 672–675. https://doi.org/10.7326/m20-2428.

53. Lowdon, J. W., Diliën, H., Singla, P., Peeters, M., Cleij, T. J., Van Grinsven, B., & Eersels, K., (2020). MIPs for commercial application in low-cost sensors and assays – An overview of the current status quo. *Sensors and Actuators B: Chemical, 325*, 128973. https://doi.org/10.1016/j.snb.2020.128973.

54. Maddox, I., (2024). *Artificial Intelligence in the Courtroom: Forensic Machines, Expert Witnesses, and the Confrontation Clause.* https://core.ac.uk/download/613830435.pdf (accessed on 9th May 2025).

55. Mbatha, E. I. T. D. S. (2018). *The Evaluation of Potential Dietary Media, Measurement Parameters and Storage Techniques for use in Forensic Entomotoxicology.* https://core.ac.uk/download/158296175.pdf (accessed on 9th May 2025).

56. McLevain, T., (2021). *The Opioid Crisis—Why Is It So Hard to Tame?* https://core.ac.uk/download/520100769.pdf (accessed on 9th May 2025).

57. Mnisi, P. Z. (2023). *Post-Mortem Toxicological Analysis of Hair in Violent Fatalities: An Investigation into Long-Term Drug Exposure.* https://core.ac.uk/download/590319313.pdf (accessed on 9th May 2025).

58. Morgan, J., (2023). Wrongful convictions and claims of false or misleading forensic evidence. *Journal of Forensic Sciences, 68*, 908–961. https://doi.org/10.1111/1556-4029.15233.

59. Muehlethaler, C., Leona, M., & Lombardi, J. R. (2015). Review of surface enhanced Raman scattering applications in forensic science. *Analytical Chemistry, 88*, 152–169. https://doi.org/10.1021/acs.analchem.5b04131 (accessed on 9th May 2025).

60. Oliveira, J. R. I. L., Rodrigues, L., Kahl, J. M. M., Berlinck, D. Z., & Costa, J. L. (2024). Green analytical toxicology procedure for determination of ketamine, its metabolites and analogues in oral fluid samples using dispersive liquid–liquid microextraction (DLLME). *Journal of Analytical Toxicology*. https://www.semanticscholar.org/paper/e8527bc0032e3ee19d70e858cdb465f3cf54516e (accessed on 9th May 2025).

61. Ossanes, D., Birk, L., Petry, A. U. S., Paz de Menezes, F., Gonzaga, A. P., Schlickmann, P. F., Eller, S., et al. (2023). Cork sheet as an efficient biosorbent for forensic toxicology: Application to vitreous humor analysis. *Journal of Analytical Toxicology*. https://www.semanticscholar.org/paper/f761ff9ecd08d3f2447d981f432f71c92fabc6cb (accessed on 9th May 2025).

62. Pardo, B., Taylor, J., Caulkins, J. P., Kilmer, B., Reuter, P., & Stein, B. D. (2019). *The Future of Fentanyl and Other Synthetic Opioids.* RAND Corporation eBooks. https://doi.org/10.7249/rr3117.

63. Peter, K. T., Tian, Z., Wu, C. L., Lin, P., White, S. M., Du, B., McIntyre, J. K., et al. (2018). Using high-resolution mass spectrometry to identify organic contaminants linked to urban stormwater mortality syndrome in Coho salmon. *Environmental Science & Technology, 52*, 10317–10327. https://doi.org/10.1021/acs.est.8b03287.

64. Pitterl, F., Pavlic, M., Liu, J., & Oberacher, H., (2024). Insights into the human metabolism of hexahydrocannabinol by non-targeted liquid chromatography–high-resolution tandem mass spectrometry. *Journal of Analytical Toxicology, 48*, 350–358. https://www.semanticscholar.org/paper/7a3893d32c6a168ae406286ea9d06a9afe8057d6 (accessed on 9th May 2025).

65. Polles, A., Bundy, C., Jacobs, W., & Merlo, L. J. (2021). Adaptations to substance use disorder monitoring by physician health programs in response to COVID-19. *Journal of Substance Abuse Treatment, 125*, 108281. https://doi.org/10.1016/j.jsat.2021.108281.

66. Popovych, V., Skrobala, V., Kopylov, V., & Kopystynskyi, Y. O. (2025). Heavy metals distribution in water and soil of the coastal zone of the Styr River (Ukraine) and its tributaries. *Journal of Ecological Engineering*. https://www.semanticscholar.org/paper/4482a902dba892abce5e545a3a138a57d0841fbb (accessed on 9th May 2025).

67. Quarta, G., Hajdas, I., Molnár, M., Varga, T., Calcagnile, L., D'Elia, M., Molnár, Á., et al. (2022). The IAEA forensics program: Results of the AMS 14C intercomparison exercise on contemporary wines and coffees. *Radiocarbon, 64*, 1513–1524. https://www.semanticscholar.org/paper/2cbe89c6e489abed7530c405a42def99df6c0ce1 (accessed on 9th May 2025).

68. Sacco, M. A., Tarzia, P., Tarallo, A. P., Lombardo, S., Princi, A., & Aquila, I., (2024). Asphyxia with a blunt instrument: Which forensic evidence to use in complex cases of murder. *La Clinica Terapeutica, 175*(Suppl 2(4)), 196–198. https://www.semanticscholar.org/paper/b018b3d216631ed4398bf9aa02c17ccf3c42b397 (accessed on 9th May 2025).

69. Santos, B. P. Dos., Birk, L., Schwarz, P., Sebben, V., Sgaravatti, Â. M., de Gouveia, G. C., Petry, A. U. S., et al. (2024). A validated dilute-and-shoot LC-MS/MS urine screening for the analysis of 95 illicit drugs and medicines: Insights from clinical and forensic Brazilian cases. *Journal of Analytical Toxicology*. https://www.semanticscholar.org/paper/127303592c115d9e5d47b203fd45165bdabc964c (accessed on 9th May 2025).

70. Seaman, W., & Whitehouse, J. H. (2001). *Florida Marine Biotechnology: Research, Development and Training Capabilities to Advance Science and Commerce*. https://core.ac.uk/download/11016354.pdf (accessed on 9th May 2025).

71. Shanks, K. G., Kurtz, S. A. K., & Behonick, G. S. (2024). Detection of the benzodiazepine bromazolam by liquid chromatography with quadrupole time-of-flight mass spectrometry in postmortem toxicology casework and prevalence in Indiana (2023). *Journal of Analytical Toxicology*. https://www.semanticscholar.org/paper/9fe67b46928b4b8c4a08d077c03a82f34ed0149d (accessed on 9th May 2025).

72. Sinha, S. K., Maji, S. R., & Roy, C., (2023). *Gas Chromatography–Mass Spectrometry (GC-MS): A Comprehensive Review of Synergistic Combinations and Their Applications in the Past Two Decades*. https://core.ac.uk/download/618379294.pdf (accessed on 9th May 2025).

73. Soltaninejad, K., (2023). Poisons and drugs used in homicidal poisoning: A systematic review. *International Journal of Forensic Sciences*. https://www.semanticscholar.org/paper/90026320c26e66d1d33c1ec3f26f6dc3491c2772 (accessed on 9th May 2025).

74. Steuer, A. E., Brockbals, L., & Kræmer, T., (2019). Metabolomic strategies in biomarker research: New approach for indirect identification of drug consumption and sample manipulation in clinical and forensic toxicology? *Frontiers in Chemistry, 7*. https://doi.org/10.3389/fchem.2019.00319 (accessed on 9th May 2025).

75. Stuck, M. M. (1996). *Comparison of Positive Screening and Confirmatory Results from Federally*

Mandated Drug Testing of Urine. https://core.ac.uk/download/217299247.pdf (accessed on 9th May 2025).

76. Teunissen, S. F., Fedick, P. W., Berendsen, B. J. A., Nielen, M. W. F., Eberlin, M. N., Cooks, R. G., & van Asten, A. C. (2017). Novel selectivity-based forensic toxicological validation of a paper spray mass spectrometry method for the quantitative determination of eight amphetamines in whole blood. *Journal of the American Society for Mass Spectrometry, 28*, 2665–2676. https://doi.org/10.1007/s13361-017-1790-0.

77. Tiapkin, A., & Lushchyk, I., (2023). Problematic issues of definition of digital forensics. *Theory and Practice of Jurisprudence*. https://www.semanticscholar.org/paper/69877a4c84a92aff7f9695f5bbb4362fcd3b8b12 (accessed on 9th May 2025).

78. Tiscione, N. B., & Alford, I., (2018). Carfentanil in impaired driving cases and the importance of drug seizure data. *Journal of Analytical Toxicology, 42*, 476–484. https://doi.org/10.1093/jat/bky026.

79. Tseng, Z. H., Olgin, J. E., Vittinghoff, E., Ursell, P. C., Kim, A., Sporer, K. A., Yeh, C., et al. (2018). Prospective countywide surveillance and autopsy characterization of sudden cardiac death. *Circulation, 137*, 2689–2700. https://doi.org/10.1161/circulationaha.117.033427.

80. Verma, P., Ujjainia, P., Moza, B., & Mukherjee, D., (2024). Nanoparticles as silent witnesses: Significance, challenges and ethical considerations in forensic analysis. *RASAYAN Journal of Chemistry*. https://www.semanticscholar.org/paper/fd7ecfa4fad5650e9c140c2f182254e28798a550 (accessed on 9th May 2025).

81. Vincenti, M., Salomone, A., Gerace, E., & Pirro, V., (2013). Application of mass spectrometry to hair analysis for forensic toxicological investigations. *Mass Spectrometry Reviews, 32*(4), 312–332. https://www.semanticscholar.org/paper/600cf4a387acdb5890fb579b11cc2a5854dc10c8 (accessed on 9th May 2025).

82. Voicu, V., Brehar, F. M., Toader, C., Covache-Busuioc, R. A., Corlatescu, A. D., Bordeianu, A., Costin, H. P., et al. (2023). Cannabinoids in medicine: A multifaceted exploration of types, therapeutic applications, and emerging opportunities in neurodegenerative diseases and cancer therapy. *Biomolecules, 13*, 1388. https://doi.org/10.3390/biom13091388.

83. Yskak, A., Chashkov, V., Daribayeva, S., & Kazbekova, K., (2024). Comprehensive assessment of heavy metals content in the water of the Verkhnetobolsky and Karatomarsky reservoirs in the northern region of the Republic of Kazakhstan. *3i Intellect Idea Innovation – Интеллект Идея Инновация*. https://www.semanticscholar.org/paper/655519e53c11535031293 78be18262b6b11b0c73 (accessed on 9th May 2025).

84. Zeppenfeld, K., Tfelt-Hansen, J., Riva, M., Winkel, B. G., Behr, E. R., Blom, N. A., Charron, P., et al. (2022). 2022 ESC guidelines for the management of patients with ventricular arrhythmias and the prevention of sudden cardiac death. *European Heart Journal, 43*, 3997–4126. https://doi.org/10.1093/eurheartj/ehac262.

85. Zerbo, S., Spanò, M., Albano, G., Buscemi, R., Malta, G., & Argo, A., (2023). A fatal suicidal sodium nitrite ingestion determined six days after death. *Journal of Forensic and Legal Medicine, 98*, 102576. https://doi.org/10.1016/j.jflm.2023.102576.

86. Zhen, L., (2017). *Effects of Filtration Sterilization on the Stability of Ketamine, Selected Benzodiazepines and Metabolites in Female Urine*. https://core.ac.uk/download/142076178.pdf (accessed on 9th May 2025).

CORROSIVE POISONS

5

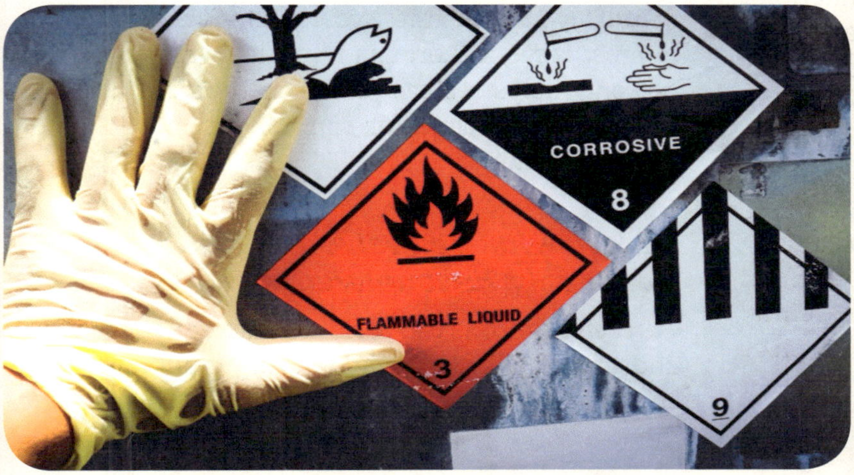

LEARNING OBJECTIVES

After studying this chapter, you will be able to:

1. Identify types of corrosive poisons
2. Understand detection and analysis techniques
3. Learn case studies in forensic toxicology
4. Focus on prevention and safety measures

Introduction

Corrosive toxins in forensic work combine chemistry with law enforcement in a way that presents some challenging issues when it comes to identifying hazardous chemicals. New psychoactive substances (NPS) keep emerging, so, generally speaking, experts are leaning hard on flexible, robust methods to track these hazards. There is also a push to not only refine the identification of these substances more precisely but also to shape legal processes that facilitate the conviction of offenders. Data sharing and ongoing collection across various agencies – as recent studies have noted (Gillies et al., 2015) – appear to significantly enhance the trustworthiness of the evidence we gather, even if the process sometimes feels somewhat disjointed. Basic tests, such as color changes in samples, often initiate the process. However, they can struggle with selectivity and sensitivity as the chemicals shift in unexpected ways (Fu et al., 2017). All in all, incorporating corrosive agents into forensic debates remains crucial for both deepening scientific insight and enhancing public safety.

Definition of Corrosive Poisons

Corrosive substances can wreak significant harm on human health—something forensic experts frequently encounter (Figure 5.1). These chemicals, which quickly damage tissue upon contact, often lead to grim outcomes that are not easily explained. You might find hydrochloric acid (HCl) and sulfuric acid (H_2SO_4) popping up in poisoning cases; generally speaking, HCl tends to cause only superficial necrosis, whereas H_2SO_4 is more likely to trigger extensive, sometimes transmural, damage that can end in organ failure (Chaurasia et al., 2024). Everyday items, such as toilet cleaners, also contribute to these injuries. There are incidents of ingestion where folks suffer widespread organ damage even without clear evidence of gastric perforation, hinting at a rather complex injury mechanism. In most cases, gaining a solid understanding of these effects and the underlying mechanisms is essential for experts attempting to diagnose and piece together forensic puzzles.

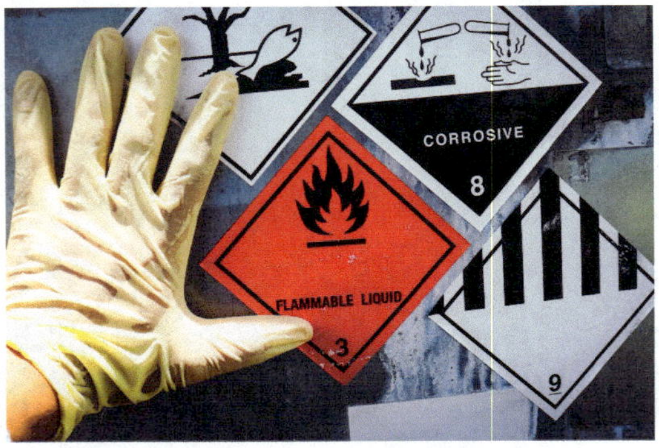

Figure 5.1. Corrosive substances.

Source: ReAgent Chemicals. (2024). *Corrosive Chemical Label.* https://www.chemicals.co.uk/wp-content/uploads/2024/06/Corrosive-chemical-label-scaled.jpg.

Importance of Forensics in Poison Analysis

Forensic science, hooked up with poison analysis, is key to figuring out what really went on during toxic exposure incidents. Cases with harsh, corrosive substances—where a quick, spot-on detection often sways legal deals and sparks community health alerts—show just how vital timely answers can be. Detailed examinations sometimes uncover recurring motifs in poisoning patterns, hinting at both unexpected accidents and deliberate overdoses. For instance, one study noted that about 7.8% of pediatric emergencies were linked to accidental drug-caustic exposure (Arslan et al., 2022). Likewise, analysis of unnatural deaths revealed that poisoning figured in roughly 19.3% of these cases (Kim et al., 2021). In most cases, a thorough forensic investigation not only helps resolve justice matters but also lays the groundwork for smarter, future public health initiatives.

Overview of Corrosive Poisons Commonly Encountered

Corrosive poisons can seriously damage tissues and organs, which is why figuring them out is so vital in forensic work (Figure 5.2).

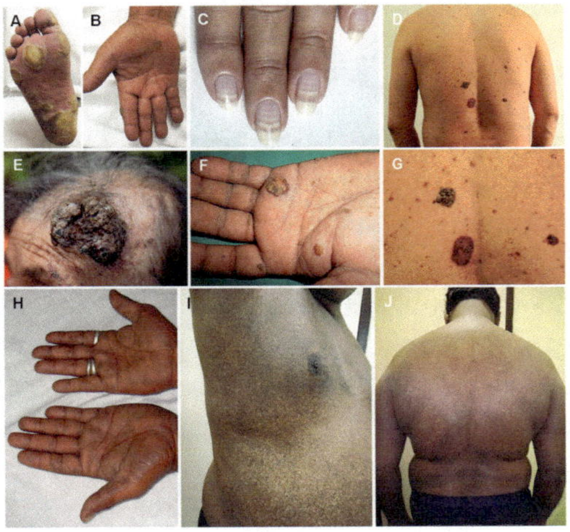

Figure 5.2. Corrosive poisons can seriously damage tissues and organs, which is why figuring them out is so important in forensic work.

Source: Pons, M., Perramon, A., Navarro, J., & Pujol, M. (2023). Description of figure if available. In *Journal of Clinical Medicine, 12*(8), Article 2591.

Strong acids—such as HCl—and bases, like sodium hydroxide, can cause harm that is both sudden and irreversible; sometimes their effects can resemble other medical issues, which can really muddle the diagnosis process. These chemicals often mess with the usual chemical profile of biological samples, which in most cases makes toxicology tests even more unpredictable. Forensic experts typically rely on inorganic analysis to identify these substances, a method that highlights the complexity of the chemical fingerprinting process (Bergeron et al., 2015). Generally speaking, understanding how these toxins behave is crucial for accurate investigations—and ultimately, for ensuring justice is served.

Historical Context of Corrosive Poisons in Criminal Cases

Corrosive poisons themselves have existed as more than just crime accessories, also seeing how forensic science itself has evolved alongside our changing ideas of justice and right and wrong. Poisons such as arsenic, lead, and mercury have been around for centuries as insidious but deadly powers, often inserting themselves into murders and betrayals where their efforts were subtle but deadly. Generally speaking, even in ancient times, these toxins were known to cause damage to major organs and disrupt fundamental bodily functions, signaling a real need for accurate and delicate identification in forensic scenarios (Machado and Dinis-Oliveira, 2023). As investigative aids improved with the passage of time, the power to choose these poisonous substances became central to unraveling mysterious deaths that would otherwise have remained unsolved. In most cases, cumulative legal principles and mounting scientific scrutiny have helped to strip away successive layers of criminal intent in addition to bringing to the forefront the inherent challenges in dealing with victims (Barnard et al., 2024).

Methodology of Forensic Analysis

When dealing with corrosive poisons, forensic analysis requires us to employ methods that are both rigorous and reliable. Techniques like thin layer chromatography (TLC) and UV-Vis spectroscopy jump in here—they have opened up new ways to spot these chemicals hidden in messy biological samples. One study, for example, combined TLC with liquid-liquid extraction to isolate chlordiazepoxide, demonstrating how adjusting solvent mixes can significantly impact retention factors and recovery rates in a range of samples, from food to beverages (Rajan et al., 2025). You may also notice that a broader forensic framework—one that, in most cases, aligns with ideas from the National Institute of Standards and Technology—helps investigators gather evidence with sufficient detail to be accepted in court (Herman et al., 2025). All in all, these approaches emphasize confirmatory testing and align well with best practices in forensic toxicology, proving themselves to be crucial when unraveling investigations involving corrosive poisons.

Significance of Understanding Corrosive Poisons

Corrosive poisons raise a range of issues within forensic science—especially in criminal cases and toxicology. Understanding what these substances do is not just about pinpointing the cause of an injury or death; it also helps sort out when a poisoning is simply an accident versus when someone has been harmed on purpose, a point that really matters in self-harm cases. In most cases, victims do not exhibit clear signs immediately, which means a detailed and careful examination is necessary to make sense of the situation. At the same time, understanding the unique properties of these poisons can significantly enhance the work of forensic toxicologists, guiding not only immediate treatment but also longer-term safety measures that benefit public health. By blending insights from both toxicology and mental health, experts can generally improve diagnostic accuracy and fine-tune their intervention strategies, addressing both the physical and psychological sides of corrosive poisoning incidents (Barnard et al., 2024) (Figure 5.3).

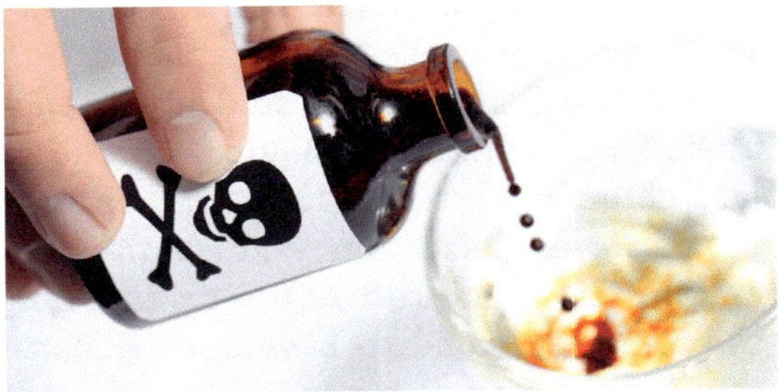

Figure 5.3. Significance of understanding corrosive poisons.

Source: Acko General Insurance. (n.d.). *First Aid Guide: Dealing with a Case of Poisoning*. https://acko-cms.ackoassets.com/First_Aid_Guide_Dealing_with_a_case_of_poisoning_8c28775984.png.

5.1. Types of Corrosive Poisons

Learning Outcome

1. Know acids and their properties
2. Explain bases and their effects
3. Identify common corrosive substances in forensics
4. Learn mechanisms of toxicity
5. Discuss symptoms of exposure
6. Focus on environmental sources of corrosive poisons
7. Identify industrial applications and risks
8. Learn case studies of corrosive poisonings
9. Focus on the legal implications of corrosive poison use

Corrosive poisons have been around forever and were pretty easy to get, which has thrown plenty of challenges at forensic investigators over time. Lots of these substances—take strong acids and alkalis, for example—can really mess up human tissues and organs, often leading to rapid and sometimes fatal outcomes if not treated quickly. Back in the 19th and early 20th centuries, poisoning cases laid bare a mix of legal and medical puzzles that made it tough to detect and adjudicate these incidents properly. Issues such as unreliable chemical tests and doctors not always recognizing the symptoms made trials even more complicated (Merry et al., 2010).

Generally speaking, understanding how each corrosive agent works is key; their damage often shifts depending on their chemical makeup and the specific manner of exposure. All of this really highlights why a deep dive into forensic toxicology matters—it not only helps identify the type of poison involved, but also provides a better understanding of just how extensive the harm might be (Mishra et al., 2020).

5.1.1. Acids and their Properties

Acid poisoning is not just about swallowing something harmful—it shows up as a mix of changes in various organs (Figure 5.4). Hydrochloric acid (HCl) tends to cause quite visible damage; it wrecks the esophagus and stomach with coagulative necrosis that lines up with autopsy findings (Chaurasia et al., 2024). Sulfuric acid (H_2SO_4), on the other hand, usually leads to even graver injuries, often producing full-thickness necrosis that not only ruins the gastrointestinal tract but also extends its damage to organs such as the liver, kidneys, and beyond. These acids, by their very nature as strong corrosives, require a careful forensic examination to fully understand how they operate. In most cases, grasping these specific characteristics is key for forensic pathologists who are trying to differentiate between cases and boost the accuracy of diagnosing corrosive poisonings.

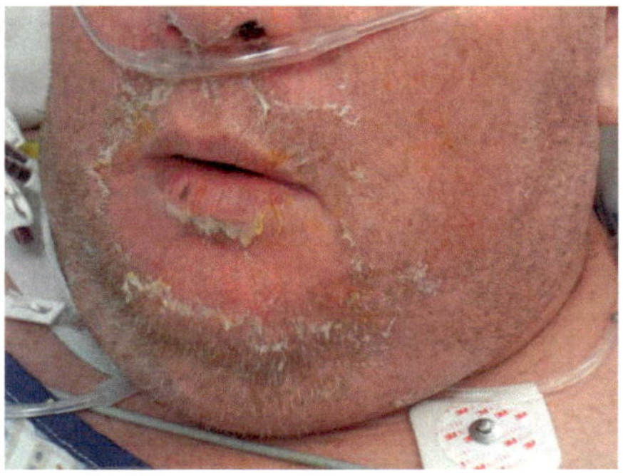

Figure 5.4. Acid poisoning.

Source: Osterhoudt, K. C., & Shannon, M. W. (2023). Acid poisoning. In *Clinical Toxicology, 61*(7), 689–696. Taylor & Francis.

5.1.2. Bases and Their Effects

Different bases and their corrosive actions play a significant role in forensic work, especially when it comes to poisonings. Forensic experts who understand how these chemicals mix with our tissues can piece together what went wrong during a poisoning event. Sometimes, caustic substances wreak havoc on mucosal membranes, sparking sudden, severe medical crises that need immediate care; a few reports have even pointed out that agricultural chemicals, common in many rural areas, often pop up as the culprit (Anas et al., 2016). At the same time, cultural factors sometimes influence the way evidence is gathered and interpreted, making it even more challenging to achieve justice. A balanced forensic method that incorporates attention to these cultural quirks typically enhances both the accuracy and reliability of evidence collection—helping ensure a more comprehensive understanding of how different poisons leave their corrosive mark (Bergeron et al., 2015).

5.1.3. Common Corrosive Substances in Forensics

Investigating corrosive substances in criminal cases reveals a quirky blend of chemistry, law, and medical practices (Figure 5.5). Strong acids, such as sulfuric and hydrochloric, as well as equally aggressive bases like sodium hydroxide, not only wreak havoc on tissues almost instantly but also make spotting evidence and prosecuting those involved a real headache. Back in the 1800s, when these chemicals were more accessible, poisoning incidents shot up; often, symptoms went unrecognized by medical experts, which muddled legal outcomes (*as noted in* Merry et al., 2010). In most cases, forensic methods have improved over time, with simple color tests, for instance, stepping in to boost detection. However, the rise of new agents and the limitations of conventional tests still leave investigators scrambling (Fu et al., 2017). All in all, understanding these intertwined challenges is crucial to advancing forensic science.

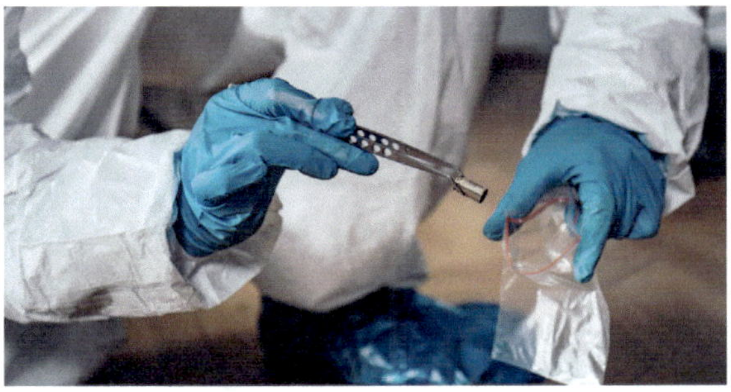

Figure 5.5. Investigating corrosive substances in criminal cases reveals a quirky blend of chemistry, law, and medical practices.

Source: SoundThinking. (2023). *CSI Hazmat Team Working in a Crime Scene.*

5.1.4. Mechanisms of Toxicity

Chemical compounds and our bodies occasionally conflict in ways that result in unforeseen harm (Figure 5.6). Corrosive toxins, for instance, tend to damage cells directly as well as upset the entire system. Formic acid is one that particularly stands out—it tends to bother the body when inhaled or absorbed through the skin, causing severe respiratory and intestinal problems. In an unfortunate case, a young man died after experiencing corrosive burns alongside out-of-the-ordinary spikes in carboxyhemoglobin levels (Baković et al., 2015). Notably, the universally recognized harmful characteristics of formic acid, with a pH of approximately 0.79 and a substantial amount of sulfuric ions, illustrate how quickly contact can damage tissues (Gillies et al., 2015). Understanding these patterns of damage is, in a majority of instances, critical to forensic analysis as it helps reconstruct injury severity and the unseemly circumstances that accompany poison deaths.

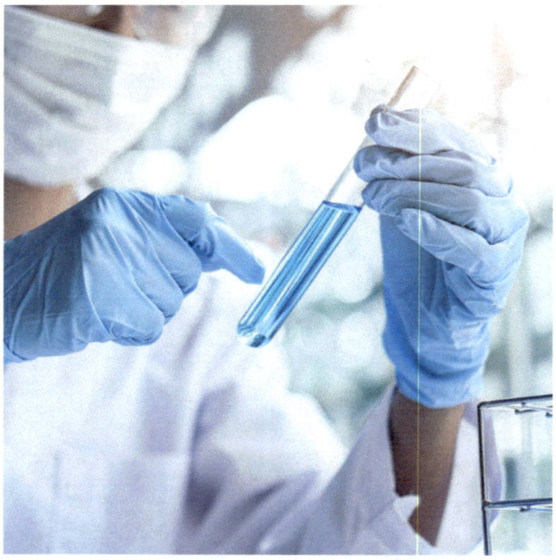

Figure 5.6. Chemical substances and our bodies sometimes clash in ways that lead to unexpected damage.

Source: Storyblok. (n.d.). *Laboratory Test Tube.* https://a.storyblok.com/f/80031/1000x1000/29bb351902/laboratory-test-tube-1000x1000.jpg.

5.1.5. Symptoms of Exposure

Symptoms of corrosive poison exposure offer key evidence in forensic analysis. Chemical weapons agents (CWAs) can trigger effects that range from minor irritation to severe physiological distress – a range that most often indicates the distinctions in substance toxicity (Kumar et al., 2022). It is essential to pinpoint exactly when these symptoms start; this helps analysts determine both the nature and duration of exposure. Now and then, a field-portable gas chromatography–mass spectrometry (GC-MS) system pops up in the field and justifies its place by identifying the toxic agent accurately, hence enabling the investigators to rebuild what could have possibly transpired (Leary et al., 2019). Forensic experts then map specific symptoms to the incriminating chemicals, piecing together exposure episodes and offering insight into the circumstances of poisoning. Stated, the investigation of symptoms not only helps us better understand deadly toxins but is also an essential consideration in solving criminal cases.

5.1.6. Environmental Sources of Corrosive Poisons

Industrial activities and ecological deterioration tend to get entangled in a knotty system that exposes individuals to toxic substances (Figure 5.7). Naturally occurring toxic heavy metals—those frequently churned up by human endeavors—appear as key culprits; for example, as Machado and Dinis-Oliveira (2023) state, substances like lead, mercury, and arsenic gradually creep into our food and drinking water. Too often, though, these toxins are simply part of nature's background hum; industrial activity adds extra quantities, piling on the danger in novel ways. In most instances, these corrosive chemicals disrupt simple cellular processes, at times even hijacking critical processes and causing severe problems such as neurological and kidney malfunction. Recent research into optical sensors, for instance, has highlighted the urgent need for enhanced surveillance of such environmental hazards (Kumar et al., 2022). In general, this blend of industry and nature reflects a sobering fact—one that is crucial to both forensic study and broader public health endeavors. Overall, it reminds us that when human endeavor is combined with natural processes, the outcomes can be complicated and far-reaching.

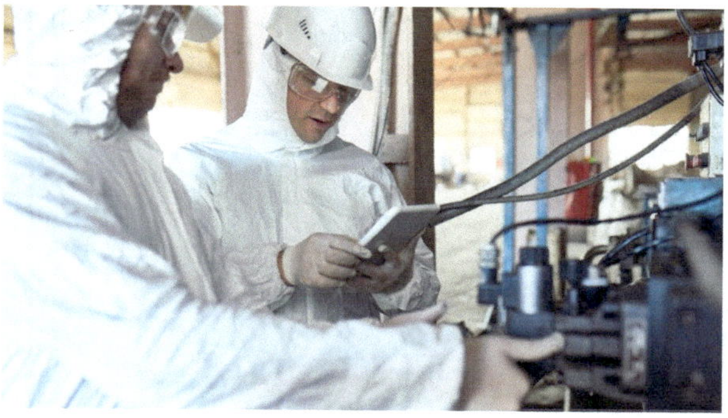

Figure 5.7. Industrial operations and environmental decay often create a tangled mess that puts people at risk from hazardous substances.

Source: VinciWorks. (2024). *Workplace Safety Compliance Illustration.*

5.1.7. Industrial Applications and Risks

Industrial progress is now closely intertwined with forensic science—a link that becomes quite clear when experts analyze corrosive substances. In manufacturing, agriculture, and other sectors, corrosive chemicals help operations run more smoothly; however, they also pose some significant health risks. Accidental misuse—or even just unintentional exposure—really drives home the need for strict safety rules and well-thought-out regulatory measures. Professionals handling these chemicals often require a solid foundation, one that is sometimes built from resources such as the EU CBRNE Glossary (Krzysztof et al., 2022); having that understanding can make a significant difference. At the same time, disruptive technologies continue to emerge, with advanced sensor systems being developed to detect and mitigate the risks associated with these agents. Generally speaking, these innovations not only enhance industrial safety but also play a crucial role in protecting public health as technology continues to transform our working landscape (Carter et al., 2021).

5.1.8. Case Studies of Corrosive Poisonings

Corrosive poisoning cases have taught us a lot about forensic work, showing up in a jumble of case studies that do not follow a neat pattern at all. Experts in the field often wrestle with identifying and analyzing these corrosive agents, with victims sometimes displaying unexpected symptoms that really depend on the specific substance in play. New tools, such as optical molecular sensors, have joined the scene to refine detection methods, making the overall forensic picture a bit clearer (Kumar et al., 2022). In many medico-legal reviews, there is a noticeable number of violent incidents tied to poison exposure, which means keeping proper records and trimming down reporting blunders becomes super important (Aktaş et al., 2018). All these bits of evidence point toward a clear need for more awareness and hands-on training for forensic teams, so they are ready to handle the messy details of corrosive poisoning cases.

5.1.9. Legal Implications of Corrosive Poison Use

Poisoning's past is full of legal twists – especially when it comes to how corrosive substances get sold and controlled. In the 1800s and early 1900s, these hazardous chemicals were introduced to the market before any comprehensive regulations could be established, often leaving authorities in a legal quandry. Usually, jurors just could not wrap their heads around the mix of medical and chemical evidence thrown into the courtroom, and that muddled the efforts to prosecute poison-related cases. The fact that these corrosive poisons were so cheap and easy to access only added fuel to the fire—providing both opportunity and motive for potential murderers. Recent forensic advances, as noted in current research on color tests, underscore the clear need for updated legal standards on poison detection and regulation to ensure justice is served in cases involving these hazardous substances (Merry et al., 2010; Fu et al., 2017) (Figure 5.8).

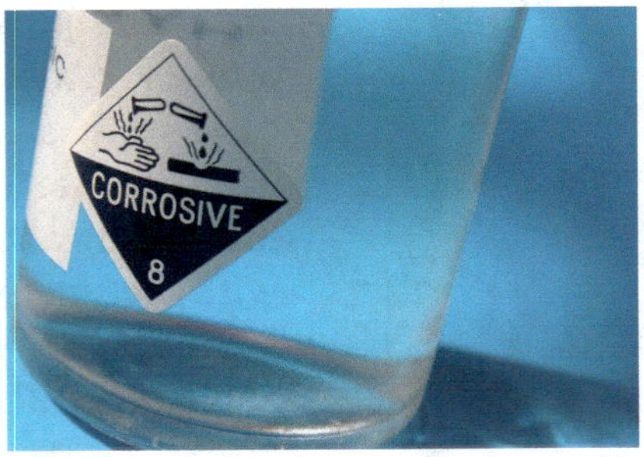

Figure 5.8. Corrosive poisons were so cheap and easy to access only added fuel to the fire—providing both opportunity and motive for potential murderers.

Source: Sky News. (2017). *Crime Scene Investigators at Work.*

Test Your Knowledge

1. What are the effects of hydrochloric acid ingestion on the body?
2. Give two examples of alkaline corrosive poisons.

5.2. Detection and Analysis Techniques

Learning Outcome

1. Learn chemical analysis methods
2. Explain spectroscopy in poison detection
3. Describe chromatography applications
4. Focus on toxicological screening processes
5. Discuss the role of mass spectrometry
6. Learn field testing kits for first responders
7. Know the limitations of current detection methods
8. Focus on advances in forensic technology
9. Describe the importance of accurate detection in legal cases

Forensic investigators often encounter challenging situations when attempting to identify corrosive toxins. Such chemicals require detection and analysis methods that must be both accurate and reliable - a challenge that science is gradually but eventually overcoming. Optical molecular sensors, for example, have garnered significant attention; they have demonstrated the ability to detect a wide range of harmful agents, including corrosive poisons that, at certain times, even resemble chemical warfare materials (Kumar et al., 2022). And then there's the work of TiO_2 electrochemical biosensors, which appears to provide an interesting means of finding biological markers associated with incidents of poisoning. In general, such biosensors are equipped with a combination of sensitivity and selectivity that is essential, particularly when human safety and juridical concerns are involved (Bertel et al., 2021). Relying on these advanced techniques, forensic experts can paint a reasonably clear picture of corrosive materials, supporting investigations as well as public health measures. All things considered, these technological advancements represent a significant step forward in mitigating toxic exposures, even if the path is not always smooth sailing.

5.2.1. Chemical Analysis Methods

Forensic work on corrosive poisons can be a tangled mess—chemical tests, for one, play a huge, almost indispensable role (Figure 5.9). These tests provide the key pieces of information needed to identify toxins and piece together what happened in the event of a poisoning incident. Sometimes, methods like chromatographic and spectrometric analyses make it possible to pick up tiny amounts of dangerous substances hiding in biological samples; in most cases, that means experts can confidently say what caused a death. For example, when pesticide residues were checked, it generally turned out that poisoning cases had decreased slightly—chemicals such as quinalfos and chlorpyrifos, for instance, have recently been attracting forensic attention (Madhavan et al., 2019).

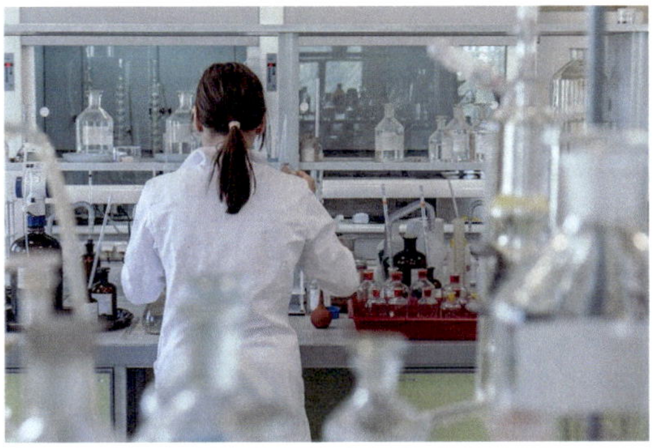

Figure 5.9. Forensic work on corrosive poisons can be a tangled mess—chemical tests, for one, play a huge, almost indispensable role.

Source: Financial Crime Academy. (2023). *Financial Crime Investigation Graphic*.

Furthermore, the recent, slight resurgence of mercuric chloride poisoning warrants a closer examination of the testing practices that govern both patient treatment and post-mortem examination procedures (Cappelletti et al., 2019). In the end, using these broad, sometimes overlapping methods not only ups the accuracy of diagnoses but also deepens our overall grasp of how corrosive poisons impact forensic science.

5.2.2. Spectroscopy in Poison Detection

Forensic labs heavily rely on cutting-edge analysis to track down toxic substances; it is not as straightforward as checking off boxes. UV-Vis spectroscopy, for example, has quickly become a favored tool—even when compounds are hidden in messy mixtures, it manages to separate them. Its sensitivity really comes in handy for confirming corrosive agents, which fit the strict standards forensic work requires. In one study, researchers found that combining TLC with UV-Vis provided a reliable method for detecting chlordiazepoxide in food samples (Rajan et al., 2025), indicating the flexibility of these methods. Systematic toxicology generally adopts a broad approach, insisting on using multiple techniques—such as inductively coupled plasma-mass spectrometry for detecting metals and liquid chromatography for identifying organic toxins—to elucidate suspected poisoning cases (Pragst, 2025). Overall, while the process might seem intricate, these diverse methods work together in a relatively natural, if not slightly unpredictable, way.

5.2.3. Chromatography Applications

Forensic science often begins with the challenging task of identifying and measuring harsh toxins, and in many cases, robust tests are necessary. Chromatography emerges as a key method—it breaks down complex mixtures to isolate and remove those hazardous chemicals. Sometimes, you will see GC-MS in action; this tool is essential for detecting substances like CWAs and other harmful compounds (Kumar et al., 2022). Then, there are instances involving herbicides such as diquat, where chromatography enables us to examine biological samples for solid post-mortem toxicology checks (Basilicata et al., 2022). In most cases, these techniques do more than pinpoint the culprit behind a fatal poisoning—they also help shape prompt, fitting clinical decisions that can significantly improve survival chances (Figure 5.10).

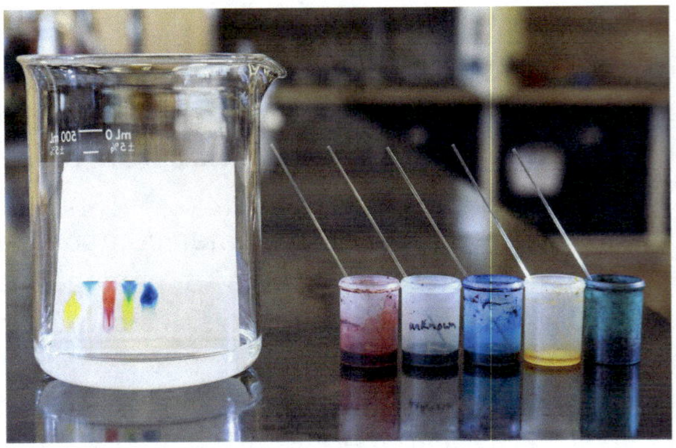

Figure 5.10. Chromatography, a key method, breaks down muddled mixtures to pull out those dangerous chemicals.

Source: Encyclopaedia Britannica. (n.d.). *Simple Paper Chromatography with Various Inks.* https://cdn.britannica.com/13/203213-050-C5F16F5C/Simple-paper-chromatography-various-inks.jpg.

5.2.4. Toxicological Screening Processes

Toxicology analysis and forensic analysis often overlap, both essential for identifying corrosive poisons that drastically impact health. The majority of toxic substances tend to cross-react at the cellular level, disrupting vital organs such as the nervous system, intestines, and even the kidneys (Machado and Dinis-Oliveira, 2023). In forensic contexts, identifying specifically which toxin is involved is crucial, especially where there is suspected poisoning and time is critical. Analysts have to depend on advanced technology—GC-MS and liquid chromatography-electrospray tandem mass spectrometry—to detect these toxic substances, sometimes emerging in criminal cases like drug-facilitated sexual assault (DFSA) (AlOtaibi et al., 2023). In general, these screening tests not only guide definitive diagnoses but also aid the criminal justice system with vital evidence in such instances related to toxic exposures.

5.2.5. Role of Mass Spectrometry

Identifying and measuring substances precisely stands at the heart of forensic work, particularly when corrosive poisons are involved. Mass spectrometry often becomes the go-to tool—its knack for detecting even the tiniest traces of toxic chemicals is hard to beat. It converts chemical substances into ions and then checks their mass-to-charge ratios, a process that helps experts unravel the complex mixtures typically found at crime scenes. Over time, this method has evolved, sometimes pairing unexpectedly with other analytical techniques to enhance the reliability of the evidence. Generally speaking, advances in the field have also sparked new developments in color test reagents and similar technologies, broadening the scope of toxicological screening for emerging psychoactive substances (Fu et al., 2017). As a cornerstone of modern forensic science, mass spectrometry not only targets corrosive poisons but also deepens our overall understanding of chemical threats in the CBRNe landscape (Krzysztof et al., 2022).

5.2.6. Field Testing Kits for First Responders

Breakthroughs in forensic science and technology mean that first responders now have a whole new set of tools for handling hazardous substances, such as corrosive poisons (Figure 5.11). Field testing kits—those handy, portable devices—allow crews to quickly identify the dangerous substances they are dealing with right at the scene. Inside these kits, you will find a mix of gadgets, including optical molecular sensors that do not just pick up typical corrosives but also scan for more intricate toxins such as nerve and blister agents (recent studies back this up, Kumar et al., 2022). Much of the progress behind these devices relies on blended research from nanoscience and other modern technology fields, providing responders with straightforward tools for on-the-spot analysis (Committee, 2023). In most cases, incorporating these innovative tools into the mix effectively highlights the importance of being prepared for chemical emergencies.

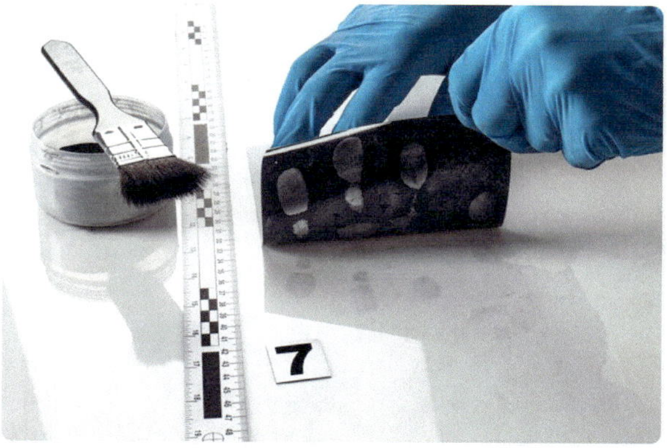

Figure 5.11. Breakthroughs in forensic science and tech mean first responders now have a whole new set of tricks for handling hazardous stuff like corrosive poisons.

Source: Shutterstock. (2019). *Forensic Handprint on a Surface.*

5.2.7. Limitations of Current Detection Methods

Identifying corrosive poisons in forensic analysis is a challenging endeavor. Most labs deal with a tangle of problems—it is not just the tech glitches, but also the dirty, complicated nature of sample matrices that gets in the way. High-performance liquid chromatography (HPLC), for instance, is a popular tool in most cases of analytical chemistry; however, its reliability can decline when interfering chemicals are present in biological samples (Granados et al., 2023). In the majority of cases, the detection processes we use do not necessarily pinpoint specificity as much as sensitivity, particularly when dealing with volatile substances that are apt to evaporate quickly. Take the DFSA, for example—volatile agents are commonly applied, and conventional toxicology tests tend to miss them since they evaporate rapidly and fall below target thresholds (AlOtaibi et al., 2023). Overall, these challenges clearly indicate that newer, more sophisticated methods are needed that can actually improve both accuracy and reliability in the detection of corrosive poisons for forensic purposes.

5.2.8. Advances in Forensic Technology

Forensic science keeps pushing forward in ways that sometimes catch you off guard. New tech keeps popping up – HPLC being one of those surprises – which now helps break down and study the messy samples we see in toxicology labs. When you combine HPLC's flexible nature with modern mass spectrometry, forensic experts can pinpoint corrosive poisons more effectively, often leading to clearer case resolutions (Granados et al., 2023). Some labs even dabble in what they call concurrent neutron and X-ray tests (NeX); this approach provides a deeper understanding of how materials behave. In most cases, NeX makes it easier to sift through complicated, multi-phase data, revealing hints about how toxic substances act and interact after exposure (Hjelm et al., 2024). All in all, these technological advances, albeit somewhat unpredictable in their own way, are at the heart of making forensic investigations faster and more precise when dealing with corrosive poisons.

5.2.9. Importance of Accurate Detection in Legal Cases

Accurate detection is crucial in legal cases involving hazardous corrosive substances (Figure 5.12). Identifying toxic compounds correctly is critical – even a small error could wrongly convict an innocent person or allow a true culprit to escape responsibility. Sometimes, modern methods, such as the endoscopic approach for post-mortem checks, reveal unexpected clues about corrosive agents. Forensic science itself digs into every detail at a crime scene, gathering and analyzing evidence so that, in most instances, the right individuals are held accountable. At the same time, the uninvolved are overlooked (Ahluwalia et al., 2023). In many cases, a steady focus on getting detection right not only strengthens the legal system's foundation but also boosts public trust in forensic practice.

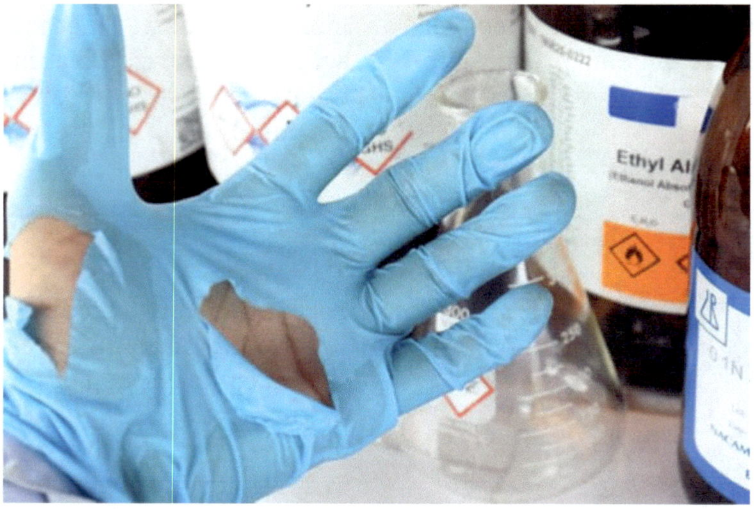

Figure 5.12. Accurate detection matters a lot in legal cases involving dangerous corrosive substances.

Source: Storemasta. (n.d.). *Corrosive Chemical Warning label.* https://blog.storemasta.com.au/hs-fs/hubfs/corrosive%20chemical.jpg?width=500&name=corrosive%20chemical.jpg.

Test Your Knowledge

1. What is the role of pH in determining the severity of corrosive poisoning?
2. Which industrial chemicals are commonly associated with corrosive burns?

5.3. Case Studies in Forensic Toxicology

Learning Outcome

1. Identify notable historical cases involving corrosive poisons
2. Focus on analysis of modern forensic cases
3. Explain the role of expert testimony in court
4. Discuss challenges faced in prosecution
5. Know the impact of forensic findings on case outcomes
6. Describe ethical considerations in forensic analysis
7. Understand public perception of corrosive poison cases
8. Lessons learned from past cases
9. Know future implications for forensic practices

Corrosive toxins have had an interesting path in forensic toxicology—one which truly reveals the way that drug use has changed over time. In the 1930s, for example, a history from Krakow revealed 69 death cases in which corrosives were utilized to take one's life (Włek et al., 2021); this obviously indicates an era when individuals tended to choose these damaging agents as their last resort. Today, however, there is a noticeable shift, with more cases now involving the combination of drugs, and drug products are nowadays likely to be the substances of choice for suicide. For instance, mercuric chloride, despite its once–ill–reputed status, continues to puzzle forensic scientists. The symptoms and evidence gathered during post-mortems are key to making the correct diagnosis, even though copious studies have for years explained its lethal properties (Cappelletti et al., 2019). Overall, this shift from corrosives to contemporary drugs requires new forensic practices, reflecting the changing trends in toxicology that we observe in our modern society.

5.3.1. Notable Historical Cases Involving Corrosive Poisons

Corrosive poisons have left their mark in unexpected ways—stories that have, over time, reshaped the world of forensic science. There have been high-profile episodes involving heavy metals and various toxic agents that, frankly, remind us just how lethal these substances can be. Some 19th-century arsenic cases, for example, not only demonstrated the raw strength of these corrosives but also highlighted how difficult it can be to detect them in biological tests. In Machado and Dinis-Oliveira (2023), it is generally noted that catching sight of a specific toxin quickly can really change the game; rapid detection, even amid uncertainty, has often been the difference between a good and a bad outcome. New tools, such as portable GC-MS, have, in most cases, altered investigative methods by enabling faster analysis in challenging—and sometimes hostile—settings, with military applications further highlighting their benefits in both civilian and armed forces contexts (Leary et al., 2019) (Figure 5.13).

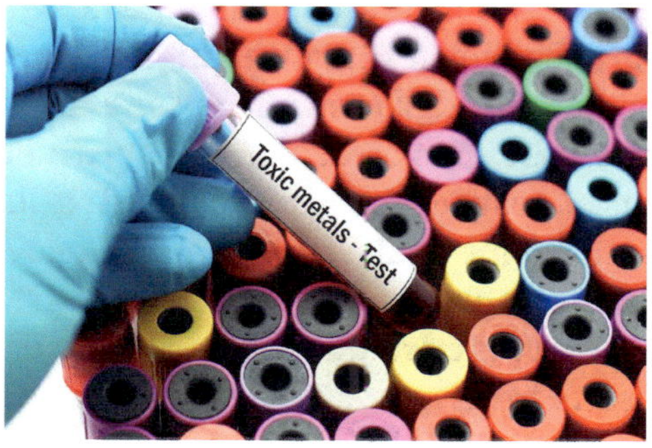

Figure 5.13. Heavy metals testing.

Source: CPTC Labs. (n.d.). *Eliminates Heavy Metals*. https://az-cdn.cptclabs.com/wp-content/uploads/Eliminates-Heavy-Metals.jpg.

5.3.2. Analysis of Modern Forensic Cases

Corrosive poisons play a significant role in forensic work today. Autopsies often reveal that acids do not behave the same way—HCl, for example, usually causes a type of coagulative cell death that you mostly see in the esophagus and stomach; meanwhile, sulfuric acid tends to create deeper, full-thickness injuries along with noticeable bleeding (Chaurasia et al., 2024). In many instances, these differences force experts to hone in on subtle clues, as their interpretation of the damage can affect both clinical decisions and legal outcomes. One also sees that methadone poisoning, with its tangled metabolic issues, adds another layer of complexity for forensic assessments (Batotsyrenov et al., 2024). When everything is considered, these cases highlight the intricate relationship between toxicology and forensic science.

5.3.3. Role of Expert Testimony in Court

Expert testimony often makes all the difference in forensic investigations—it is the kind of clarity and trust that can sway a case in court (Figure 5.14). When things get messy with dangerous substances like mercury, experts step in to simplify technical data for judges and juries who, frankly, might not have the specialized background. Take one domestic violence case (Sinha et al., 2023): a detailed look into procedures such as gastric lavage and even vomit analysis ended up uncovering alarmingly high mercury levels. Experts not only conduct meticulous tests but also explain the results in terms that are easily understood in the real world. In most cases, this kind of straightforward explanation helps bridge that ever-present gap between raw forensic data and legal decisions, subtly outlining the nuances of toxicology (Ahluwalia et al., 2023). Ultimately, when expert testimony is solid—even if it is not always perfectly polished—it reinforces the integrity of the forensic evidence and nudges the judicial process toward a more informed outcome.

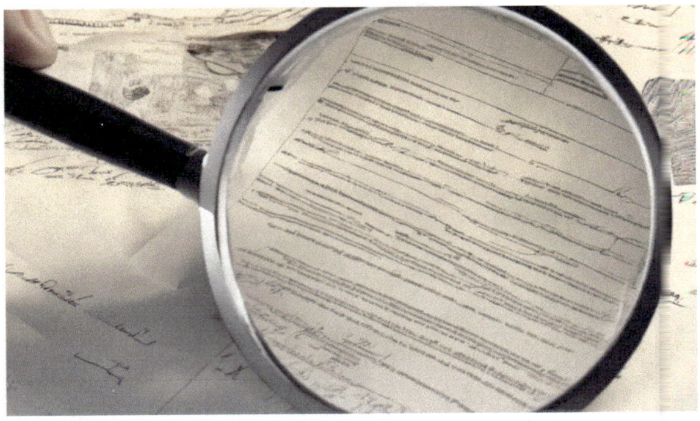

Figure 5.14. Expert testimony often makes all the difference in forensic investigations—it is the kind of clarity and trust that can sway a case in court.

Source: Litili Group. (2023). *Handwriting Analysis*.

5.3.4. Challenges Faced in Prosecution

Poisoning cases tend to throw a curve into prosecutions, particularly when corrosives are involved. Toxicology tests almost inevitably wind up being the key to determining what really happened, albeit waiting on the viscera reports can really slow things down. When the death is suspected to be due to poisoning, the professionals usually go into chemical analysis for detecting poisons; however, these analyses—most of the time—yield no results, making the situation all the more confusing (Dixit et al., 2024). Acute acid corrosive ingestion, however, makes things even more complicated; pathologists see enormous, occasionally mottled, fields of tissue destruction that render it difficult to pinpoint intent or the complete circumstances of the death (Chaurasia et al., 2024). Overall, these obstacles do not just delay legal proceedings but also undermine the overall evidentiary foundation required for a sound prosecution, illustrating just how complicated the intersection of forensic science and legal accountability can be.

5.3.5. Impact of Forensic Findings on Case Outcomes

Forensic findings are crucial when it comes to how cases are resolved, especially those involving corrosive poisons. Expert testimony that comes from digging into forensic details can change everything—it might tip the scales so that a matter ends up in criminal court or sometimes, surprisingly, gets handled civilly. In areas where acid attacks occur frequently, weaving forensic results into everyday legal work has been a gamechanger for coming up with laws and preventive measures. Generally speaking, evidence shows that places such as Bangladesh have seen a marked drop in acid attack incidents, thanks to strict penalties and local public awareness projects built around forensic data (Calcini et al., 2022). Equally, having a team of seasoned medical toxicologists is beneficial—they significantly enhance the ability to interpret toxicological results and provide greater precision to legal decisions in poisoning cases (Marks et al., 2020). All in all, the combination of forensic work and legal outcomes clearly demonstrates the importance of solid forensic practices in addressing crimes involving corrosive substances.

5.3.6. Ethical Considerations in Forensic Analysis

Forensic work often throws up some really tricky ethical issues, especially when it comes to dealing with harsh, corrosive poisons (Figure 5.15). Experts in the field have to balance—often in a pretty messy way—the need to gather accurate data against the real emotional fallout for those involved, like victims and their families. It is not always cut and dry; in many cases, trying to figure out if a poisoning happened on purpose or by accident turns into a real challenge. Take, for example, how suicidal poisoning among women keeps coming up as a significant concern (Kholeif, 2023). Then, there is the possibility that even a slight bias in reading toxicology reports might compromise a criminal case, which suggests that we generally need solid ethical guidelines to keep things on track (Althobaiti et al., 2023). All in all, mixing ethical duties with the pursuit of forensic accuracy is not just about legal outcomes—it also plays a massive part in how much people trust forensic science as a tool for fair justice.

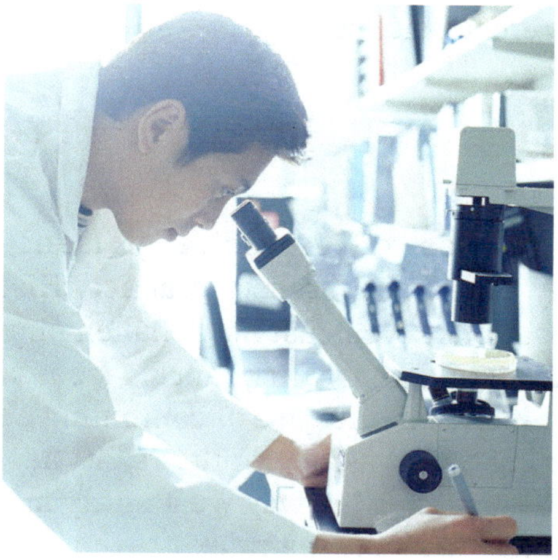

Figure 5.15. Forensic work often throws up some tricky ethical issues, especially when it comes to dealing with harsh, corrosive poisons.

Source: ExploreHealthCareers. (2016). *Forensic Toxicologist at Work.* https://explorehealthcareers.org/wp-content/uploads/2016/11/forensic_toxicologist.jpg.

5.3.7. Public Perception of Corrosive Poison Cases

Poison-related crimes from the past have left their mark on how we see corrosive substances being used in mischief. Cases from the 1800s and early 1900s suddenly shed light on a host of problems – weak medical tests and juries that struggled to comprehend complex scientific concepts. It turns out that, in many instances, poisoning symptoms were misread, letting these crimes slip by undetected, and this really fed the idea that such incidents happened way more frequently than most people thought (Merry et al., 2010). Sometimes, poisoning becomes entangled with other misdeeds, such as product tampering, which further complicates how people understand harmful contamination; naturally, this raises numerous questions about both intent and consequence (Kilbane et al., 2016). All in all, this murky history still stokes a lingering fear about corrosive poisons—a feeling that, generally speaking, continues to color modern discussions on criminal behavior and forensic science.

5.3.8. Lessons Learned from Past Cases

Classic cases of corrosive poisons have actually redefined forensic practice. Historical investigations reveal just how challenging it was to identify and analyze chemicals from various environments. In the case of combining neutron scattering with X-ray methods, it has been critical—it refines the way we identify materials and demystifies the complexity when multiple chemical substances interact in a single case of poisoning (Hjelm et al., 2024). A deep excavation of ancient stories of mysterious disappearances, in the majority of instances, indicates that a meticulous examination of toxic hints can lay bare layers that aren't immediately apparent (Klein, 2023). In aggregate, these situations typically emphasize the importance of having world-class scientific equipment in conjunction with a sound method of analysis, one that, in the majority of cases, renders forensic findings related to corrosive poisons considerably more reliable.

5.3.9. Future Implications for Forensic Practices

Current advances in forensic science are shaking up how corrosive poison cases get handled, both in investigations and in court. What's striking is the push for better standardization and a boost in professionalism—a point many experts agree is key to reducing mistakes. You often hear in forensic anthropology talks that adhering to strict educational guidelines and proper accreditation tends to reduce legal errors (Langley et al., 2025). Then, there is the role of Artificial Intelligence; AI is not just a buzzword, but a real force in streamlining tasks such as toxicological testing and gathering evidence (Rajasekar et al., 2024). With machine learning combined with detailed data analysis, forensic professionals can now identify harmful substances more reliably. In most cases, this blend of solid science and cutting-edge technology appears poised to transform our legal system into something both more efficient and, ultimately, more just (Figure 5.16).

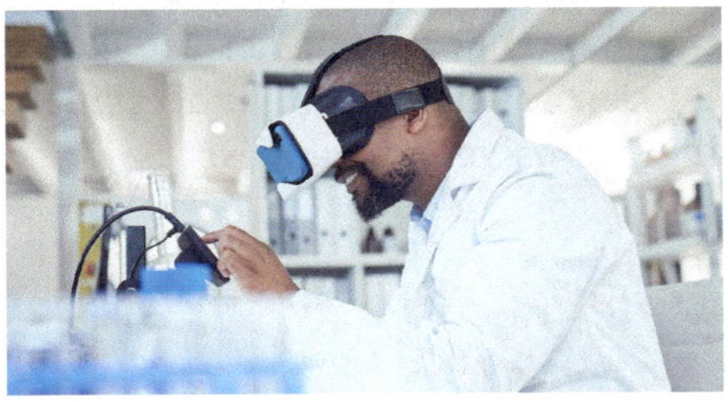

Figure 5.16. The role of artificial intelligence in forensic practices.

Source: University of Alabama at Birmingham. (n.d.). *AI in Medicine.* https://www.uab.edu/degrees/images/hero/ai-medicine-gc.jpg.

Test Your Knowledge

1. How does media coverage affect public perception of corrosive poisoning cases?
2. What role does public awareness play in preventing corrosive substance misuse?

5.4. Prevention and Safety Measures

Learning Outcome

1. Understand regulations surrounding corrosive substances
2. Explain safety protocols in laboratories
3. Discuss public awareness campaigns
4. Focus on training for first responders
5. Learn emergency response strategies
6. Discuss the role of education in prevention
7. Learn workplace safety standards
8. Identify community resources for poison control
9. Describe the importance of reporting and monitoring incidents

Corrosive poisons have a significant impact on public health, so implementing solid prevention and safety measures is not just useful—it is essential. Poison Control Centers (PCCs) provide immediate help, offering quick advice from preventing an incident to diagnosing and treating it, which is something we really rely on. Research, in most cases, indicates that only about 47% of WHO member states have established these key facilities (Prodanchuk et al., 2024), leaving a significant gap in our overall safety net for managing chemical risks. This missing piece could, arguably, enhance our ability to monitor toxic substances and develop more effective chemical safety plans. At the same time, incorporating advanced technologies like Artificial Intelligence can be a real game-changer, helping us foresee potential hazards and reduce emergency response times (Kahla, 2024). And, of course, ongoing education and training are crucial—ensuring both the public and first responders know what to look for and how to react when corrosive poisons emerge.

5.4.1. Regulations Surrounding Corrosive Substances

Handling dangerous chemicals—particularly those corrosives that require special handling—comes under a web of regulations established to safeguard the public and our planet (Figure 5.17). These regulations, far from being presented in the form of a tidy checklist, combine directives on how to handle, store, and dispose of hazardous chemicals with suggestions on their value in forensic applications. For instance, there are specific container label requirements that enable forensic experts to quickly identify and address such materials during investigations. For the most part, it is required to adhere to safety data sheets (SDS), which explicitly detail the hazards associated with each chemical, be it corrosive poisons that may unexpectedly appear at a crime scene. Strictly adhering to these guidelines not only ensures the safety of forensic professionals but also maintains the integrity of evidence, thereby adding credibility to the justice system in instances of intentional harm (Mšlin et al., 2023; Tamba et al., 2024).

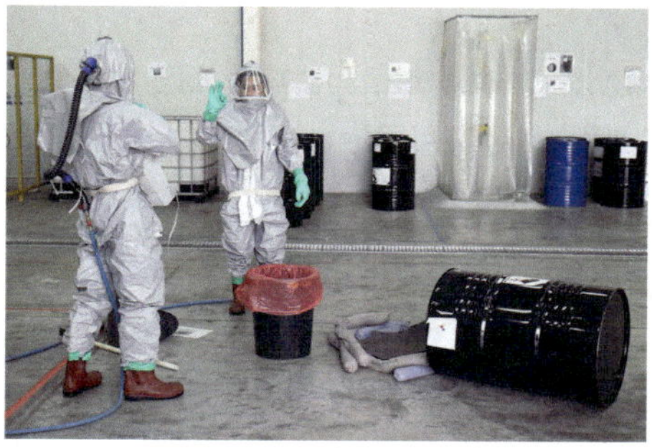

Figure 5.17. Managing hazardous materials—especially those corrosive substances that require demand extra care—falls under a network of strict rules established to protect both the public and the environment.

Source: Human Focus. (n.d.). *Safe Handling of Hazardous Substances at Work.* https://humanfocus.co.uk/wp-content/uploads/Safe-handling-of-hazardous-substances-at-work.jpg.

5.4.2. Safety Protocols in Laboratories

Forensic labs that handle corrosive chemicals come with a fair share of hazards, making strict safety measures a must. Generally speaking, you need to manage these risks carefully—a minor slip-up can not only cause serious injuries but also taint critical evidence. It all starts with hands-on training in using everyday protective gear, such as gloves, goggles, and lab coats; these items serve as your first line of defense. Additionally, adhering to guidelines for storing and disposing of corrosives properly goes a long way in preventing accidents and environmental harm. A well-ventilated lab, complete with safety showers and eyewash stations, further reduces exposure—even though such details are sometimes overlooked. In short, all these practices work together to protect both the people on site and the credibility of forensic analyses, since even minimal contamination can compromise the validity of outcomes (Krzysztof et al., 2022).

5.4.3. Public Awareness Campaigns

Public awareness campaigns are a significant concern when it comes to handling corrosive poisons—a challenge that frequently arises in forensic studies and interventions (Figure 5.18). They do not merely list dangers; instead, they help people grasp how to manage hazardous substances safely, generally aiming to reduce the number of poisoning cases, particularly among children, who are often the hardest hit. Recent observations reveal that accidental poisonings crop up more than one might expect among young patients, with drugs frequently playing the leading role (Oto et al., 2023). Some research even nudges public health initiatives toward safety education, suggesting that teaching proper storage and use of chemicals can really make a difference (Al-Khattabi, 2023). A mix of channels—social media, schools, local events—is used to draw in communities in a relaxed, sometimes slightly offbeat way, which adds a human touch to these campaigns. Ultimately, increased awareness not only empowers individuals but also fosters a sense of shared, albeit imperfect, responsibility to prevent poisoning incidents in forensic contexts.

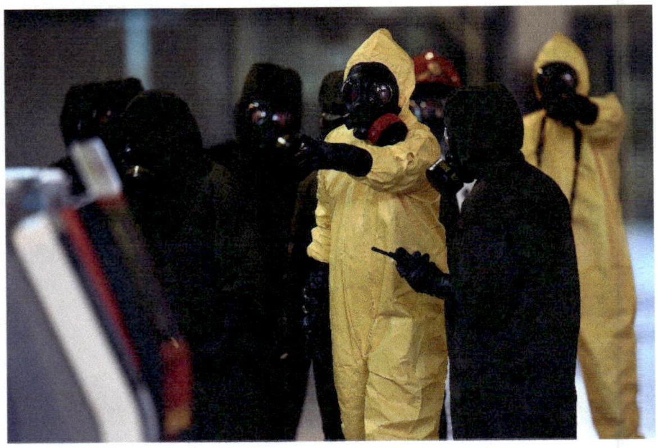

Figure 5.18. Public awareness campaigns are a significant concern when it comes to handling corrosive poisons—a challenge that frequently arises in forensic studies and interventions.

Source: Center for Strategic and International Studies (CSIS). (n.d.). *PONI Nuclear Policy Image.* https://csis-website-prod.s3.amazonaws.com/s3fs-public/PONI_1.jpg.

5.4.4. Training for First Responders

Often, the success of forensic work with corrosive toxins hinges on how well first responders are prepared. These individuals usually arrive on the scene first—and they need more than a textbook grasp of safety rules; they must quickly get a feel for the unique quirks of each chemical. Training is not just about memorizing protocols; it is about recognizing early signs of exposure, selecting the right protective gear, and implementing effective decontamination steps. Generally speaking, incorporating basic toxicology concepts helps them assess the risks that these agents may pose. Interestingly, lessons gathered from research into CWAs sometimes find their way into everyday safety strategies, showing that the link between field training and forensic methods is both crucial and complex. All in all, the overlap between laboratory techniques and on-scene expertise remains crucial to maintaining investigations that are both safe and effective (Kumar et al., 2022; Ahluwalia et al., 2023).

5.4.5. Emergency Response Strategies

Timely emergency help is key when corrosive poisons hit, especially if someone gets badly hurt by chemicals like benzalkonium chloride (BAC) (Figure 5.19). One striking case—generally speaking—involved a young child who ended up with severe breathing problems after accidentally swallowing a disinfectant with BAC; rapid med intervention, paired with supportive care, really made a difference in his full recovery (Vțescu et al., 2024). In most cases, having a solid, if not slightly patchy, poisoning reporting system plays a significant role in identifying risky trends. Take, for example, the broad monitoring set up in Saudi Arabia—it not only paves the way for quick medical responses but also backs public health efforts to cut down on poisoning, particularly among vulnerable kids (Al-Khattabi, 2023).

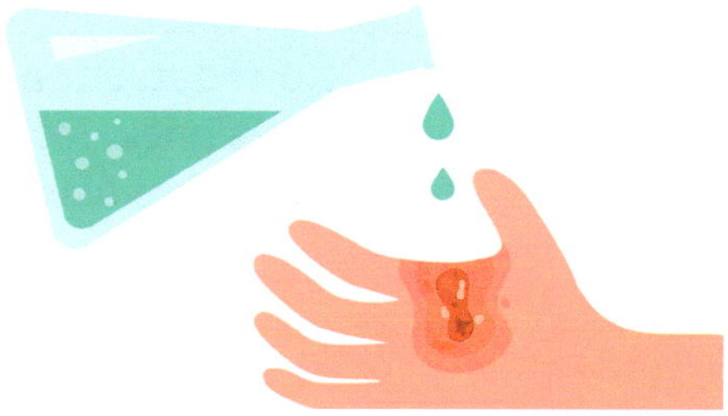

Figure 5.19. Timely emergency help is key when corrosive poisons hit, especially if someone gets badly hurt by chemicals like benzalkonium chloride (BAC).

Source: Acko General Insurance. (n.d.). *First Aid Guide: Chemical Burn.* https://acko-cms.ackoassets.com/First_Aid_Guide_Chemical_Burn_022dc80ab3.png.

All in all, mixing swift treatment protocols with a dependable reporting setup forms the backbone of handling corrosive poison incidents in forensic settings.

5.4.6. Role of Education in Prevention

Providing people with straightforward, accurate advice plays a significant role in reducing the risks associated with corrosive chemicals. When parents, caregivers, and others really get that everyday item—like cleaning supplies or medications—can be risky, they are more likely to take basic steps to keep kids safe. The numbers do show, for instance, that many poisoning cases involve young children who accidentally grab these accessible products (Singh et al., 2023). At the same time, there is a growing sense that better training for medical personnel and social workers—so they can spot early signs of self-harm or suicidal behavior—might help curb intentional poisonings. Generally speaking, when communities share practical knowledge through targeted outreach, folks become more vigilant, and that extra bit of awareness can make a real difference in lowering these tragic incidents.

5.4.7. Workplace Safety Standards

Forensic labs must take safety seriously—especially when handling corrosive toxins that can cause serious harm to health (Figure 5.20). Dangerous substances, which sometimes show up in illicit liquors (Kaur et al., 2024), demand tight protocols to keep exposure low and contamination at bay; even a small mistake might lead to severe, even fatal, poisoning. Cases with methanol and other risky chemicals show, in most cases, that testing needs extra care, as research on illicit liquors (Kaur et al., 2024) indicates. It is also crucial that safety measures encompass aspects such as altrenogest, as it is used in horse therapies but can sometimes mask harmful steroid impurities (Elbourne et al., 2024). Overall, setting up broad, protective workplace guidelines not only helps forensic teams guard themselves but also keeps their analyses steady, ultimately boosting the trustworthiness of their findings.

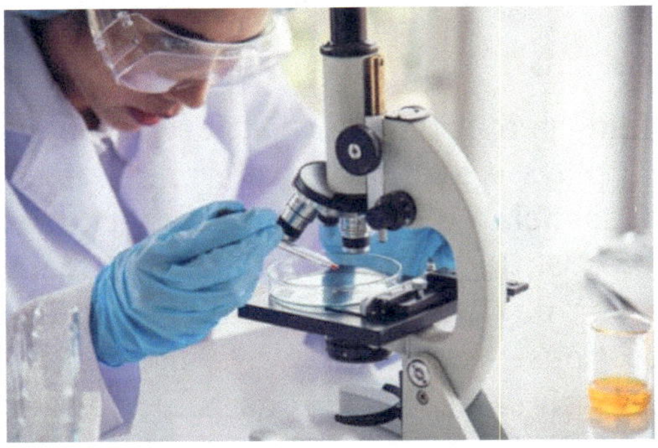

Figure 5.20. Forensic labs must take safety seriously—especially when handling corrosive toxins that can cause serious harm to health.

Source: Storemasta. (n.d.). *Lab Technician Viewing Sample Under Microscope.* https://blog.storemasta.com.au/hubfs/Blog%20images/All%20New%20blog.storemasta%20images/lab%20technician%20viewing%20sample%20under%20microscope.jpg.

5.4.8. Community Resources for Poison Control

Corrosive poisons can be particularly damaging, and prompt medical attention can make all the difference. Local poison centers and dedicated hotlines offer fast, practical support—guiding both healthcare professionals and everyday individuals when things go awry. They are not just about crisis management; these centers also dish out clear advice on treatment options and the potential nastiness of toxic effects, even if it sounds a bit direct. In many cases, increasing public know-how and sharing these crucial tips seems to lower poisoning incidents while boosting overall community health. Sometimes, weaving the insights from these centers into forensic work sheds new light on how common corrosive substances really are, which, in turn, leads to more brilliant prevention tactics. At the end of the day, forensic experts and poison control teams joining forces establish a working model for addressing health issues related to toxic exposures (Churchill, 2022; Barnard et al., 2024).

5.4.9. Importance of Reporting and Monitoring Incidents

Corrosive poisons in forensic work present numerous challenges. In 2004, over 45,000 kids and teens lost their lives to acute poisoning (Althobaiti et al., 2023)—a stark reminder of why we need to track these incidents carefully. Setting up a clear, if not downright straightforward, way to record these poisoning cases gives us a better idea of what is really happening and how it affects public health, generally speaking. Detailed incident reports not only help us identify trends associated with specific toxins but also foster a collaborative effort between law enforcement and health officials, who ultimately work together to address these issues. New detection tools—such as optical sensors designed for CWAs—further emphasize the importance of monitoring hazardous substances, thereby enhancing preparedness and response plans (Kumar et al., 2022). All in all, a solid, sometimes imperfect, framework for reporting and monitoring really goes a long way toward mitigating the risks associated with corrosive poisons in forensic investigations.

Test Your Knowledge

1. What are the key strategies to prevent corrosive poison exposure in households?
2. Why is it essential to store corrosive substances in properly labeled containers?
3. How can education help reduce the incidence of acid attacks?

SUMMARY

Forensic work involving corrosive poisons is not simple—it truly requires careful methods and rigorous oversight. Lately, we are noticing more drug-facilitated crimes that use volatile chemicals like chloroform, which ends up exposing pretty significant gaps in the way things are usually done; these gaps, in most cases, need to be addressed right away. Sometimes investigators even rely on sophisticated tools, such as GC-MS, to detect even the slightest traces of these corrosive agents (AlOtaibi et al., 2023), a clear indication of just how complex and layered criminal forensics has become. Trying to trace residues after blasts or explosive events shows you cannot afford to take shortcuts with precision. Comprehensive screening and analytical routines prove to be vital, especially since evidence can become contaminated, and the mix of chemicals ultimately plays a significant role in the outcomes (Dhananjoy et al., 2022). In the end, stepping up our regulatory frameworks around managing these corrosive substances seems absolutely key to refining forensic practices and keeping our justice system on point.

Corrosive poisons matter a great deal in forensic science, especially when legal cases are on the line. Figuring out these tricky substances—and their impact on our health—really tends to jumble case outcomes, so every little detail seems to count. Lately, studies have shown that New Psychoactive Substances (NPS) appear at varying rates in different regions, which generally prompts us to gather more detailed data. For example, one inquiry (Gillies et al., 2015) suggests that increasing our efforts to collect NPS data may sharpen our understanding of the complex and toxic situations we face. Additionally, the overall picture of NPS—its connection to forensic investigations—still leaves some important gaps in evidence that need to be addressed to support public health, in most cases (Gillies et al., 2015). All in all, taking a closer, albeit imperfect, look at these issues is crucial to improving forensic practices surrounding corrosive poisons.

KEY TERMS FROM THIS CHAPTER

- Acid poisoning
- Acids
- Alkalis
- Bases
- Carboxyhemoglobin
- Chemical tests
- Chemical warfare agents
- Exposure
- Gas chromatography
- Hydrochloric acid (HCl)
- Mass spectrometry
- Mucosal membranes
- Sulfuric acid

CRITICAL THINKING QUESTIONS

1. **Which of the following is an example of an acidic corrosive poison?**
   a. Sodium hydroxide
   b. Hydrochloric acid
   c. Ammonia
   d. Lye
2. **What is the primary effect of alkali poisoning on tissue?**
   a. Burning of the mucous membranes and esophagus
   b. Causing protein coagulation
   c. Liquefaction and deep tissue necrosis
   d. Immediate destruction of the stomach lining
3. **Which of the following is a common source of acidic corrosives in poisoning cases?**
   a. Vinegar
   b. Sulfuric acid
   c. Baking soda
   d. Bleach
4. **What is the most common outcome of severe corrosive poisoning?**
   a. Renal failure
   b. Respiratory arrest
   c. Cardiac arrest
   d. Multisystem organ failure due to shock and sepsis
5. **Why is vomiting not recommended after the ingestion of corrosive poisons?**
   a. It could increase the absorption of the toxin.
   b. It could cause more damage to the esophagus and mouth.
   c. It could worsen symptoms like diarrhea.
   d. It has no effect on the toxic process.

Short Answer Questions

1. What is a corrosive poison?
2. Name two common types of corrosive poisons.
3. What is the difference between acid and alkali corrosives in terms of tissue damage?
4. Give two examples of acid corrosives and their familiar sources.
5. What are the clinical features of acid poisoning?
6. What are the signs and symptoms of alkali poisoning?
7. Why is vomiting contraindicated in corrosive poisoning?
8. What are the complications of corrosive ingestion?
9. How do corrosive poisons cause death?
10. What postmortem findings are typical in corrosive poison cases?
11. How can one differentiate between acid and alkali poisoning at autopsy?

Answers to Critical Thinking Questions

1. (b); 2. (c); 3. (b); 4. (d); 5. (b)

REFERENCES

1. Ahluwalia, J. K., & Sharma, R., (2023). The role of forensic science in criminal investigation. *International Journal for Multidisciplinary Research, 5*. https://doi.org/10.36948/ijfmr.2023.v05i06.9530.
2. Aktaş, N., Gülaçtı, U., Lök, U., Aydın, İ., Börta, T., & Çelik, M., (2018). Characteristics of the traumatic forensic cases admitted to emergency department and errors in the forensic report writing. *Bulletin of Emergency and Trauma, 6*, 64–70. https://doi.org/10.29252/beat-060110.
3. Al-Khattabi, G. H. (2023). *An Overview of the Chemical and Drug Overdose Poisoning Reporting System as a Surveillance System, Makkah, Saudi Arabia 2018–2019*. https://doi.org/10.20944/preprints202311.1179.v1.
4. AlOtaibi, S. O., Althinyan, G. K., Alzakari, Z. A., Mohamed, F. A., & Menezes, R. G. (2023). The use of volatile substances in drug-facilitated sexual assault: A systematic review. *Cureus*. https://doi.org/10.7759/cureus.33430.
5. Althobaiti, B. M., El-Readi, M. Z., Althubiti, M., Alhindi, Y., Alzahrani, A. R., Alghamdi, S., Ayoub, N., et al. (2023). Patterns of acute poisoning for children during outbreak of coronavirus in Makkah region, Saudi Arabia. *Frontiers in Pediatrics, 11*. https://doi.org/10.3389/fped.2023.1087095.
6. Anas, M. K. P. (2016). *A Study of Observation in Treatment Modality of Acute and Chronic Poisoning Cases by Analyzing Clinical Laboratory Parameters and its Outcome in Tertiary care Hospitals*. https://core.ac.uk/download/235660891.pdf (accessed on 9th May 2025).
7. Arslan, I., & Demir, K., (2022). Evaluation of forensic cases presented to the pediatric emergency department. *Turkish Journal of Emergency Medicine, 22*, 137–142. https://www.semanticscholar.org/paper/98cf495c0272d23df557ab3c98771a42d0210ab6 (accessed on 9th May 2025).
8. Baković, M., Mayer, D., & Nestić, M., (2015). *Suicidal Chemistry: Combined Intoxication with Carbon Monoxide and Formic Acid*. https://core.ac.uk/download/130165591.pdf (accessed on 9th May 2025).
9. Barnard, C. C., & Carpenter, E., (2024). *A Classification for Medical and Veterinary Libraries*. https://doi.org/10.56920/lshtmp-1.
10. Basilicata, P., Pieri, M., Simonelli, A., Capasso, E., Casella, C., Noto, T., Policino, F., et al. (2022). Diquat poisoning: Care management and medico-legal implications. *Toxics, 10*, 166. https://doi.org/10.3390/toxics10040166.
11. Batotsyrenov, C. B., Kuznetsov, S., Lodyagin, A. H., Reinuk, V. L., Molin, Y. A., Litvincev, B. S., Klimanov, D. V., et al. (2024). Thanatogenesis and forensic assessment of severe acute methadone poisoning. *Russian Journal of Forensic Medicine*. https://www.semanticscholar.org/paper/9f67cd402bfc269831d4119b28d72243a551ea43 (accessed on 9th May 2025).
12. Bergeron, W. P., & Taylor, S. K. (2015). *Cultural Considerations in Forensic Science in the United States*. https://core.ac.uk/download/198422999.pdf (accessed on 9th May 2025).
13. Bertel, L., Miranda, D. A., & García-Martín, J. M. (2021). Nanostructured titanium dioxide surfaces for electrochemical biosensing. *Sensors, 21*, 6167. https://doi.org/10.3390/s21186167.
14. Brzozowski, K., Daoust-Maleval, I., Geypens, B., Goulart de Medeiros, M., Iatan, A. E., Lequarre, A. S., & Santopolo, D., (2022). *EU CBRNe Glossary*. https://core.ac.uk/download/642865393.

pdf (accessed on 9th May 2025).

15. Calcini, G., (2022). *Acid Attacks: An Overview of Legal Measures and Motivation Trends in India, Pakistan, Bangladesh, Colombia, and Cambodia*. https://core.ac.uk/download/548486229.pdf (accessed on 9th May 2025).
16. Cappelletti, S., Piacentino, D., Fineschi, V., Frati, P., D'Errico, S., & Aromatario, M., (2019). Mercuric chloride poisoning: Symptoms, analysis, therapies, and autoptic findings. A review of the literature. *Critical Reviews in Toxicology, 49*, 329–341. https://doi.org/10.1080/10408444.2019.1621262.
17. Carter, C. M., Hood, J. P., Jackson, M., Lonstein, R., et al. (2021). *Disruptive Technologies with Applications in Airline & Marine and Defense Industries*. https://core.ac.uk/download/386944514.pdf (accessed on 9th May 2025).
18. Chaurasia, S., Tomar, M. S., Ganvir, R., & Singh, S., (2024). Acute corrosive acid ingestion: A case series of four autopsies. *Indian Journal of Forensic Medicine & Toxicology*. https://www.semanticscholar.org/paper/bc711fc22673a86850637ad593092234ecbb4d48 (accessed on 9th May 2025).
19. Churchill, W., (2022). An interplay of shadows and light: The decolonial potential of red-black unity (Part I). *Zanj: The Journal of Critical Global South Studies, 3*. https://doi.org/10.13169/zanjglobsoutstud.3.1.0004.
20. Dixit, P., & Kumari, M., (2024). Challenges in viscera analysis: Addressing errors in forensic reporting and their medico-legal implications. *Indian Internet Journal of Forensic Medicine and Toxicology*. https://www.semanticscholar.org/paper/92f73203c17266faa2ab4cb227dc8516d35bd3d8 (accessed on 9th May 2025).
21. Elbourne, M., Keledjian, J., Cawley, A., & Fu, S., (2024). Administration route differentiation of altrenogest via the metabolomic LC-HRMS analysis of equine urine. *Molecules, 29*. https://www.semanticscholar.org/paper/59c437acb3f9e3e617b60eda6bea8a92843b4914 (accessed on 9th May 2025).
22. Fu, S., & Philp, M., (2017). *A Review of Chemical 'Spot' Tests: A Presumptive Illicit Drug Identification Technique*. https://opus.lib.uts.edu.au/bitstream/10453/123158/4/DTA_submitted%20revision.pdf (accessed on 9th May 2025).
23. Gillies, A., (2015). *Closing Evidence Gaps on the Prevalence and Harms of New Psychoactive Substances in Scotland*. https://core.ac.uk/download/132846011.pdf (accessed on 9th May 2025).
24. Gillies, A., (2015). *Mapping Current and Potential Sources of Routine Data Capture on New Psychoactive Substances in Scotland*. https://core.ac.uk/download/132846012.pdf (accessed on 9th May 2025).
25. Granados, M., Di Gaudio, F., Cucina, A., Indelicato, S., Hefnawy, M., El-Gamal, A. A., El-Gendy, M. A., et al. (2023). *High Performance Liquid Chromatography – Recent Advances and Applications*. IntechOpen eBooks. https://doi.org/10.5772/intechopen.105269.
26. Herman, R. U., & Prasetyo, A., (2025). Analysis of Address Resolution Protocol poisoning attacks on Mikrotik routers using live forensics methods. *International Journal of Engineering Business and Social Science*. https://www.semanticscholar.org/paper/90bbc22aa5d62f70efbff2f23cd138f7bd2bf75a (accessed on 9th May 2025).

27. Hjelm, R. P., Weber, J., Hussey, D. S., Bockstaller, M. R., Vogel, S. C., Khaykovich, B., Siebenbürger, M., et al. (2024). *The Scientific Case for Concurrent Neutron and X-Ray Scattering and Spectroscopy.* https://doi.org/10.2172/2350626.

28. Kahla, L. Z. (2024). Leveraging artificial intelligence for crime detection and prevention. *International Journal of Scientific Research in Engineering and Management.* https://www.semanticscholar.org/paper/51508319c003c5aedabfdb1285ef692949114167 (accessed on 9th May 2025).

29. Kaur, G., Thakur, A., Mukherjee, D., & Moza, B., (2024). Forensic analysis of illicit liquors in Himachal Pradesh: Assessing toxicity and composition for public health safety. *Indian Journal of Forensic and Community Medicine.* https://www.semanticscholar.org/paper/6447bc8ebfa6f900b4a747fa7cdf4d8c2ff8ab69 (accessed on 9th May 2025).

30. Kholeif, W., (2023). Acute poisoning among adult females admitted to Alexandria Poison Center – Egypt. *Zagazig Journal of Forensic Medicine,* https://doi.org/10.21608/zjfm.2023.198765.1145.

31. Kilbane, S. C., & Wilson, M. A. (2016). *Criminal Poisoning and Product Tampering: Toward an Operational Definition of Malicious Contamination.* https://core.ac.uk/download/74244105.pdf (accessed on 9th May 2025).

32. Kim, J., Kim, D., Kim, T. G., Na, J., Park, M., Park, J. H., Lee, N., et al. (2021). A statistical analysis of forensic autopsies performed in the Jungbu Province of Korea in 2020. *Korean Journal of Legal Medicine.* https://www.semanticscholar.org/paper/71b9b0135b7b63e99684298bee31154c083548ae (accessed on 9th May 2025).

33. Klein, N. M. (2023). *1. Bleeding Through.* Transcript Verlag eBooks. https://doi.org/10.1515/9783839465592-002.

34. Kumar, V., Kim, H., Pandey, B., James, T. D., Yoon, J., & Anslyn, E. V. (2022). Recent advances in fluorescent and colorimetric chemosensors for the detection of chemical warfare agents: A legacy of the 21st century. *Chemical Society Reviews, 52,* 663–704. https://doi.org/10.1039/d2cs00651k.

35. Langley, N. R., Tersigni-Tarrant, M., Passalacqua, N. V., Crowder, C. M., Garvin, H., McQuade, W. E. P., Soto, M. M., et al. (2025). The future of forensic anthropology practice and education: Competencies, certification, and licensure. *American Journal of Biological Anthropology, 186*(3), e70034. https://www.semanticscholar.org/paper/46c6d0db49080ec883590df1c7c82f7cac293a24 (accessed on 9th May 2025).

36. Leary, P. E., Kammrath, B. W., Lattman, K. J., & Beals, G. L. (2019). Deploying portable gas chromatography–mass spectrometry (GC-MS) to military users for the identification of toxic chemical agents in theater. *Applied Spectroscopy, 73,* 841–858. https://doi.org/10.1177/0003702819849499.

37. Machado, C. de C., & Dinis-Oliveira, R. J. (2023). Clinical and forensic signs resulting from exposure to heavy metals and other chemical elements of the periodic table. *Journal of Clinical Medicine, 12,* 2591. https://doi.org/10.3390/jcm12072591.

38. Madhavan, I., Balan, R. K., Asokan, B. N., Andrews, A. M., & Valliot, A., (2019). A retrospective analysis of pattern of suicide in autopsied cases in a tertiary care hospital. *Asia Pacific Journal of Medical Toxicology, 8,* 45–49. https://doi.org/10.22038/apjmt.2019.13175.

39. Marks, C. J. (2020). *The Core Competencies Required by Toxicology Students in Order to Function Effectively in a Poisons Information Center: A Delphi Study.* https://core.ac.uk/download/328346641.pdf (accessed on 9th May 2025).

40. Merry, K. J. (2010). *Murder by Poison in Scotland During the 19th and Early 20th Centuries.* https://core.ac.uk/download/282378.pdf (accessed on 9th May 2025).

41. Mishra, A., (2020). *Forensic Chemistry and Toxicology.* https://core.ac.uk/download/322580838.pdf (accessed on 9th May 2025).

42. Nițescu, V., Lescaie, A., Boghițoiu, D., & Ulmeanu, C., (2024). Benzalkonium chloride poisoning in pediatric patients: Report of case with a severe clinical course and literature review. *Toxics, 12*, 139. https://doi.org/10.3390/toxics12020139.

43. Oto, A., KILIÇ, S., & Şahin, M., (2023). Acute poisonings requiring intensive care in childhood and a hidden threat, suicide attempts: A single-center experience. *The European Research Journal, 9*, 1105–1113. https://doi.org/10.18621/eurj.1341860.

44. Pragst, F., (2025). Systematic toxicological analysis in forensic and clinical laboratories: A challenging task of analytical chemistry. *ChemTexts.* https://www.semanticscholar.org/paper/9ea88b3c70dafdaff6c1dfe3569b42da439bc82f (accessed on 9th May 2025).

45. Prodanchuk, M., & Basanets, A., (2024). The role of national toxicology centers in addressing issues of prevention, diagnosis and treatment of poisoning, toxicovigilance and chemical safety. *Ukrainian Journal of Military Medicine.* https://www.semanticscholar.org/paper/335bfab6ba968e27d9aa471eb1024a8e848d69f0 (accessed on 9th May 2025).

46. Rajan, S., & Neole, N., (2025). Green forensic toxicology: Optimizing chlordiazepoxide detection in milk, whiskey, and whiskey cream matrices. *Indian Journal of Forensic Medicine & Toxicology.* https://www.semanticscholar.org/paper/394699352df614680e98fa8548f44abe4686419d (accessed on 9th May 2025).

47. Rajasekar, K., & Vezhaventhan, D., (2024). Artificial intelligence revolutionizing legal and forensic practices: A comprehensive analysis. In *2024 15th International Conference on Computing Communication and Networking Technologies (ICCCNT).* https://www.semanticscholar.org/paper/b26e733f0a81aaef427eb2d0e3f321ccafbf3bb5 (accessed on 9th May 2025).

48. Saha, D., Dhabal, S., & Sen, D. J. (2022). Forensic science deals with safety armor during warfare explosives. *Journal of Forensic Science and Research, 6*, 24–41. https://doi.org/10.29328/journal.jfsr.1001033.

49. Singh, R. K., Singh, S., Sunil, S., & Rani, M., (2023). Household poisoning in children: Case series. *IP International Journal of Forensic Medicine and Toxicological Sciences, 7*, 148–151. https://doi.org/10.18231/j.ijfmts.2022.033.

50. Sinha, S., Rao, K. A., & Rawat, A., (2023). Forensic approach towards criminal use of mercury in domestic violence. *Sri Lanka Journal of Forensic Medicine Science & Law, 14*, 24–31. https://doi.org/10.4038/sljfmsl.v14i1.7909.

51. Tamba, A. W., & Purnomo, H., (2024). Causality teachings in planned murder crimes. *Policy Law Notary and Regulatory Issues (POLRI), 3*, 197–206. https://doi.org/10.55047/polri.v3i1.1012.

52. The Scientific Committee. (2023). Proceedings of the workshop NANO23@uniVR – 8–9 June 2023, University of Verona, Italy. *European Journal of Histochemistry, 67.* https://doi.org/10.4081/ejh.2023.3778.

METALLIC POISONS

6

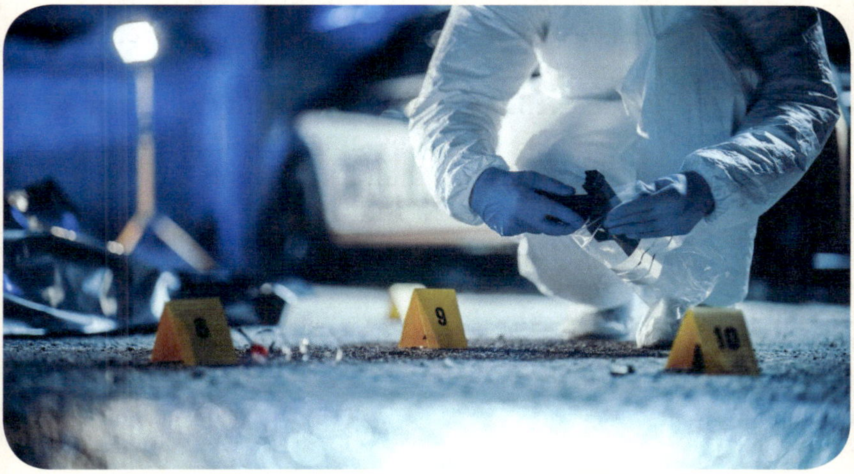

LEARNING OBJECTIVES

After studying this chapter, you will be able to:

1. Understand types of metallic poisons
2. Learn detection methods in forensics
3. Focus on case studies involving metallic poisons
4. Explain health implications and legal consequences

Introduction

Forensic science and the study of metallic toxins now seem way more intertwined in criminal justice than ever before. How these metals interact with our bodies often lights up clues during forensic exams—even if they seem small at first—shaping the direction of an investigation. Sometimes the very method used to spot these poisons can shift a case from a supposed accident to a potential homicide or even a suicide, which really shows why a careful look is so important. Police records and lab tests keep coming up as key pieces that help sketch out the patterns and behaviors behind poisoning incidents. Research emerging from places like Gilgit-Baltistan generally indicates that a step-by-step, methodical analysis can untangle cause from effect in cases where a combination of different groups and pressures leads to unfavorable outcomes (Yousafzai et al., 2024). At the same time, as modern weapons evolve—and sometimes even unintentionally carry metallic toxins—the entire forensic picture becomes even murkier, prompting experts to scrutinize every potential piece of evidence (Mulani et al., 2024).

Definition of Metallic Poisons

Environmental factors and human health have long been intertwined, and metallic pollutants have emerged as a particularly concerning aspect of that relationship. Often originating from industrial spills or natural mineral deposits, these metals tend to accumulate in living organisms and cause significant toxic issues. In simple terms, arsenic, lead, and mercury are considered metals that can significantly damage biological systems—they are infamous for their detrimental effects on both our bodies and the environment. Studying them is not just an academic matter; in most cases, it is a practical concern for forensic science, where being able to detect and measure these metals in biological samples is crucial in poisoning investigations (Merry et al., 2010). Recent strides in food safety have also highlighted how important it is to grasp how these metal risks affect our health (Dave et al., 2021). Overall, this research clearly demonstrates the urgent need for reliable detection methods in forensic work, even if the process sometimes appears somewhat complex (Figure 6.1).

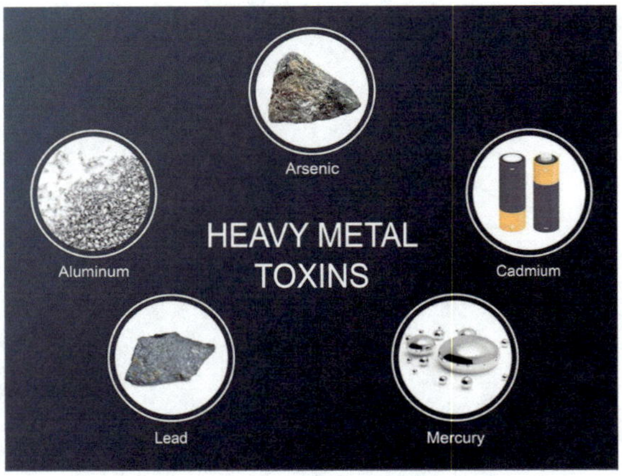

Figure 6.1. Metallic poisons are toxins.

Source: Samaterials. (n.d.). *Heavy Metals in Material Testing.* https://www.samaterials.com/img/cms/heavy-metals-1500-x-1125-opti.jpg.

Importance of Forensics in Detecting Metallic Poisons

Exploring metallic toxins in forensic science reveals a complex interplay of legal and medical concerns—especially when tests were relatively basic. In the past, poisoning events often slipped under the radar, creating big headaches for doctors and legal folks alike. Chemical tests were not really sufficient and juries, not always clued into forensic details, meant that a lot of cases ended up unsolved or misjudged (Merry et al., 2010). Generally speaking, forensic chemistry and toxicology have made significant advancements, enhancing our ability to identify these toxins and providing a more nuanced understanding of their effects on the body (Mishra et al., 2020). All in all, this evolution not only sheds light on old mysteries but also cements the essential role of forensic science in today's efforts to serve justice when dealing with metallic toxins.

Overview of Common Metallic Poisons

Metallic poisons are found everywhere, which is a significant concern for forensic work. It is kind of surprising that metals like lead, arsenic, and mercury—yes, those everyday troublemakers—can sneak into things like blood and urine, affecting human health in more ways than one. These substances slowly build up in our bodies, and in most cases, that gradual accumulation leads to chronic issues that further complicate forensic investigations. New techniques, like solid-phase microextraction or even paper-based sensors (Bordbar et al., 2021; Câmara et al., 2022), are now being used to spot these trace elements in very complex samples, and generally speaking, that is changed the game for detection. And, really, pinning down these toxins is not just about solving an individual case—it ultimately shapes public health policies and environmental safety measures, highlighting just how intertwined forensic science is with our broader societal well-being.

Historical Context of Metallic Poisons in Criminal Cases

Metallic poisons have undergone a significant shift in how courts view them, thanks in large part to decades—and even centuries—of forensic advancements. Back in the day, everyday metals like arsenic or lead got used in shady murder plots, which is why they earned a grim nickname as invisible killers. Their dangerous reactivity and toxicity, well known in both medical circles and legal cases, made these substances a longstanding concern. Examining various cases from the 19th century reveals that identifying these toxins was not straightforward; the symptoms often mimicked those of more natural illnesses, complicating investigations. In most cases, recent reviews even point out that these poisons originate from various sources, including rough mining operations and common household items (Machado and Dinis-Oliveira, 2023). All in all, this layered historical background—generally speaking—sheds light on how today's forensic methods are a lot more effective at identifying and solving poisoning cases (Barnard et al., 2024) (Figure 6.2).

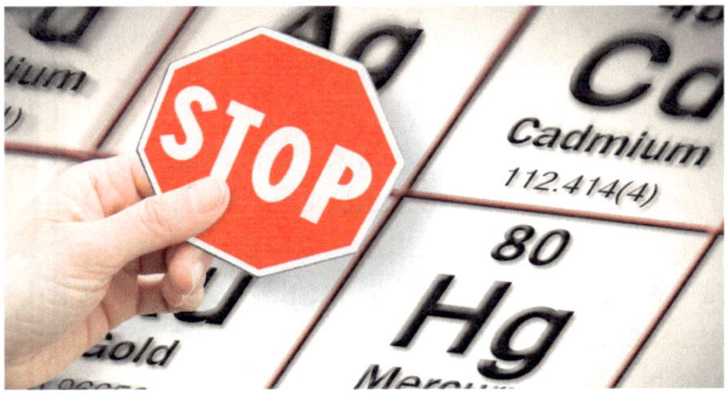

Figure 6.2. Everyday metals like arsenic or lead got used in shady murder plots, which is why they earned a grim nickname as invisible killers.

Source: Mind Your Fitness. (2020). *Heavy Metal Poisoning*. https://mindyourfitness.in/wp-content/uploads/2020/10/Heavy-Metal-Poisoing-2.png.

Scope of the Discussion

Metallic poisons in forensics are not just about identifying a substance; they have become part of a multifaceted approach that combines traditional methods with new technologies. Scientists are now busy figuring out not only how toxic these metals can be but also the many routes they take into the body—details that often turn out to be crucial clues in cracking a case. Lately, portable gadgets like biosensors and hand-held assays have begun to shake things up, giving investigators the ability to check for metals on site almost as precisely as the more cumbersome lab tests (Pohanka, 2020). In many cases, these quick methods hold their own against traditional techniques. It is also worth noting that, alongside the technical aspects, discussions about these poisons naturally drift into debates about environmental impacts and ethical concerns surrounding their use. All in all, this topic extends beyond the nuts and bolts of science, touching on broader social and ecological issues and, in turn, adding an extra layer to the forensic narrative surrounding metallic poisons.

Methodologies Used in Forensic Analysis

Forensic work relies on combining a range of advanced methods to detect metal toxins in biological samples. Mass spectrometry, for example, is a real workhorse—it detects even the tiniest traces of harmful elements and provides investigators with data they can rely on. This tool enables experts to identify distinct metal signatures in a sample, which often helps them narrow down the potential poisoning culprit. In many cases, analysts also incorporate multivariate techniques; recent studies (Casparsen, 2024) suggest that these methods help untangle complex toxicology data, making it easier for experts to interpret. Food forensics has been showing a similar trend—strict testing is necessary to detect pollutants, which clearly underscores why accredited practices matter (Banerjee, 2024). Continually finetuning these approaches is pretty essential for ramping up public safety and keeping the legal process robust, even if there are some quirks along the way.

Significance of Understanding Metallic Poisons

Metallic toxins in forensic work are not just about identifying them; they also have implications for public health and environmental safety (Figure 6.3). Technology continues to push the envelope, and with it, our methods for finding and studying these harmful substances have become significantly more effective—lab-on-a-chip devices, for example, now deliver results that are both fast and reliable. In most cases, this progress is particularly significant because it helps us identify risks associated with food safety and environmental issues, as recent studies have demonstrated by examining how metallic pollutants interact with living systems (Apostu et al., 2008).

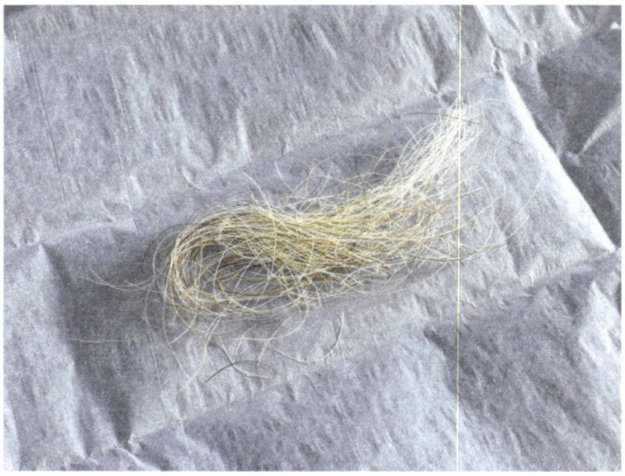

Figure 6.3. Metallic toxins in forensic work are not just about identifying them; they also have broader implications for public health and environmental safety.

Source: StoryMD. (n.d.). *Medical Research and Diagnostics.* https://cdn.storymd.com/optimized/Rda5GeQSXd/original.jpg.

It is also interesting to note that exploring how these poisons act under various conditions, ranging from typical farming practices to what occurs during food processing, provides scientists with the opportunity to develop strategies that better manage these risks (Dave et al., 2021). All in all, engaging in this type of research not only enhances forensic investigations but also helps inform public policy in ways that aim to safeguard consumers and maintain a healthy food supply.

6.1. Types of Metallic Poisons

Learning Outcome

1. Explain lead and its toxicological effects
2. Focus on mercury and its sources
3. Learn the historical and modern relevance of arsenic
4. Explain cadmium and its industrial applications
5. Describe thallium and its use in criminal cases
6. Describe barium and its health implications
7. Analyze antimony and its detection methods
8. Know chromium and its environmental impact
9. Compare the toxicity levels of various metallic poisons

Metallic toxins like lead, arsenic, and mercury have a peculiar connection with forensic analysis—it is all about understanding what makes each one tick. You might notice that these poisons, by nature, present different challenges. Take lead poisoning, for instance; in most cases, it comes from everyday exposures at work or from environmental contamination, which can lead to long-term health issues and, when doses are high, sudden, acute toxicity. Arsenic, carrying a dark history in cases of homicide, ends up serving both as a poison and a forensic marker because it is usually found in body tissues—a fact that turns it into a kind of double-edged tool. Mercury, often associated with industrial settings and its tendency to accumulate over time, raises serious concerns about its impact on the nervous system and overall bodily functions. New lab methods—such as pairing SEM with EDS—have enhanced our ability to detect these metals in biological samples, thereby refining forensic investigations and legal decisions (Nunziata et al., 2025). All in all, the study of these metallic toxins remains a key research area, supported by statistically significant data on poisoning death rates and shifting demographic trends (Bartoshyk, 2024).

6.1.1. Lead and Its Toxicological Effects

Lead contaminates our surroundings in ways that pose real health risks, especially when forensic tests need to spot metallic toxins (Figure 6.4).

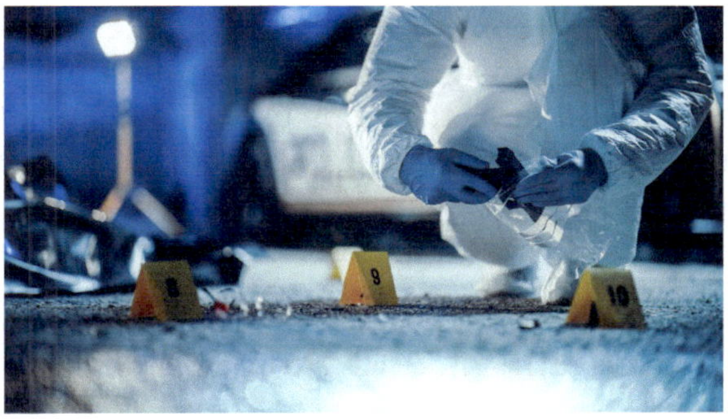

Figure 6.4. Lead contaminates our surroundings in ways that pose real health risks, especially when forensic tests are needed to detect metallic toxins.

Source: Alarid, M. (n.d.). *Forensics Mistakes.* https://irp.cdn-website.com/caf4330a/dms3rep/multi/forensics+mistakes+-+Michael+Alarid.jpeg.

Once it enters our system, it disrupts key bodily functions – including nerve signals, blood production, and even kidney function. Its effects on the brain can pop up as lapses in thinking and odd behavior in severe cases, it might even trigger something like encephalopathy, which is particularly worrisome for kids with still-developing brains. Even low doses seem to leave noticeable marks on intelligence and mood, suggesting that no exposure level is entirely safe. Forensic work often relies on detecting traces of lead in samples, underscoring its close connection to toxicology and investigative practices. Recent studies (Mishra et al., 2020) demonstrate that when toxins like lead are grouped together, the serious health dangers become clear—so detecting them early and acting promptly is key.

6.1.2. Mercury and Its Sources

Mercury played a curious role in history, combining its ready availability with the emerging field of forensic science. Back in the late 1800s, people used mercury as a common remedy—primarily for syphilis—which meant it was easy to get in the medical world. Yet, this ready access came at a steep cost; sadly, its toxic side effects soon reared their head, triggering a host of health issues like mercury poisoning that experts could not ignore. Over time, as people began to grasp the dangers of various toxins, trailblazers in toxicology—Thomas Scattergood being one of them—began documenting these troubling cases involving mercury and other harmful substances (Sellers et al., 2019). Soon, legal rules surrounding poisons shifted, leaving both jurors and doctors in most cases perplexed about how to distinguish between mercury poisoning and other ailments (Merry et al., 2010). All in all, the combination of easy access, rising toxicity, and evolving forensic methods effectively highlights just how intricately mercury became entwined in the story of forensic science.

6.1.3. Arsenic: Historical and Modern Relevance

Arsenic has intrigued people for centuries—long before modern labs existed, folks recognized its dangerous side. In fact, it was not just known as a poison; it found its way into everyday remedies and even served as a pigment in art, an unexpected twist in its colorful history. Some notorious cases, especially those involving high-society intrigue, really put it in the spotlight as a deadly substance. Today, we still worry about arsenic because traces of it end up contaminating our water supplies and the environment; recent studies have attempted to clarify just how complex the issues of ecological health and toxin exposure can be. Generally speaking, arsenic's harmful impact on cell processes has been linked to major disorders across various systems—a fact that keeps forensic toxicologists busy (Machado and Dinis-Oliveira, 2023). All in all, learning about arsenic not only uncovers quirky historical facts but also informs how modern science addresses public health challenges in an ever-changing world (Figure 6.5).

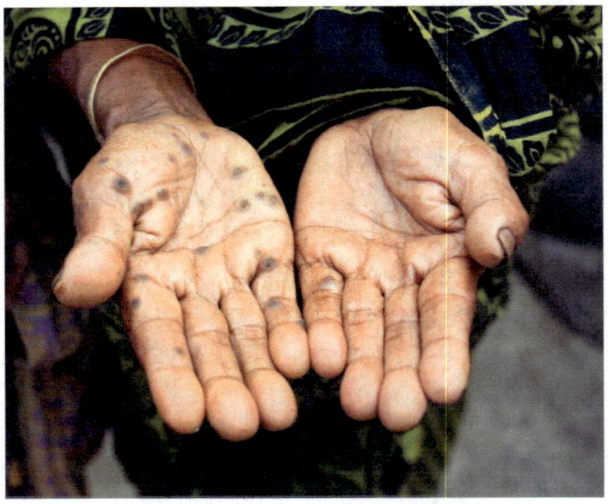

Figure 6.5. Arsenic toxins.

Source: Wikipedia Contributors. (n.d.). *Arsenic Poisoning.* https://upload.wikimedia.org/wikipedia/commons/thumb/2/24/Arsenic_Poisoning.jpg/800px-Arsenic_Poisoning.jpg.

6.1.4. Cadmium and Its Industrial Applications

Industrial activities can impact our health and the world we live in in ways that may not always be apparent. Take cadmium, for example—a heavy metal used in various applications, such as electronics, batteries, and pigments—which, despite its usefulness, poses serious toxic issues. Cadmium's benefits sometimes hide its risks; exposure is linked to problems like kidney damage and a higher chance of cancer, a fact that keeps health experts and environmental agencies on high alert. Research has shown that in many water samples, cadmium levels end up far exceeding the safety thresholds set by organizations like the U.S.E.P.A, which is pretty concerning. It does not end there: this metal also tends to accumulate in food crops, meaning that even small amounts in our food can become a problem (Awasthi et al., 2022). Generally speaking, cadmium appears to play a dual role—as a useful industrial tool and, at the same time, a hazardous pollutant—and understanding its use is crucial when developing strategies in both forensics and public health. Ultimately, examining the application of cadmium in industry helps us strike a balance between its practical benefits and the risks it poses, a crucial consideration for protecting both human health and the environment.

6.1.5. Thallium and Its Use in Criminal Cases

Thallium is a curious heavy metal that has had its share of involvement in criminal forensics over the years. It pops up in everyday industrial settings, but in certain homicide cases, quietly does its work as a poison. Generally speaking, victims might show a mix of symptoms – from upset stomachs to nerve troubles – that often resemble common illnesses or less alarming issues, making it tricky for investigators. Usually, doctors only catch on once an autopsy uncovers unexpectedly high levels of the metal (Machado and Dinis-Oliveira, 2023). In most cases, forensic specialists rely on detailed toxic tests, which can ultimately tip the scales in a case (Barnard et al., 2024). All in all, understanding thallium's elusive behavior is crucial, as its sneaky nature can mask problems until it is almost too late, leaving everyone a little off balance in the investigation (Figure 6.6).

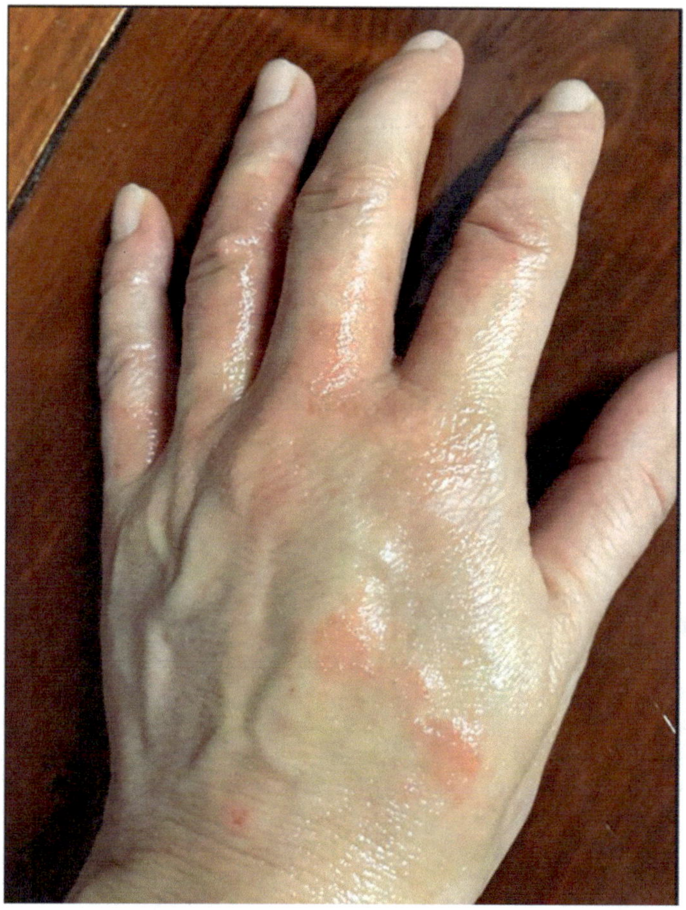

Figure 6.6. *Thallium* poisoning.

Source: MDPI. (2025). *Chemical Structure and Properties.* https://www.mdpi.com/applsci/applsci-15-01732/article_deploy/html/images/applsci-15-01732-g001.png.

6.1.6. Barium and Its Health Implications

Barium is present in nearly every aspect of our environment, and it is beginning to raise significant concerns—especially in areas where mining and intensive farming are prevalent. People usually end up exposed to it through water and food that have been tainted, and in turn, this exposure can lead to a host of problems, like trouble breathing and upset stomachs. Research now and then shows that barium levels in soils can exceed safe limits, a pattern notably observed in areas such as the Pine Ridge Reservation (Kant et al., 2013), where a long history of mining has significantly altered both the soil and the plants. Even more, barium's toxic behavior is quite complex; generally speaking, figuring out exactly how it moves and messes with health calls for a close, forensic-style look. When experts uncover barium as a likely toxic culprit in investigations—especially in puzzling cases of illness or unexpected deaths—it becomes clear that more in-depth studies of poisonous exposure are in order (Sylvia et al., 2017). Altogether, these issues remind us that environmental science, public health, and forensic medicine are surprisingly, and perhaps inevitably, intertwined.

6.1.7. Antimony and Its Detection Methods

Antimony detection is a key player in forensic work—this metal's toxic properties and its tendency to contaminate various sites make it a constant concern (Figure 6.7). People have long relied on methods such as atomic absorption spectroscopy (AAS) and inductively coupled plasma mass spectrometry (ICP-MS) to measure antimony in biological and environmental samples; these approaches, in most cases, provide the precision and sensitivity required for forensic analysis. Lately, there has been some notable progress on the electrochemical front, where detection techniques are becoming increasingly sophisticated enough to detect even the smallest traces of this hazardous element. For instance, innovative microelectrodeposition methods that utilize bubble walls have, quite interestingly, shown that they can rapidly detect trace amounts—a finding that adds a fresh twist to toxicology in criminal investigations. Additionally, new real-time monitoring systems now enable experts to check antimony levels on-site, which may impact legal outcomes and public health strategies. All in all, these mixed approaches highlight why having flexible, robust detection systems are so important when dealing with stubborn metal toxins like antimony (Fahemi et al., 2024; Herman et al., 2025).

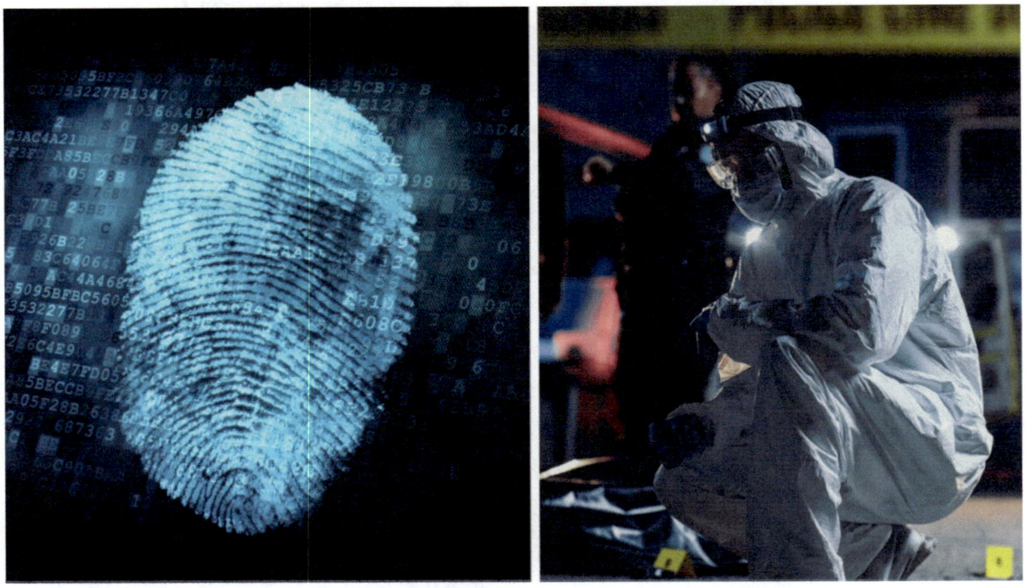

Figure 6.7. Antimony detection is a real key player in forensic work.

Source: Interesting Engineering. (2024). *Antimony Chemical Structure*. https://cms.interestingengineering.com/wp-content/uploads/2024/09/antimony-7.png?w=1920.

6.1.8. Chromium and Its Environmental Impact

Chromium appears in many environments, which alone makes it something we need to examine closely in forensic work. This metal, classified as a transition element, is highly toxic—especially when it is in its hexavalent state—and it often contaminates soil and water due to industrial leaks and improper waste disposal practices. Such pollution can severely impact ecosystems and even human populations, so experts tend to check environmental samples for any trace of chromium. Its harmful effects on water life only add to the complexity, meaning we have to dig a bit deeper into how it moves through nature and affects living systems. For instance, everyday human activities release chromium into the environment, which then disrupts key nutrient and carbon cycles essential for aquatic health. Looking back at chromium's long use in public health, it is clear that updating classification methods can help forensic research better allocate necessary resources (Barnard et al., 2024). All in all, chromium is not just another number in a lab test—it ties together industrial practices, ecosystem balance, and public safety in ways that we cannot afford to ignore.

6.1.9. Comparison of Toxicity Levels Among Metallic Poisons

Understanding how different metallic toxins affect our system is a significant concern in forensic toxicology—exposure can, in most cases, be extremely hazardous. Heavy metals like lead and mercury disrupt cell functions; they even displace essential minerals, which only exacerbates their harmful effects. Mercury poisoning, for example, can cause deep neurological issues and even organ failure, making affected animals unsafe for human consumption because of the risk these toxins pose (Acheampong et al., 2023).

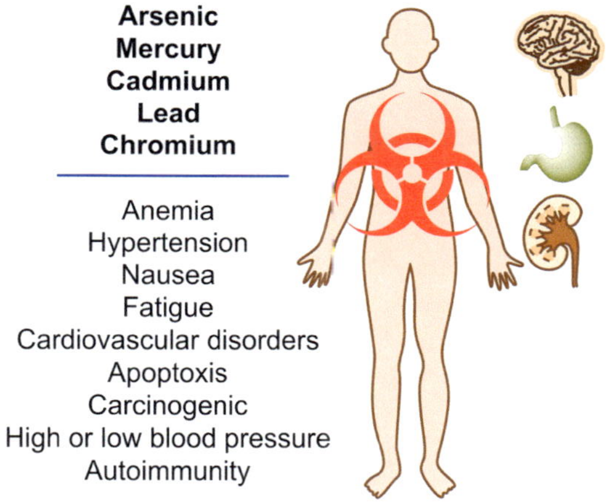

Figure 6.8. Heavy metals like lead and mercury mess with cell functions; they even shove essential minerals out of place, which only ramps up their harmful effects.

Source: ResearchGate. (2023). *Adverse Health Effects of Heavy Metals: Mercury, Cadmium, and Lead.*

On the other hand, lead exposure ends up being linked to problems in cognitive development and has been tied to a host of health issues in both kids and adults. Since forensic investigations tend to assess not only the presence of these poisons but also their potential impact on a living system, comparing toxicity levels in a nuanced manner becomes essential for gauging risks and fine-tuning remediation efforts in contaminated environments (Krzysztof et al., 2022) (Figure 6.8).

Test Your Knowledge

1. What is a metallic poison?
2. Name four common metallic poisons.

6.2. Detection Methods in Forensics

Learning Outcome

1. Learn analytical techniques for identifying metallic poisons
2. Explain the role of mass spectrometry in forensic analysis
3. Know the use of atomic absorption spectroscopy
4. Focus on the application of x-ray fluorescence
5. Know the importance of sample preparation
6. Identify challenges in detecting metallic poisons
7. Describe advances in detection technology
8. Discuss case studies showcasing detection methods
9. Understand future trends in forensic detection

Forensics has come a long way in identifying metallic toxins that are often undetectable on standard tests. These poisons often evade normal detection, so experts have had to develop specialized methods to catch them. One interesting approach utilizes electrochemical analysis to detect even the tiniest traces; for example, a steady bubble barrier can facilitate the microelectrodeposition of metallic films, making sample analysis significantly more sensitive (Fahemi et al., 2024). Live forensic techniques also come into play—using tools like Wireshark on network data demonstrates that forensic science is not limited to the lab, blending technology with traditional methods (Herman et al., 2025). In most cases, combining these modern tactics not only speeds up and sharpens the detection of metallic poisons but also gives criminal probes and public safety a much-needed boost.

6.2.1. Analytical Techniques for Identifying Metallic Poisons

Forensic labs often face a challenging task when it comes to detecting metallic toxins (Figure 6.9). Experts sometimes rely on ultra-sensitive methods—take ICP-MS, for example—that can pick up even the tiniest trace elements in a biological sample, which really ups the trustworthiness of toxicology tests. Other approaches, such as atomic absorption spectrophotometry (AAS) and gas chromatography-mass spectrometry (GC-MS), also provide clues about the chemical composition of poisons like mercuric chloride.

The way mercuric chloride poisoning shows up in patients is often pretty complex, making it all the more important to have methods that can tell different types of intoxication apart so clinicians and legal teams can respond more effectively. In most cases, recent studies have also pointed to the promise of nanomaterials—platinum nanoparticles, for instance, with their unique properties offer new angles for detecting metallic contaminants (Jeyaraj et al., 2019). All in all, combining these robust analytical techniques is indispensable when tackling the challenges that metallic poisons pose in forensic investigations (Cappelletti et al., 2019).

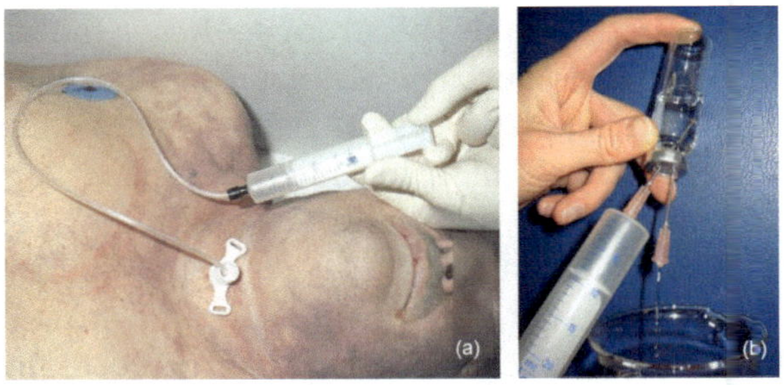

Figure 6.9. Forensic labs often face a tough job when it comes to spotting metallic toxins.

Source: Springer Nature. (2024). *Figure Illustrating Research Findings*. https://media.springernature.com/lw685/springer-static/image/art%3A10.1007%2Fs40828-024-00197-w/MediaObjects/40828_2024_197_Fig18_HTML.jpg.

6.2.2. Role of Mass Spectrometry in Forensic Analysis

Forensic science has come a long way, and now it needs sharper tools for toxicology tests. Mass spectrometry, for example, has increasingly become a go-to method—especially when trying to track down metallic toxins like arsenic and mercury, which can be particularly challenging at times. It pinpoints molecular details and measures quantities so effectively that the whole process becomes smoother, often yielding results that feel both dependable and robust. Back in the day, even before the Marsh test was established, heated debates about detecting arsenic led people to recognize the value of expert input in forensic work (Caudill et al., 2009). Today, as questions about expert competence continue to arise in legal cases, there is a growing push for rigorous methods and a system that demands accountability (Caudill et al., 2009). With its refined capabilities, mass spectrometry not only helps find these metallic poisons but also reinforces the trust we place in forensic evidence.

6.2.3. Use of Atomic Absorption Spectroscopy

Metallic poisons in forensic science are notoriously complex, and they require methods that are remarkably precise in both detection and quantification. Atomic absorption spectroscopy (AAS) often excels in this area, thanks to its impressive sensitivity in detecting even trace amounts of harmful metals. This technique is based on a straightforward idea—that free atoms absorb light—, allowing analysts to gauge metal levels in a variety of materials, from blood and other biological fluids to environmental samples. In many cases, its rapid turnaround and minimal sample prep give labs a leg up in getting results fast—something no one really wants to miss. Occasionally, through wedded integration with additional steps, such as liquid-liquid extraction, the overall precision of the analysis receives a noticeable boost, ensuring that metallic toxins do not slip by unnoticed (Rajan et al., 2025). Forensic toxicology is receiving increased attention these days, which generally points to AAS as a key tool in unraveling poisoning cases and in holding toxic substances legally accountable in criminal investigations (Tekin et al., 2023) (Figure 6.10).

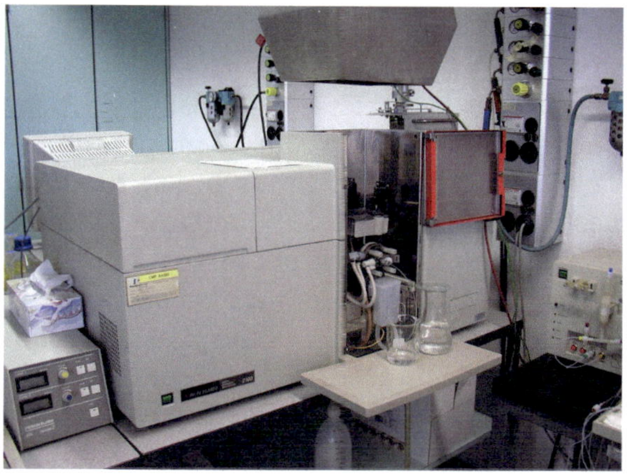

Figure 6.10. Atomic absorption spectroscopy (AAS).

Source: Wikipedia Contributors. (n.d.). *Flame Atomic Absorption Spectrometry.* https://upload.wikimedia.org/wikipedia/commons/thumb/5/51/FlammenAAS.jpg/1200px-FlammenAAS.jpg.

6.2.4. Application of X-Ray Fluorescence

Advanced analytical methods have significantly enhanced the examination of forensic materials. X-ray fluorescence (XRF) is a prime example—it identifies the elements present in a sample without damaging it, which comes in handy when searching for metallic toxins in various specimens. In most cases, this approach enables lab experts to detect even tiny amounts of heavy metals that are known to harm the environment and accumulate in food chains, thereby disrupting the ecological balance (Joseph et al., 2023). Its sharp accuracy also helps reveal toxic substances in biological samples, offering clues about possible exposure routes, especially in individuals who might have encountered organophosphorus compounds (Shajhutdinova et al., 2022). All these factors, taken together, show just how vital the role of XRF is in linking environmental toxins to human health outcomes.

6.2.5. Importance of Sample Preparation

Forensic work on metallic toxins largely depends on how you handle the sample preparation—it is a stage that can make or break the entire investigation (Figure 6.11). Generally speaking, getting a sample ready is not just about isolating the compounds you need; it also sharpens the sensitivity and selectivity of the tests that follow. New ideas, such as GreETs (green extraction techniques), are emerging as innovative ways to accelerate and improve the process, aligning with today's green chemistry principles (Câmara et al., 2022).

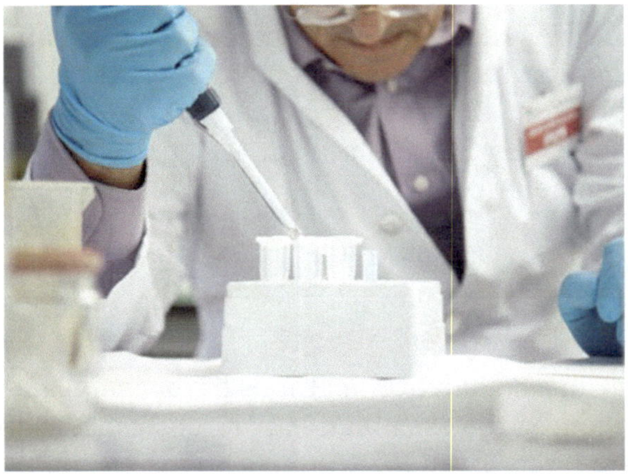

Figure 6.11. Forensic work on metallic toxins largely depends on how you handle the sample preparation—it is a stage that can make or break the entire investigation.

Source: Labcompare. (n.d.). *Laboratory Analysis Equipment.* https://media.labcompare.com/m/53/article/577530.jpg.

There is also a growing interest in using nanoparticles—particularly platinum ones (PtNPs)—due to their exceptional catalytic abilities, which aid in the detection of toxic metals during analysis (Jeyaraj et al., 2019). In most cases, paying careful attention to how samples are prepped is not just a minor detail; it is a critical step that underpins the trustworthiness and accuracy of later results when it comes to pinpointing metallic poisons in different settings.

6.2.6. Challenges in Detecting Metallic Poisons

Forensic work on metallic poisons is not exactly straightforward. There is a jumble of issues when trying to flag these compounds—each metal behaves in its own quirky way when it comes to toxicity, meaning that a standard detection approach often falls short. Old-school methods sometimes struggle to capture nuance, which can lead to misidentifications. And then you have factors like natural degradation or even a bit of contamination muddying the waters in biological samples, making it all even more uncertain. Some folks are turning to newer ideas—biosensors, for example. These nifty devices, which blend nanotech magic with everyday chemistry, are enhancing our ability to detect heavy metals with greater sensitivity and accuracy. Even so, despite these cool strides forward, there is still a long road ahead before we have biosensors that are both simple to use and really effective across the board, as noted by (Gao, 2024). At the end of the day, getting reliable results hinges not just on having fancy tech but also on setting up solid protocols that can handle all these messy variables, as Likitha et al. (2025) remind us. In most cases, that mix of inventive devices and well-thought-out methods is what will eventually clear up this challenging landscape.

6.2.7. Advances in Detection Technology

Forensic science has come a long way – it is no longer just about old methods, but a richer mix of techniques now helps spot metallic poisons in unexpected ways. Take ambient ionization mass spectrometry (AIMS); it quickly analyzes samples in their natural state, so you do not need to spend hours on tedious preparation or slog through chromatographic separation (Henderson et al., 2024). This jump in technology speeds up the detection of toxic substances and allows investigators to check things on the spot, rather than waiting in the lab. In most cases, forensic dentistry has also stepped up, offering additional, dependable ways to identify cases when traditional approaches are insufficient (Emam, 2024). Together, these breakthroughs signal a significant turning point in how metallic poisons are detected, boosting both the overall efficiency and precision of forensic investigations (Figure 6.12).

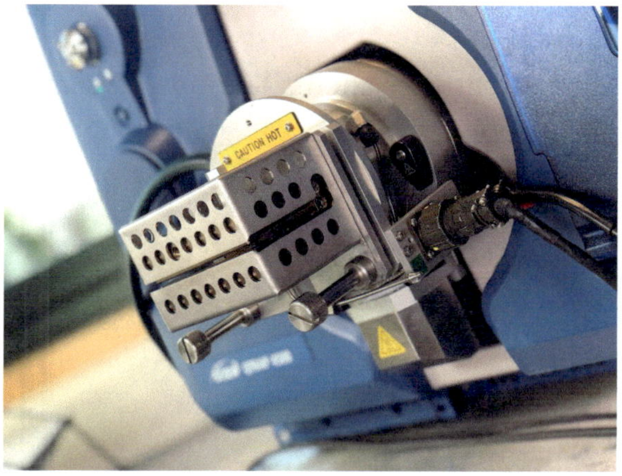

Figure 6.12. Ambient ionization mass spectrometry (AIMS).

Source: Mass Spec Analytical. (2019). *Mass Spec® and SCIEX® Share Fast Forensic Solutions.* https://www.msaltd.co.uk/getattachment/4503106c-4dbd-4476-93db-e6e5fff5bed6/Mass-Spec%C2%AE-and-SCIEX%C2%AE-Share-Fast-Forensic-Solution.aspx.

6.2.8. Case Studies Showcasing Detection Methods

Early efforts to pinpoint metallic poisons sparked both notable scientific fixes and heated debates in forensic science. Historical accounts reveal that experts once struggled to detect substances like arsenic—long before reliable methods, such as the Marsh test, were developed. Critics generally argued that these professionals lacked the necessary expertise during trials, and they were, at times, even called "mad alchemists," a label that hints at the uneasy mix between fresh scientific breakthroughs and public doubt. Examining things from different angles reveals that the varied approaches and underlying divisions in understanding have long influenced forensic practices. These echoes from the past remain relevant today, with modern detection methods in cases of metallic poisoning sometimes drawing similar charges of pride and moral uncertainty (Caudill et al., 2009).

6.2.9. Future Trends in Forensic Detection

Forensic detection has come a long way—especially when it comes to metallic poisons, those elusive substances that used to trip up investigators because they hide so well, and chemical tests are really complicated. Back in the day, detecting these toxins was a major challenge, but now methods like mass spectrometry and upgraded chromatographic techniques enable labs to detect even the tiniest traces in biological samples (Merry et al., 2010). In many cases, the mix of artificial intelligence and machine learning into everyday forensic routines has made it easier to pinpoint toxic compounds and cut down on human slip-ups, generally speaking making the whole process a bit more reliable. With growing concerns over food safety—contaminants sometimes slipping in during processing—food toxicologists have become increasingly important, bridging the gap between rigid legal standards and emerging scientific advances. All in all, these shifts point to a lively, ever-changing scene in forensic science, where detecting metallic poisons in various scenarios continues to become more effective, even if things are not always perfectly neat and tidy (Figure 6.13).

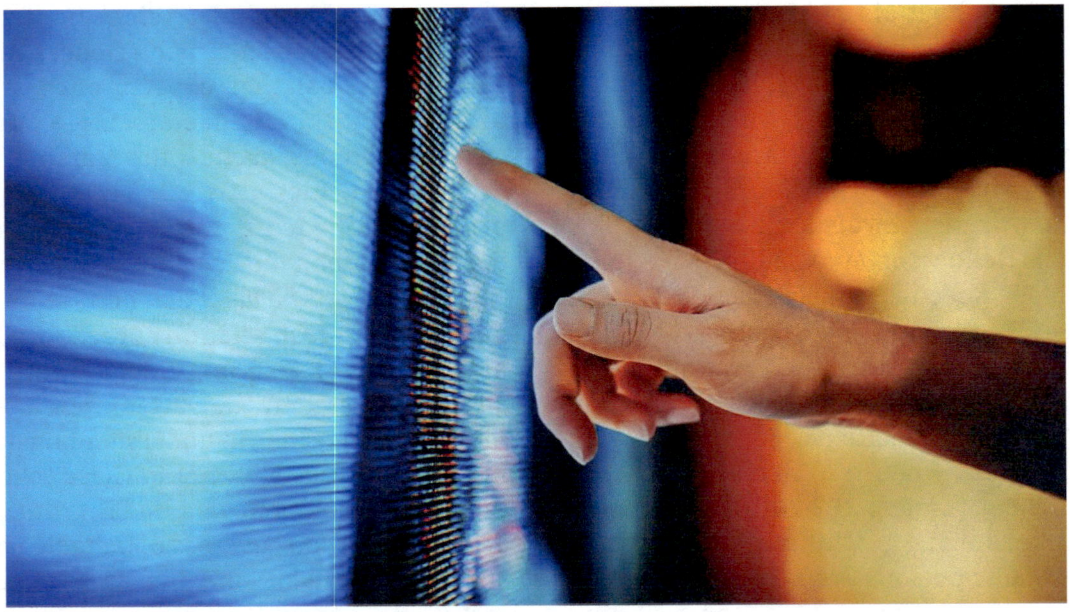

Figure 6.13. The mix of artificial intelligence and machine learning into everyday forensic routines has made it easier to pinpoint toxic compounds and cut down on human slip-ups, generally speaking, making the whole process a bit more reliable.

Source: Telefónica Tech. (2025). *Modern SOC Cyber Auto.* https://media.telefonicatech.com/telefonicatech/uploads/2025/2/modern-soc-cyber-auto_telefonica-tech.jpg.

Test Your Knowledge

1. What is the principle behind atomic absorption spectroscopy (AAS) in metal detection?
2. Which technique is commonly used for screening multiple heavy metals simultaneously?

6.3. Case Studies Involving Metallic Poisons

Learning Outcome

1. Discuss notable historical cases of arsenic poisoning
2. Explain modern cases involving lead poisoning
3. Learn about thallium poisoning in criminal investigations
4. Know mercury exposure in environmental cases
5. Understand cadmium-related health crises
6. Describe forensic analysis in high-profile cases
7. Know the legal implications of metallic poison cases
8. Discuss the role of forensic experts in court
9. Focus on lessons learned from case studies

Metallic poisoning investigations mix fields in a way that can really catch you off guard. One striking example is that of a young, large-breed dog discovered dead—clearly it had endured both physical abuse and a dose of poison. Lab tests later picked up rodenticide levels in its liver; this showed, in most cases, that a deliberate attack and toxic exposure were tangled up together (Pesce et al., 2025).

Other reports even hint that different bio-toxic compounds can lead to unusually intricate poisoning scenarios. Take toad toxin: it has been used in medicine for its heart-protecting, anti-inflammatory perks, yet under certain conditions it can flip to dangerous territory, blurring the line between therapy and toxicity (Liu et al., 2025). All in all, these examples generally emphasize the need for solid forensic expertise to detect metal-based toxins—helping to inform criminal probes and spark a broader conversation about how such poisons affect both animals and humans.

6.3.1. Notable Historical Cases of Arsenic Poisoning

Arsenic has a dark reputation, having appeared in a range of historical accounts where its deadly effects are unmistakably demonstrated. You might recall the early 1900s—George Joseph Smith, for instance, murdered his own scheme by using arsenic to get rid of them in a cash bid, a clear display of its use for very personal ends. Cases like this generally reveal not only the bad intentions behind such poisonings but also the real struggles forensic experts face when trying to catch every trace. Over time, the ways we pick up arsenic have shifted, mirroring our clumsy yet growing grasp of toxins, as far back as Paracelsus, who noted how dose makes the poison centuries ago (Saganuwan, 2017). And as forensic science continues to untangle the messy details of metal poisons, old episodes like Smith's remind us that arsenic's role in crime and even in medicine has always been insidious, offering us a peek into how society tends to react when faced with such dangerous substances (Siddall, 2018) (Figure 6.14).

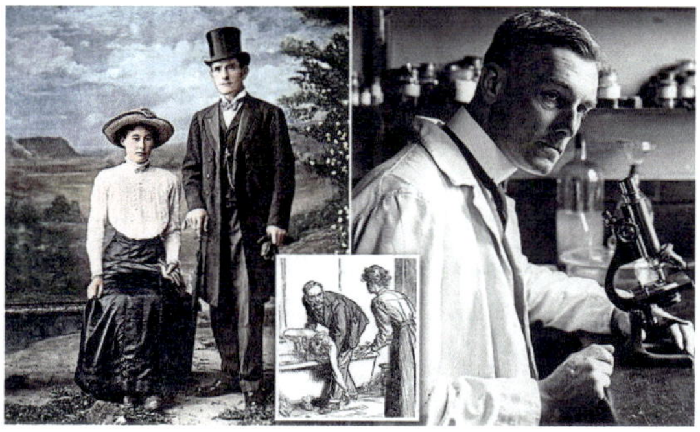

Figure 6.14. In the early 1900s, George Joseph Smith wedded his own scheme by using arsenic to get rid of his wives in a bid for cash, a clear display of its use for very personal ends.

Source: Daily Mail. (2020). *Image of a Person with Protective Gear*. https://i.dailymail.co.uk/1s/2020/04/20/01/27397764-0-image-a-140_1587344214222.jpg.

6.3.2. Modern Cases Involving Lead Poisoning

Analytical chemistry has a long history in forensics, and it is key when dealing with lead poisoning cases today. Lead, which often appears due to crumbling pipes or old lead-based paint, presents its own set of challenges that keep forensic teams on their toes. In many cases, experts don't just grab a sample and run a test—they work carefully to gather evidence and mix modern toxic tests with old-school techniques, aiming to figure out where the lead started and how far it has spread. In urban areas, sources of lead can appear unexpectedly, ranging from faulty plumbing to emissions from nearby factories, making the issue even more complex. And since lead sticks around in the environment for ages—making it harder to tell if poisoning happened suddenly or over time—comprehensive, sometimes repeated analyses become a must. Forensic professionals, who must thoroughly understand the nuances of metallic toxins, especially lead, must work through these puzzles to determine if a case is accidental, self-inflicted, or a deliberate act (Verma, 2018; Paixão, 2019).

6.3.3. Thallium Poisoning in Criminal Investigations

Thallium poisoning in criminal cases can really upend an investigation (Figure 6.15). The toxin creeps in with these subtle, almost sneaky effects, making you scratch your head over what is really happening. Exposure may trigger a complex array of neurological issues, leaving doctors and forensic teams to piece together clues, and sometimes, things can be misinterpreted (Blain et al., 2024). It is not unusual for symptoms caused by different toxins to be overlooked, resulting in delayed diagnosis and treatment. Often, the real struggle is matching a messy clinical picture with hard lab evidence—especially when thallium is not even suspected at first glance. Some past studies have even suggested that cases we would attribute to agricultural chemicals may actually conceal a thallium component, highlighting the complexity of toxicology (Anas et al., 2016). As detection methods continue to improve, identifying thallium as the culprit could make a significant difference in solving these complex cases.

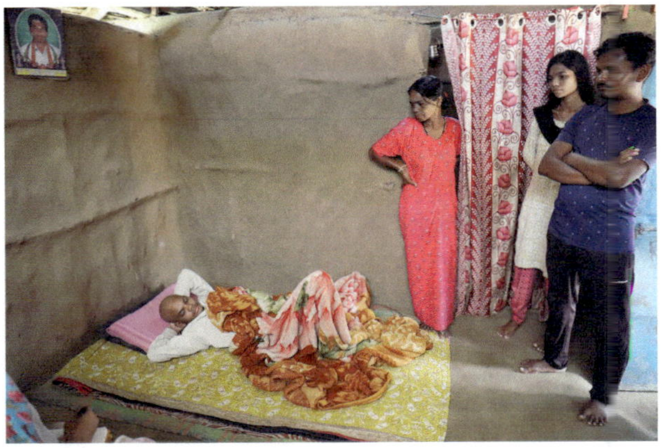

Figure 6.15. Thallium poisoning in criminal investigations.

Source: The Hindu. (n.d.). *Photograph of Unidentified Subject.* https://th-i.thgim.com/public/incoming/8gv2x5/article67467106.ece/alternates/FREE_1200/IMG_1227.JPG.

6.3.4. Mercury Exposure in Environmental Cases

Mercury poisoning has a profound impact on communities—especially those already vulnerable. Take the English-Wabigoon River in Ontario, for example; decades ago, Dryden Chemical Company casually dumped waste there, and soon local fish began carrying dangerously high levels of methylmercury, leaving the Grassy Narrows First Nations community to bear the brunt of the fallout. Generally speaking, research by Mergler et al. shows that mercury's nasty aftereffects can ripple through families, with mental health issues and even a boost in suicide risk cropping up over three generations—a sign of just how intertwined cultural practices and local diets are with the state of the environment (Rothenberg, 2023). In most cases, mercury's extensive damage draws uneasy parallels with arsenic exposure, which has been linked to gene mutations and developmental issues (Li et al., 2022). All in all, these troubling findings prompt a more in-depth forensic investigation into mercury toxicity and a serious call for environmental cleanup and broader public awareness.

6.3.5. Cadmium-Related Health Crises

Cadmium contamination illustrates how unchecked industrial practices can significantly impact our environment (Figure 6.16). Industries growing too fast—with little oversight—have led places like the Sonoran Desert to face unsettling metal pollution; local ecosystems end up caught in the fallout of these massive industrial moves.

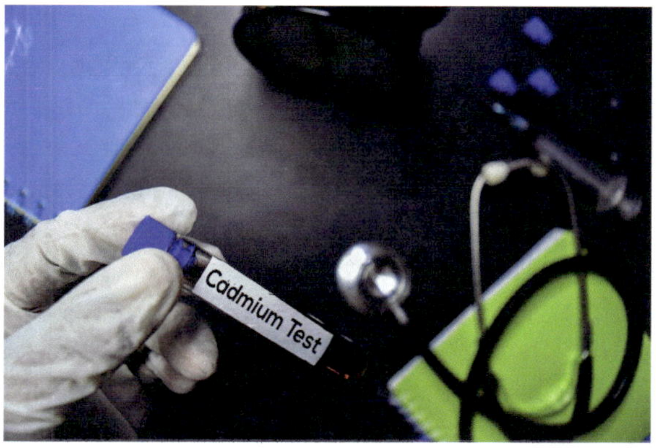

Figure 6.16. Cadmium-related health crises.

Source: GrassrootsHealth. (2020). *Cadmium Test Image.* https://www.grassrootshealth.net/wp-content/uploads/2020/06/cadmium-test.jpg.

Research generally tells us that cadmium, known for being seriously harmful, tends to hit the most vulnerable folks even harder, causing issues like kidney problems and a boost in cancer risks. The backstory here is also quite troubling: urban sprawl and industrial expansion, often driven by economic pressures that sometimes prioritize profit over public safety, have paved the way for this toxic legacy. At the same time, as rules and regulations slowly catch up, cadmium's legal status remains murky, which only makes cleanup efforts even tougher on communities already struggling (Kamel et al., 2023). All in all, these intertwined challenges truly necessitate a multifaceted, multidisciplinary approach to mitigate the toxic effects of cadmium exposure.

6.3.6. Forensic Analysis in High-Profile Cases

High-profile legal cases often rest on forensic work that zeroes in on metallic poisons. When poisoning is even suspected—such as in instances involving organophosphorus compounds—a detailed forensic investigation becomes absolutely essential to determine whether toxins are present. Generally speaking, studies suggest irritant poisons, particularly those encountered in farming settings, play a significant role in fatal outcomes. It is important to remember that past struggles with subpar testing methods and jurors' occasional difficulty in grasping toxic details further muddle these cases; forensic experts, therefore, must sometimes juggle complex explanations to deliver clear, scientifically backed evidence in court (Merry et al., 2010). All in all, forensic analysis in these poisoning cases not only tilts legal verdicts but also shines a light on broader issues about how we manage and regulate dangerous substances.

6.3.7. Legal Implications of Metallic Poison Cases

Forensic science has long navigated the complex world of legal disputes, particularly when cases involve toxic metals—think of the debates that erupted over expert testimony. Courts began relying heavily on scientific evidence, so ensuring that arsenic-detection methods worked as claimed became crucial. Back in the day, critics pointed out serious flaws in these techniques; before the Marsh test even showed up, such shortcomings often undermined legal cases built on shaky science. Today, you will still hear heated conversations about the expertise of experts and the heavy ethical burdens they carry. In most cases, when overconfident professionals make mistakes, it is not just their own standing that is at risk, but the entire legal process can suffer, occasionally leading to grave miscarriages of justice. Interestingly, the tug-of-war between complex empirical data and more personal interpretations still lingers, proving that controversies of the past—like those tied to metallic poisons—continue to echo in modern discussions on forensic evidence and its legal fallout (Caudill et al., 2009).

6.3.8. Role of Forensic Experts in Court

Forensic know-how and courtroom drama get pretty tangled up, especially when heavy poisons like arsenic are involved. In many cases, when toxicology becomes particularly complex, experts step in to untangle the details; they translate a jumble of lab findings into something the court can actually use. Looking back, there were times—long before tests like Marsh's became the norm—when debates over arsenic detection showed just how tricky it was to juggle solid science and the demands of legal proof. Some critics, generally speaking, remind us that relying too heavily on these expert accounts can backfire; they point to recurring hints of overconfidence and questionable moral judgment from early 19th-century trials right up to today's forensic discussions (Caudill et al., 2009). All of this kind of underscores the need to really scrutinize how forensic methods are carried out—because even a minor slip-up in expertise might throw off a trial's balance, and that can seriously derail the quest for justice when toxic metals are on the line (Caudill et al., 2009) (Figure 6.17).

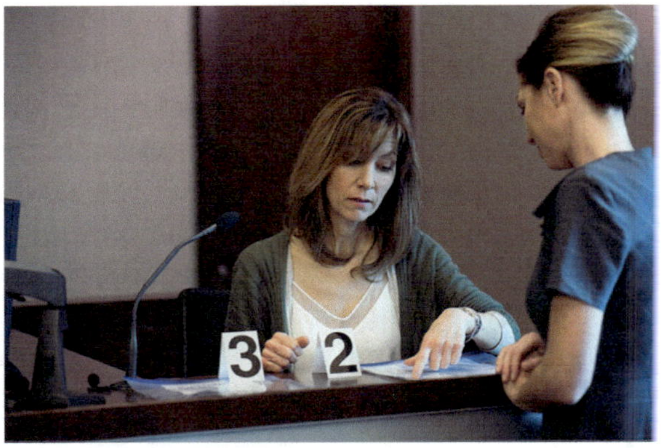

Figure 6.17. Role of forensic experts in court.

Source: Wiley Interdisciplinary Reviews. (n.d.). *Front Cover Image for WIREs Forensic Science*. Wiley Online Library. https://wires.onlinelibrary.wiley.com/cms/asset/4b95d08c-d015-4bf5-8e8f-4c66a601465d/wfs21320-toc-0001-m.jpg.

6.3.9. Lessons Learned from Case Studies

Metallic toxin analysis in forensic cases can get surprisingly tricky—case studies, for one, throw a lot of light on just how much we need a blend of different expert insights. Each investigation offers its own unique perspective on how these substances behave in living systems, and they continually remind us that relying on cutting-edge detection methods is essentially a necessity. For example, running neutron and X-ray experiments simultaneously has, in many cases, opened up new ways to understand how these materials interact (Hjelm et al., 2024). Sometimes the data turns out to be ambiguous, which highlights the need for solid frameworks that encompass both the detailed chemical aspects and the broader context (Gurr et al., 2023). Ultimately, the main takeaway is that a thorough analysis is not only key to understanding the exact nature of these metal toxins, but also crucial for establishing preventive measures against such toxic risks in society.

Test Your Knowledge

1. What are the key clinical features in a case of acute arsenic poisoning?
2. How can forensic toxicologists confirm chronic lead exposure in a deceased individual?

6.4. Health Implications and Legal Consequences

Learning Outcome

1. Understand short-term effects of metallic poison exposure
2. Explain long-term health consequences
3. Focus on vulnerable populations at risk
4. Learn legal definitions of poisoning
5. Focus on criminal charges associated with metallic poisons
6. Describe role of forensic evidence in legal proceedings
7. Identify public health policies regarding metallic poisons
8. Know ethical considerations in forensic investigations
9. Discuss advocacy for stricter regulations

Metallic toxins, like arsenic, mix up public health problems with legal concerns in ways that are not always immediately clear. When investigators dig into poisoning cases, these substances do more than harm one person—they shake up legal processes and even change how folks see forensic science. It is interesting to recall that back in the day, before tests like the Marsh test became reliable, people often put too much trust in expert opinion; this misplaced confidence sometimes resulted in wrongful convictions based on evidence that was not all that solid. Generally speaking, such overreliance on imprecise forensic insights raised some pretty serious ethical questions about expertise and its limits. Science continues to unveil new findings, while legal standards appear to lag behind, prompting a more thorough, hands-on review of forensic methods. Even now, as experts strive to keep pace with evolving challenges, accusations of hubris and a hint of incompetence continue to emerge—suggesting that a more nuanced approach may be needed to strike a balance between justice and public health (Caudill et al., 2009).

6.4.1. Short-Term Effects of Metallic Poison Exposure

Metallic poison exposure is not just a legal matter—it also forces us to notice how the body immediately copes (Figure 6.18). When someone comes in contact with metals like arsenic or lead, for instance, they might suffer from an upset stomach, muscle and nerve troubles, or even fuzzy thinking. These signs often get confused with other health issues, which makes it challenging for forensic experts to determine what is really going on. If you look back at history, things become even more complicated; during the 19th and early 20th centuries, doctors often missed poisoning cues because their chemical tests were not yet reliable (Merry et al., 2010). The ongoing debates over arsenic detection further show that forensic science is still wrestling with how to balance specialized knowledge and ethical considerations best (Caudill et al., 2009). Generally speaking, noting these quick bodily responses is pretty key when trying to solve a forensic case. It is a tangled scenario where today's challenges echo past oversights, and that mix of immediate bodily effects keeps forensic evaluations on their toes. Recognizing these early signals—even if the symptoms are confusing—remains central to piecing together the complete picture.

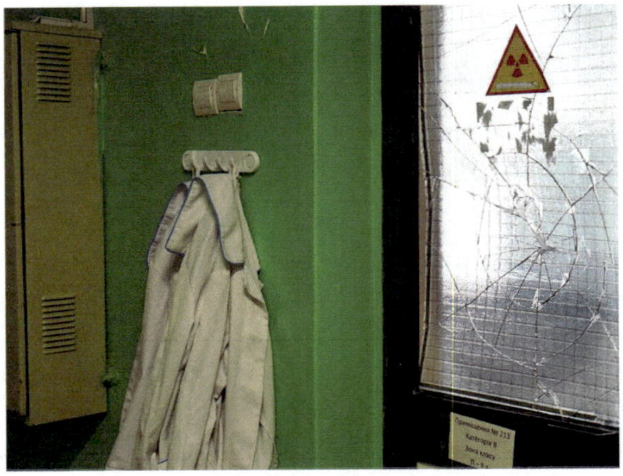

Figure 6.18. Metallic poison exposure is not just a legal matter—it also forces us to notice how the body immediately copes.

Source: RVO Health. (2023). *Radiation Concept – Chernobyl* https://media.post.rvohealth.io/wp-content/uploads/2023/05/radiation-concept-chernobyl-732x549-thumbnail-732x549.jpg.

6.4.2. Long-Term Health Consequences

Forensic science is not only about cracking cases—it is also entwined with the long-term harm that metal toxins can cause. In the past, when detection methods were still in development, heated debates raged about identifying arsenic before the Marsh test became available (Caudill et al., 2009). In most cases, prolonged exposure to metals like lead or arsenic can trigger a whole range of health issues, from nerve problems to damage in vital organs. What is more, these symptoms often creep up slowly over the years, leaving folks unsuspecting that their current health troubles might trace back to past exposure. Sometimes, a bit of overconfidence among forensic experts muddies the waters even further, stirring up ethical concerns over the duty to nail accurate diagnoses and step in when needed (Caudill et al., 2009). All in all, this highlights the urgent need for robust and trustworthy forensic practices that prioritize public health.

6.4.3. Vulnerable Populations at Risk

Forensic science, when combined with public health, can uncover risks that often hide in plain sight—especially for communities already struggling and exposed to toxic metals. In many areas where economic pressures are high and resources are scarce, research has shown that these harmful elements take a toll on people, a fact that forensic work continues to uncover. Groups in such environments usually face steep risks because healthcare support is scarce and available resources just do not cut it, making it really tough to deal with the fallout from this toxic exposure. Treatment options—such as maggot therapy—often highlight a pressing need for creative, sometimes unconventional solutions suitable for low-resource settings. Ultimately, acknowledging these repeated vulnerabilities is crucial for developing forensic practices that safeguard at-risk populations from the dangers of metallic poisons (Figure 6.19).

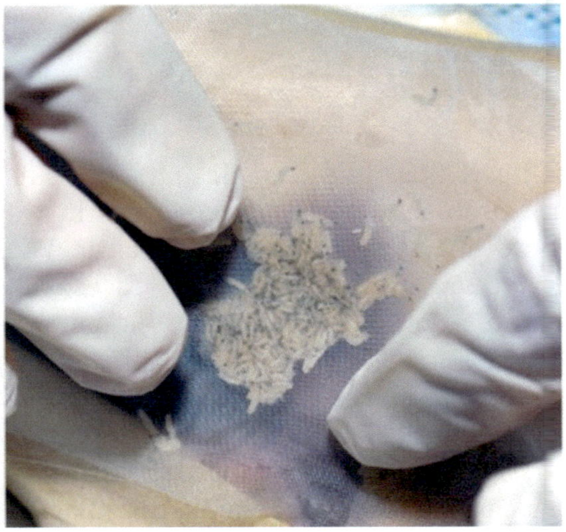

Figure 6.19. Maggot therapy.

Source: RCNi. (n.d.). *Cover Image from Primary Health Care*. https://dm3omg1n1n7zx.cloudfront.net/rcni/static/journals/phc/19/4/phc.19.4.13.s23/graphic/phc_v19_n4_23_0001.jpg.

6.4.4. Legal Definitions of Poisoning

Law and forensic science often become entangled in how we define something as seemingly straightforward as poisoning. The word, especially when metallic toxins are involved, is not as cut-and-dried as one might think. Each jurisdiction tends to paint poisoning in its own way, so the charges can swing widely depending on where you are. Because these definitions are somewhat ambiguous, forensic tests often step in to verify the presence of substances like heavy metals in biological samples – a crucial factor in determining whether exposure was an accident or something more sinister. It is interesting how lab results end up not only backing up claims of foul play or unintended exposure but also nudging the whole investigation in new directions (Ahluwalia et al., 2023; Emam, 2024). All in all, the shifting legal take on poisoning does not just clear up charges—it actually guides the tools and techniques used in forensic inquiry.

6.4.5. Criminal Charges Associated with Metallic Poisons

Arsenic and other metallic poisons have long made it tough to nail down criminal cases, a reality history keeps reminding us of. Forensic science has slowly advanced over time, and in most cases, people began to look twice at methods like the Marsh test – that pivotal procedure really shook things up. That test not only exposed the grave dangers of these toxins but also sparked debates about whether the experts handling these cases truly understood what they were dealing with. Critics argue that such controversies extend beyond a single test, reflecting broader issues within the legal system, including the influence of expert testimony and the risk of incorrect verdicts due to unreliable science. As noted, these longstanding criticisms of forensic expertise generally serve as a reminder that using scientific evidence in court is always somewhat shaky – with hints of overconfidence and a dash of moral ambiguity still coloring today's forensic landscape (Caudill et al., 2009).

6.4.6. Role of Forensic Evidence in Legal Proceedings

Legal cases can get pretty messy, especially when metallic poisons are involved and evidence reliability becomes a huge deal. The early days of arsenic tests—long before the famous Marsh test—reveal how science and legal rules have often been at odds in their own way. Back in the early 1800s, criminal trials often erupted over whether expert witnesses were up to the task; people doubted not just their technical expertise but also their moral integrity. Some folks pointed out, sometimes quite pointedly, that a bit too much expert pride might lead to more mix-ups than clear answers. You can still feel that tension today as courts grapple with the rapid advances in forensic technology. In most cases, understanding both the historical context and today's challenges is crucial to accurately assessing whether forensic evidence in metallic poison cases is reliable (Caudill et al., 2009).

6.4.7. Public Health Policies Regarding Metallic Poisons

Metallic toxins continue to appear in our environment, prompting us to reassess how we protect public health from their harmful effects (Figure 6.20). Mercury, for instance, is a significant concern—its toxic nature and widespread presence (thanks largely to industries that disrupt its natural flow) make it hard to ignore. Research indicates that local conditions significantly influence the movement of mercury, making it clear that monitoring groundwater and soil is crucial (Zouhri et al., 2025). Then there is the uptick in pesticide use—mainly in farming hotspots like Bangladesh—which only muddies the public health picture by adding a range of health risks, from sudden poisoning to more lingering issues with nerves and reproduction (Wakiluzzaman, 2025). Essentially, effective policy needs to combine steady monitoring, farmer education, and strict rule enforcement to address the multiple issues posed by metallic toxins and keep our communities safe.

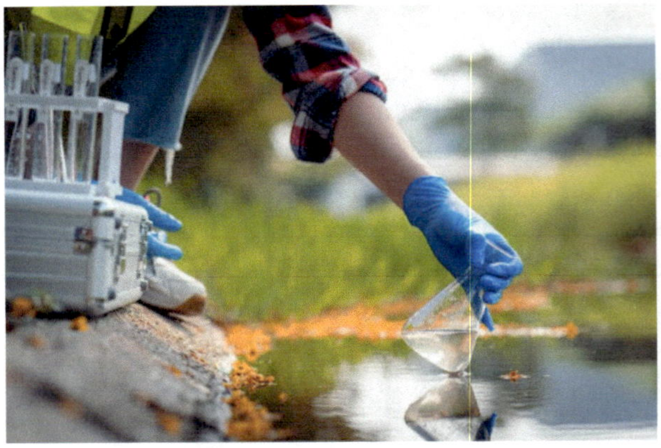

Figure 6.20. Metallic toxins continue to appear in our environment, prompting us to reassess how we safeguard public health from their harmful effects.

Source: Augusta University. (2024). *Scientist Collecting Water Sample.* https://insider.augusta.edu/wp-content/uploads/sites/25/2024/01/scientist-collecting-water-sample.jpg.

6.4.8. Ethical Considerations in Forensic Investigations

Metallic poisons in forensic cases raise a host of ethical challenges, often putting fairness and public trust at risk. Figuring out who the victims are in poisoning incidents can get messy; it is a real juggling act between giving due respect to the deceased and handling sensitive details with care. When you peek into forensic human identification, you see that professionals—torn between varied cultural views and the next-of-kin's desire to honor their loved ones (Reid et al., 2025)—face some tough calls. Forensic DNA analysis in these poisoning situations, in most instances, reveals a complex web of legal and moral issues that necessitate stringent data handling to protect individual rights and privacy (Smith et al., 2024). At the end of the day, balancing scientific progress with ethical duties remains a delicate act; many forensic experts agree that ongoing, albeit sometimes imperfect, conversations are key to maintaining both sound and just practices.

6.4.9. Advocacy for Stricter Regulations

Metallic poisons have become a significant sticking point between forensic science and criminal justice—a connection marked by surprising complexity. Scientific progress races ahead so fast that the law, in many cases, ends up trailing behind—which, frankly, leaves noticeable gaps in the forensic evidence brought to court. Calls for more rigid rules surge as a response, aiming not only to keep lab practices in line with modern science but also to prevent wrongful convictions stemming from fuzzy or misinterpreted evidence. It is a messy and sometimes overheated debate that tries to bridge a vast gulf between rapid scientific breakthroughs and legal systems that cling to finality over evolving truths. Add in the pressing need for broader research and steady funding to explore the full scope of metallic poisons, and you have a strong push to refine how these substances are detected and analyzed (Venter et al., 2020). Researchers continue to argue that addressing these gaps is, all things considered, crucial for maintaining a robust and fair judicial process (Andrea et al., 2015).

Test Your Knowledge

1. Under what circumstances can the use of metallic poisons lead to charges of attempted murder?
2. What evidence is required to prove intent in a case involving deliberate metallic poisoning?

SUMMARY

Metallic toxins weave deeply into forensic work—it is a complex mix that reminds us of the importance of understanding their full impact. It is not just about a single case; these elements, which infiltrate soil and even the food we eat, spread their influence across both land and water ecosystems (Joseph et al., 2023). In fact, trace elements found in everyday substances can quietly harm our environment, making things more complicated than a simple lab test might suggest. Forensic science, then, has to take a step back and consider these broader ecological ties when sorting out metallic poisons. In some studies, insect evidence has also emerged as a valuable component of the puzzle for estimating postmortem intervals, combining toxicology with entomology in a way that sheds new light on the entire process (Lutz et al., 2021). All things considered, combining different approaches appears to be the key to understanding metallic toxins, enhancing forensic methods, and safeguarding both public health and the environment.

Metallic poisons in forensics mix things up in a way that is not always obvious—think toxicology rubbing elbows with crime-solving techniques and even what we learn after someone is passed. It turns out that nailing down the chemical make-up in a victim, especially when suicide is on the table, is pretty key. Research generally shows that suicide cases often come with traces of toxins; things like prescription meds and even certain pesticides (yes, they sometimes get lumped in as metallic poisons) tend to pop up (Martins et al., 2022). On another note, a related field like forensic entomology—using clues from blow fly development, for example—offers hints about when decomposition began, as well as details of maggot growth stages (Roe et al., 2023). All of these clues, loosely tied together, help forensic experts eventually piece out the cause of death and possible poisoning routes, which, in most cases, steer both detective work and public health measures.

KEY TERMS FROM THIS CHAPTER

- Antimony
- Atomic absorption spectroscopy
- Batteries
- Electronics
- Lead
- Metallic toxins
- Pigment
- Arsenic
- Barium
- Cadmium
- Kidney
- Mercury
- Nerve signals
- Pigments

CRITICAL THINKING QUESTIONS

1. **Which of the following is a classical sign of chronic lead poisoning?**
   a. Mees' lines on nails
   b. Burton's line on gums
   c. Garlic odor on breath
   d. Cherry red skin
2. **Which chelating agent is used in the treatment of lead poisoning?**
   a. Deferoxamine
   b. BAL (British Anti-Lewisite)
   c. EDTA (ethylenediaminetetraacetic acid)
   d. DMSA (dimercaptosuccinic acid)
3. **Arsenic poisoning is associated with which of the following symptoms?**
   a. Hyperpigmentation and raindrop depigmentation
   b. Tinnitus and visual halos
   c. Bradycardia and hypotension
   d. Jaundice and ascites
4. **What is the characteristic odor associated with arsenic poisoning?**
   a. Rotten eggs
   b. Almonds
   c. Garlic
   d. Bitter almonds
5. **Which of the following is not typically considered a heavy metal poison?**
   a. Arsenic
   b. Lead
   c. Iron
   d. Potassium

Short Answer Questions

1. What are the significant sources of lead exposure?
2. How does mercury poisoning affect the nervous system?
3. What is the difference between organic and inorganic arsenic compounds?
4. Which type of anemia is commonly associated with lead poisoning?
5. How is cadmium poisoning typically acquired?
6. What are the signs and symptoms of chronic arsenic poisoning?
7. What is the role of chelating agents in treating metallic poisoning?
8. How is lead poisoning diagnosed in the laboratory?

Answers to Critical Thinking Questions

1. (b); 2. (c); 3. (a); 4. (c); 5. (d)

REFERENCES

1. Abbas, K., Aregbe, Y., Avenhaus, R., Aymanns, K., Bencardino, R., Burrows, B., Cagno, S., et al. (2023). *Nuclear Safeguards and Non-Proliferation – ESARDA Course Syllabus.* https://core.ac.uk/download/642864821.pdf (accessed on 9th May 2025).
2. Acheampong, S., (2023). *Heavy Metals' Poisoning in Farm Animals.* https://core.ac.uk/download/588400993.pdf (accessed on 9th May 2025).
3. Ahluwalia, J. K., & Sharma, R., (2023). The role of forensic science in criminal investigation. *International Journal for Multidisciplinary Research, 5.* https://doi.org/10.36948/ijfmr.2023.v05i06.9530.
4. Anas, M. K. P. (2016). *A Study of Observation in Treatment Modality of Acute and Chronic Poisoning Cases by Analyzing Clinical Laboratory Parameters and Its Outcome in Tertiary Care Hospitals.* https://core.ac.uk/download/235660891.pdf (accessed on 9th May 2025).
5. Apostu, S., Botar, A., & Socaciu, C., (2008). *Lab-on-a-Chip and Food Safety: Biosensors and Biocomposites to Identify Foodborne Pathogens and Chemicals.* https://core.ac.uk/download/287196999.pdf (accessed on 9th May 2025).
6. Awasthi, G., Awasthi, K. K., Vanisree, C. R., et al. (2022). *Heavy Metal Contamination of Food Crops: Transportation via Food Chain, Human Consumption, Toxicity and Management Strategies.* https://core.ac.uk/download/492702723.pdf (accessed on 9th May 2025).
7. Banerjee, S., (2024). Importance of food forensics and its mandatory implications in health safety and compliance. *IP International Journal of Forensic Medicine and Toxicological Sciences.* https://www.semanticscholar.org/paper/943142dbc4a1fb9a7335940f721e2ab6d232ca78 (accessed on 9th May 2025).
8. Barnard, C. C., & Carpenter, E., (2024). *A Classification for Medical and Veterinary Libraries.* https://doi.org/10.56920/lshtmp-1 (accessed on 9th May 2025).
9. Bartoshyk, N., (2024). Analysis of the number of deaths due to poisoning by the most common poisonous substances in the Lviv region in 2018–2023. *Forensic-Medical Examination.* https://www.semanticscholar.org/paper/11ab7886efe10b9fb28d671682ea7cd842c27417 (accessed on 9th May 2025).
10. Blain, P. G., & Vonberg, F. W. (2024). *Neurotoxicology: A Clinical Systems-Based Review.* https://core.ac.uk/download/613849271.pdf (accessed on 9th May 2025).
11. Bordbar, M. M., Sheini, A., Hashemi, P., Hajian, A., & Bagheri, H., (2021). Disposable paper-based biosensors for the point-of-care detection of hazardous contaminations—A review. *Biosensors, 11*, 316. https://doi.org/10.3390/bios11090316.
12. Brzozowski, K., Daoust-Maleval, I., Geypens, B., Goulart de Medeiros, M., Iatan, A. E., Lequarre, A. S., & Santopolo, D., (2022). *EU CBRNe Glossary.* https://core.ac.uk/download/642865393.pdf (accessed on 9th May 2025).
13. Câmara, J. S., Perestrelo, R., Berenguer, C. V., Andrade, C., Gomes, T. M., Olayanju, B., Kabir, A., et al. (2022). Green extraction techniques as advanced sample preparation approaches in biological, food, and environmental matrices: A review. *Molecules, 27*, 2953. https://doi.org/10.3390/molecules27092953.
14. Cappelletti, S., Piacentino, D., Fineschi, V., Frati, P., D'Errico, S., & Aromatario, M., (2019).

Mercuric chloride poisoning: Symptoms, analysis, therapies, and autoptic findings. A review of the literature. *Critical Reviews in Toxicology, 49*, 329–341. https://doi.org/10.1080/10408444.2019.1621262.

15. Casparsen, C., (2024). The role of toxicology in forensic investigations. *International Journal of Forensic Medicine*. https://www.semanticscholar.org/paper/da3c2ea594c2d9e2608a802503025b50e5cb0849 (accessed on 9th May 2025).
16. Caudill, D. S. (2009). *Arsenic and Old Chemistry: Images of Mad Alchemists, Experts Attacking Experts, and the Crisis in Forensic Science*. https://core.ac.uk/download/229258057.pdf (accessed on 9th May 2025).
17. Dave, P., & Dutta, G., (2021). *Detection of Pesticides in Food by CDs Blue Luminescent Material with the Help of Fluorescence Quenching Study*. https://core.ac.uk/download/595875514.pdf (accessed on 9th May 2025).
18. De Luca, A., & Sevini, F., (2015). *ESARDA 37th Annual Meeting Proceedings*. https://core.ac.uk/download/38630617.pdf (accessed on 9th May 2025).
19. Emam, ⍰ A. N. M. (2024). Role of forensic odontology in identification of persons: A review article. *Cureus*. https://doi.org/10.7759/cureus.56570 (accessed on 9th May 2025).
20. Fahemi, N., Angizi, S., & Hatamie, A., (2024). Integration of ultrathin bubble walls and electrochemistry: Innovation in microsensing for forensic nitrite detection and microscale metallic film deposition. *Analytical Chemistry*. https://www.semanticscholar.org/paper/889bd37cbf5a5494eb5d800bbf9dcb531f75b55f (accessed on 9th May 2025).
21. Gao, A., (2024). Advances in biosensors for poison detection applications. *E3S Web of Conferences*. https://www.semanticscholar.org/paper/936186f7c381c230226f330e91ce1a15f983463d (accessed on 9th May 2025).
22. Gurr, J. M., & Klein, N. M. (2023). *Norman M. Klein's "Bleeding Through: Layers of Los Angeles."* transcript Verlag eBooks. https://doi.org/10.1515/9783839465592.
23. Henderson, A., Heaney, L. M., & Rankin-Turner, S., (2024). Ambient ionization mass spectrometry for drug and toxin analysis: A review of the recent literature. *Drug Testing and Analysis, 16*, 1323–1344. https://doi.org/10.1002/dta.3644.
24. Herman, R. U., & Prasetyo, A., (2025). Analysis of address resolution protocol poisoning attacks on Mikrotik routers using live forensics methods. *International Journal of Engineering Business and Social Science*. https://www.semanticscholar.org/paper/90bbc22aa5d62f70efbff2f23cd138f7bd2bf75a (accessed on 9th May 2025).
25. Hjelm, R. P., Weber, J., Hussey, D. S., Bockstaller, M. R., Vogel, S. C., Khaykovich, B., Siebenbürger, M., et al. (2024). *The Scientific Case for Concurrent Neutron and X-Ray Scattering and Spectroscopy*. https://doi.org/10.2172/2350626.
26. Jeyaraj, M., Gurunathan, S., Qasim, M., Kang, M. H., & Kim, J. H. (2019). A comprehensive review on the synthesis, characterization, and biomedical application of platinum nanoparticles. *Nanomaterials, 9*, 1719. https://doi.org/10.3390/nano9121719.
27. Joseph, D., Ahuja, P., Dockrell, M. E. C., Purchase, D., Price, R., Krishna, S., García-Muñoz, J., et al. (2023). *Trace Metals in the Environment*. IntechOpen eBooks. https://doi.org/10.5772/intechopen.1001530.

28. Kant, J. M. (2013). *Heavy Metals in Traditionally Used Fruits Among the Lakota.* https://core.ac.uk/download/215600281.pdf (accessed on 9th May 2025).

29. Li, B., Xu, W., Luo, R., Zhuo, S., Guo, X., Cheng, K., Yun, K., et al. (2022). Estimation of the frequency and time of human exposure to arsenic by single hair analysis. *International Journal of Environmental Research and Public Health, 19.* https://www.semanticscholar.org/paper/f588994217544b26c0f0aa53695119211cb8b62b (accessed on 9th May 2025).

30. Likitha, V., Rajesh, A., Ameta, A., & Aich, S., (2025). Beyond snakes: Exploring zootoxins in invertebrates and lower vertebrates. *Uttar Pradesh Journal of Zoology.* https://www.semanticscholar.org/paper/aca94b362cb11c49a8924d11ce328d017c8b3b2a (accessed on 9th May 2025).

31. Liu, Y., Zhang, J., Wang, B., Zheng, F., & Yan, J., (2025). Epidemiological patterns and therapeutic approaches of toad toxin poisoning in a retrospective case study. *Scientific Reports, 15.* https://www.semanticscholar.org/paper/6dbb347e000126d867d45969e9a126d380b8a336 (accessed on 9th May 2025).

32. Lutz, L., Zehner, R., Verhoff, M. A., Bratzke, H., & Amendt, J., (2021). It is all about the insects: A retrospective on 20 years of forensic entomology highlights the importance of insects in legal investigations. *International Journal of Legal Medicine, 135,* 2637–2651. https://doi.org/10.1007/s00414-021-02628-6.

33. Machado, C. de C., & Dinis-Oliveira, R. J. (2023). Clinical and forensic signs resulting from exposure to heavy metals and other chemical elements of the periodic table. *Journal of Clinical Medicine, 12,* 2591. https://doi.org/10.3390/jcm12072591.

34. Mannocchi, G., Pantano, F., Romolo, F. S., Tittarelli, M., et al. (2015). *Recreational Use, Analysis and Toxicity of Tryptamines.* https://core.ac.uk/download/54534388.pdf (accessed on 9th May 2025).

35. Martins, C., Lemos, Y. V., Teodoro, M., & Drummond-Lage, A. P. (2022). Epidemio-toxicological profile of suicide cases: Analysis from a forensic unit in Brazil. *Forensic Sciences Research, 7,* 643–649. https://www.semanticscholar.org/paper/151bdc233c520ed619d646fa207a2e1bc7ada9dd (accessed on 9th May 2025).

36. Merry, K. J. (2010). Murder by poison in Scotland during the nineteenth and early twentieth centuries. https://core.ac.uk/download/282378.pdf (accessed on 9th May 2025).

37. Mishra, A., (2020). *Forensic Chemistry and Toxicology.* https://core.ac.uk/download/322580838.pdf (accessed on 9th May 2025).

38. Mulani, K., Kadam, M., Patil, S., Gosavi, N., & Ghumatkar, S., (2024). Forensic firearm identification of an ingeniously modified air rifle-firearm. *The Egyptian Journal of Forensic Sciences and Applied Toxicology.* https://www.semanticscholar.org/paper/9169d8918a47a3ad4ec82f69b10985d67f68f403 (accessed on 9th May 2025).

39. Nunziata, C., Rotter, G., & Nunziata, F., (2025). Formal relationship between the firearm "memory effect" and the decay time of the GSR particles present on the shooter's hands. *Forensic Sciences.* https://www.semanticscholar.org/paper/526959a90ce1b1e996da8e2220a132ff2ec79afa (accessed on 9th May 2025).

40. Nwachukwu, F. C., Salawu, K., et al. (2014). Determination of Selected Heavy Metals in Seasonal River in Maru Town, Zamfara State, Nigeria. *Journal of Environment and Earth Science.* https://core.ac.uk/download/234663705.pdf (accessed on 9th May 2025).

41. Paixão, T. R. L. C. (2019). Portable analytical techniques for forensic applications. *Brazilian Journal of Analytical Chemistry*. https://www.semanticscholar.org/paper/42f14adee570e8ef42f7eab23f7c2533ea3638ca (accessed on 9th May 2025).

42. Pesce, F., Sannino, E., Ragosta, E., Marigliano, L., Picazio, G., Esposito, M., Dimatteo, M., et al. (2025). Overkilling in a dog: A case report. *Animals: An Open Access Journal from MDPI, 15*. https://www.semanticscholar.org/paper/c96158be6d0b3543f7da7367888d5d3dd21e50f1 (accessed on 9th May 2025).

43. Pohanka, M., (2020). Colorimetric hand-held sensors and biosensors with a small digital camera as signal recorder: A review. *Reviews in Analytical Chemistry, 39*, 20–30. https://doi.org/10.1515/revac-2020-0111.

44. Rajan, S., & Neole, N., (2025). Green forensic toxicology: Optimizing chlordiazepoxide detection in milk, whiskey, and whiskey cream matrices. *Indian Journal of Forensic Medicine & Toxicology*. https://www.semanticscholar.org/paper/394699352df614680e98fa8548f44abe46864d9d (accessed on 9th May 2025).

45. Reid, K., Suwalowska, H., Martin, L. J., & Heathfield, L., (2025). Ethical considerations in the routine identification of human remains in forensic mortuaries. *Wellcome Open Research*. https://www.semanticscholar.org/paper/91c0dc5beb099ba83315408cfab3b43ddb9d39f1 (accessed on 9th May 2025).

46. Roe, A. L., & Higley, L. G. (2023). Stage transitions in *Lucilia sericata* and *Phormia regina* (Diptera: Calliphoridae) and implications for forensic science. *Insects, 14*. https://www.semanticscholar.org/paper/b8b9b294f14097dc222e31776f3da70748e8f833.

47. Rothenberg, S., (2023). Invited perspective: Linking the intergenerational impacts due to mercury exposure in Grassy Narrows First Nation, Canada. *Environmental Health Perspectives, 131*. https://www.semanticscholar.org/paper/d45a722067d2012d982c046447de5f20346e7c06 (accessed on 9th May 2025).

48. Saganuwan, S. A. (2017). Toxicity studies of drugs and chemicals in animals: An overview. *Bulgarian Journal of Veterinary Medicine, 20*, 291–318. https://doi.org/10.15547/bjvm.983.

49. Sellers, L. M., & Watson, K. D. (2019). *The Construction of Forensic Knowledge in Victorian Yorkshire: Dr Thomas Scattergood and his Casebooks, 1856–1897*. https://core.ac.uk/download/228168115.pdf (accessed on 9th May 2025).

50. Shajhutdinova, Z., Pashirova, T. N., & Masson, P., (2022). Kinetic processes in enzymatic nanoreactors for in vivo detoxification. *Biomedicines, 10*, 784. https://doi.org/10.3390/biomedicines10040784.

51. Siddall, R., (2018). Mineral pigments in archaeology: Their analysis and the range of available materials. *Minerals, 8*, 201. https://doi.org/10.3390/min8050201 (accessed on 9th May 2025).

52. Smith, J. H., & Singh, M., (2024). Forensic DNA profiling: Legal and ethical considerations. *Journal of Scientific Research and Reports*. https://www.semanticscholar.org/paper/30c2411eb968e68b332f37a253d3eb7fbd0ba08f (accessed on 9th May 2025).

53. Srinivasa, K., Madyastha, S., & Yadukul, M., (2016). *Study of Profile of Poisoning Cases Reported to District Hospital, Chamarajanagar, Karnataka, India*. https://core.ac.uk/download/543133903.pdf (accessed on 9th May 2025).

54. Sylvia, S., (2017). *A Retrospective Study of Deaths Due to Poisoning, Among the Autopsies Conducted at Government Kilpauk Medical College and Hospital, Chennai.* https://core.ac.uk/download/235661760.pdf (accessed on 9th May 2025).

55. Tekin, G., Seyhan, E., Aydin, I., & Aydın, F., (2023). GSR analysis by spectrophotometry method in forensic chemistry. *Dicle Üniversitesi Fen Bilimleri Enstitüsü Dergisi.* https://www.semanticscholar.org/paper/b80e9da10fd492d122cbe049554c4698174a8c2f (accessed on 9th May 2025).

56. Venter, C. H. (2020). *A Critical Review of the Current State of Forensic Science Knowledge and Its Integration in Legal Systems.* https://core.ac.uk/download/334609821.pdf (accessed on 9th May 2025).

57. Verma, A., (2018). Forensic aspect of metal poisoning: A review. *International Journal for Research in Applied Science and Engineering Technology, 6*, 1089–1092. https://www.semanticscholar.org/paper/75ea1b772fe5adc8b70fb824cbeefed883ff34e5 (accessed on 9th May 2025).

58. Wakiluzzaman, S. M. (2025). Public health implications of pesticide use in Bangladesh: A comprehensive review. *International Journal of Research and Scientific Innovation.* https://www.semanticscholar.org/paper/a07ddd67208f4ea83494c4e02b61a4ab7d7b5e69 (accessed on 9th May 2025).

59. Yousafzai, A., Aziz, M., Yousuf, S., Bano, S., & Khan, M. M. (2024). Suicide patterns in northern Pakistan: A 10-year analysis of police records from three districts of Gilgit-Baltistan. *Archives of Suicide Research: Official Journal of the International Academy for Suicide Research.* https://www.semanticscholar.org/paper/441690dc27dd80f465957832d7a7327daa79befb (accessed on 9th May 2025).

60. Zouhri, L., Delépine, J., & Zouhri, L., (2025). Assessment of mercury contamination in the chalk aquifer of the Pays de Caux and its implications for public health (France). *Water.* https://www.semanticscholar.org/paper/9dba565b2d4950d5dc9b92bdc456a302398f1645 (accessed on 9th May 2025).

NEUROTOXIC POISONS

7

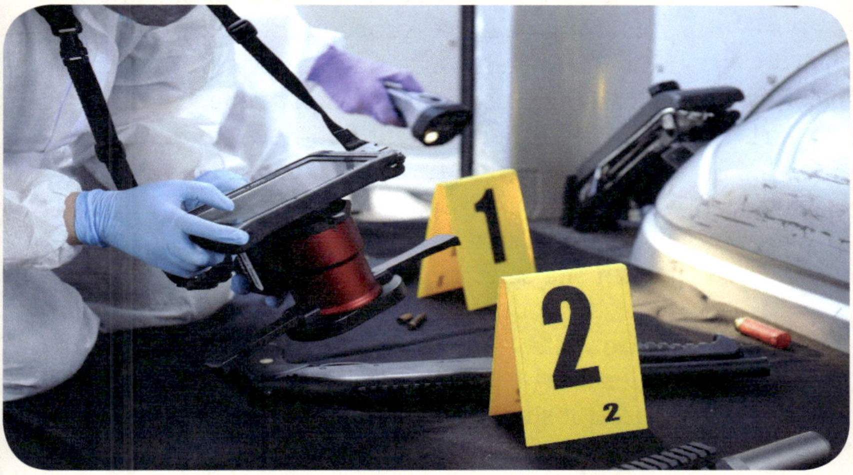

LEARNING OBJECTIVES

After studying this chapter, you will be able to:

1. Discuss types of neurotoxic poisons
2. Explain mechanisms of action
3. Focus on detection and analysis in forensic
4. Learn legal and ethical considerations

Introduction

Forensic science keeps changing, and these neurotoxic poisons have suddenly grabbed more attention in many toxicology cases. New analytical methods are popping up, and in most cases, being aware of the effects these substances have is crucial for both legal and medical systems. Consider synthetic cannabinoids—they try to mimic the effects of natural cannabis. Still, they are often much stronger, which has been linked to a worrying surge in severe poisoning and even deaths worldwide (Alves et al., 2020). Then there is the trend of chemsex, where people mix various psychoactive drugs to intensify sexual experiences; this practice, in its own way, highlights the social risks associated with neurotoxic agents (Giorgetti et al., 2017). Looking closely at these compounds does not just reveal their chemical properties; it also reminds us why they are so important in forensic investigations, and, generally speaking, understanding them can help guide more effective policies and preventive measures.

Definition of Neurotoxic Poisons

Neurotoxic poisons affect many areas, most notably in forensic labs. These agents simply attack nerve tissues, upsetting normal cell function and, in worst cases, causing nerve cells to die. A variety of culprits can be involved, ranging from heavy metals found in the environment to certain pharmaceuticals manufactured in laboratories.

Detecting these toxic substances is crucial when trying to piece together poisoning events, as understanding how they operate provides valuable clues about what went wrong. New analytical methods like DART-MS let experts spot these toxins really fast, often without the need for heavy sample prep—this speed is vital when every minute counts (Krzysztof et al., 2022). In most cases, understanding the effects of these poisons helps improve forensic work and supports legal processes. Overall, a clearer picture of these harmful agents enhances both investigations and the eventual pursuit of justice (Figure 7.1).

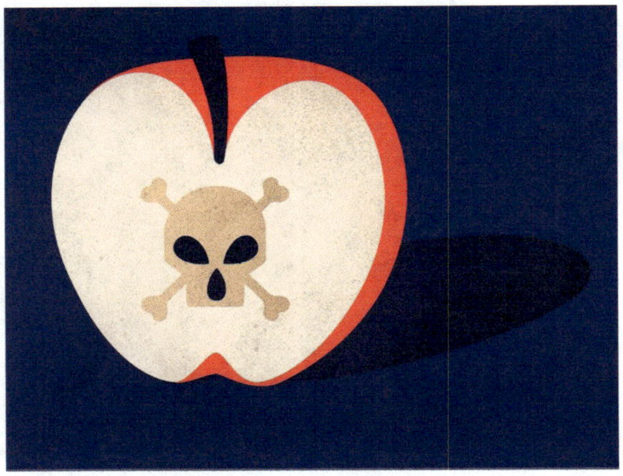

Figure 7.1. Neurotoxic poisons.

Source: The Atlantic. (2014). *Prison Interior with Inmates*. https://cdn.theatlantic.com/thumbor/C0CoaKLAWj8ZbhhwcHj9TphsqjY=/457x19:1657x919/1200x900/media/img/mt/2014/03/opener/original.jpg.

Overview of Neurotoxic Substances

Neurotoxic substances have become a real headache lately, and forensics is not handling it too easily—these compounds are baffling in their complexity and seem to evolve at lightning speed. Synthetic cannabinoids, for instance, grab a lot of attention since they are usually way more potent than what you would find in natural cannabis; they often pop up on the market with names like Spice or K2, which can really throw people off. Cases of acute intoxication, poisoning, and a subsequent jump in ER visits (and sadly, even fatalities) have become increasingly common. In most reports, nearly 50% of the newly identified new psychoactive substances (NPS) turn out to be these synthetic variants (Miliano et al., 2016; Alves et al., 2020); this trend raises serious alarms about public health and safety. Forensic experts, while doing their best to untangle and assess these tricky neurotoxins, generally agree that more research is needed—both to improve the way we detect these substances and to get a better handle on their toxicological profiles.

Historical Context of Neurotoxic Poisons in Criminal Cases

Neurotoxic poisons have long left their mark on criminal investigations. They come from a mix of sources—plants and even some animals—and early forensic experts got pretty inventive with them. Historical records often show that these toxins mimic natural illness symptoms, which muddled diagnoses and allowed some culprits to slip away. As forensic science evolved, methods such as Ultra-High-Performance Liquid Chromatography (UHPLC) and High-Resolution Mass Spectrometry (HRMS) began to identify these compounds with far greater precision (Zakaria et al., 2025). That legacy of shadowy uses not only hints at secret acts but also sparks ongoing debates about ethics and the relentless chase for justice in today's forensic world (Saucedo, 2024).

Scope of Neurotoxic Poisons in Forensic Investigations

Neurotoxic poisons are now a significant concern in forensic work—they sneak up on the central nervous system in ways that might go unnoticed yet prove deadly. Toxicology tests have gotten so much better that, in most cases, investigators can find these toxins and tie a suspect to a scene, even if the link is not immediately apparent. In traumatic incidents, these nerve-affecting substances tend to complicate the clinical story, so a precise, speedy diagnosis and treatment become crucial for survivors. At the same time, legal experts wade through tricky questions of responsibility (Singh et al., 2025). DNA phenotyping and other cutting-edge techniques are emerging in labs to help identify potential victims or suspects, thereby widening the investigative net in cases of neurotoxic exposure (Marsico et al., 2024). By blending modern approaches with time-tested methods, forensic scientists can piece together richer, more detailed profiles that address cases tainted by neurotoxic agents—this inevitably boosts the field's overall ability to deliver justice. Generally speaking, even though minor oversights (or an occasional stray punctuation mark) may slip through, the mix of old and new strategies ensures that these complex situations are handled as naturally and flexibly as real-life demands (Figure 7.2).

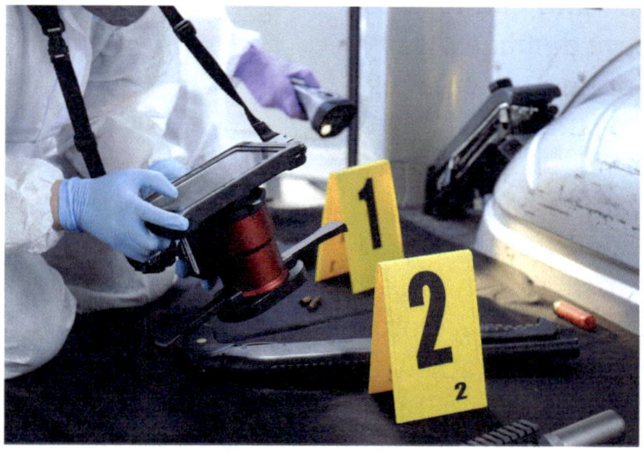

Figure 7.2. Neurotoxic poisons in forensic investigations.

Source: Foster + Freeman. (2022). *Forensic Lab Analysis Using Specialized Equipment.* https://fosterfreeman.com/wp-content/uploads/2022/01/DSC2935-scaled.jpg.

Relevance to Modern Forensic Science

Forensic science is on a constant upward trajectory, and innovative research models are crucial these days. Neurotoxic poisons have gotten more intricate, which means our old methods just will not cut it when it comes to effective investigation. Nowadays, many researchers are turning to zebrafish (Danio rerio) – these little creatures are now seen as a surprisingly affordable and flexible option, especially in low- and middle-income countries where available resources can be pretty limited (Mukherjee et al., 2024). Their distinct body makeup lets scientists observe live, non-invasively, which helps uncover both the behavioral quirks and developmental shifts caused by neurotoxins. In many cases, these fish even expose metabolites that our standard methods miss, thereby enhancing our overall understanding of human neurotoxic exposure. Forensic labs are increasingly incorporating advanced biochemical techniques, and it appears that integrating models like zebrafish may just set the stage for a new era of efficiency and accuracy in addressing neurotoxic substances (Abrosimova, 2024).

7.1. Types of Neurotoxic Poisons

Learning Outcome

1. Understand organophosphates, heavy metals, and botulinum toxin
2. Explain cyanide, strychnine, carbon monoxide, and methanol
3. Focus on pesticides
4. Discuss fentanyl and synthetic opioids

Understanding neurotoxic substances is key for forensic work—these poisons, in most cases, disrupt normal body functions and can lead to both sudden and lingering nerve damage. Heavy metals like lead and mercury, organophosphates, and even some mushroom toxins each have their own quirks when it comes to interfering with nerve signals; for example, one might see anything from rapid seizures to bouts of paralysis. It is essential to pick up on these agents in samples like blood or tissue, since doing so often helps determine if a death was accidental or possibly the result of foul play. In some instances, analyzing even the tiniest trace evidence can unexpectedly reveal what happened at a scene—indeed, these insights prove crucial for building a strong legal case. Forensic investigations often integrate concepts from pathology, toxicology, and mycology, a complexity that, frankly, makes every case both challenging and, sometimes, a bit of a head-scratcher (Kharmate et al., 2024; Wankhede, 2024).

7.1.1. Organophosphates

Agrochemicals are popping up everywhere, and there is growing concern about how they might be affecting nerve health – organophosphates, for instance, often top the list. Chlorpyrifos shows up again and again in different parts of the environment, and in most cases, it ends up harming creatures it was never meant to touch, with fish and other aquatic life taking a hit. Researchers have found that, generally speaking, chlorpyrifos slows down acetylcholinesterase (AChE)—the enzyme that normally breaks down acetylcholine—so acetylcholine accumulates at nerve junctions, disrupting normal signaling and potentially leading to fish deaths (Ambareen et al., 2023). While studies on organophosphate-induced neurotoxicity are still limited, some emerging work suggests that a neuroprotective approach—such as using caffeic acid phenyl ester—might help mitigate these effects after glyphosate exposure (Basarslan et al., 2023). All in all, this line of inquiry really highlights our need for more rigorous forensic methods to determine the implications of these toxins for public health and the environment (Figure 7.3).

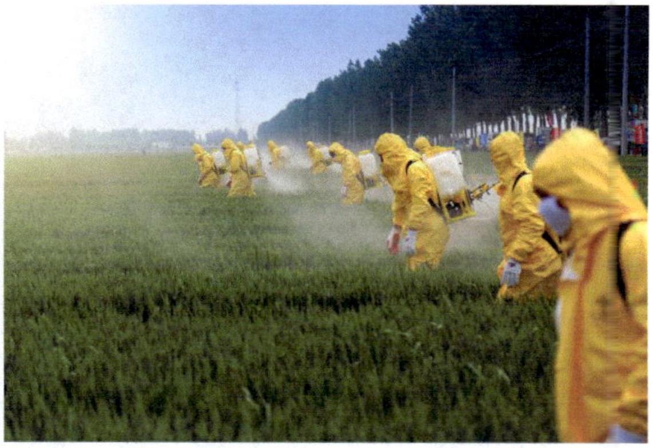

Figure 7.3. Agrochemicals.

Source: I Am Renew. (2018). *Pesticides Ban*. https://www.iamrenew.com/wp-content/uploads/2018/12/Pesticides-Ban.jpg.

7.1.2. Heavy Metals (e.g., Lead, Mercury)

Human activities have intertwined our environment and health in unexpected ways, often revealing some alarming signs. Heavy metals – think lead and mercury – sneak into nature, and they're no small fry when it comes to causing neurotoxic problems. These substances infiltrate ecosystems and work their way through food chains, sometimes disrupting the natural balance and even affecting human populations. In most cases, elevated levels of these metals have been tied to issues like cognitive slowdowns and developmental hiccups, especially in vulnerable groups like children. Research generally shows that the trouble does not end with immediate poisoning; these elements can also compromise soil and water quality, ultimately disrupting how farming works and the overall stability of communities (Joseph et al., 2023). When investigators dig into unexplained deaths – for example, cetacean strandings that might be linked to quick poisoning or long-term exposure – figuring out the part heavy metals play becomes key to identifying the underlying causes (Ulloa et al., 2024). Altogether, examining these complex interactions provides a clearer, albeit sometimes unsettling, view of neurotoxic risks across both human health and the environment.

7.1.3. Botulinum Toxin

Botulinum toxin is a big deal in forensic work—it is tied to risky food poisoning cases that can turn deadly. This neurotoxin, wedded to the bacterium Clostridium botulinum, can cause paralysis and, in many cases, even death, so pathologists tend to watch such cases very closely.

Often, clues during an autopsy do not come out clearly, making it harder to pinpoint botulism; experts therefore have to look for those subtle, unusual signs of exposure, as Devers et al. (2010) point out. Food safety concerns are growing, too, especially with home-canned foods that frequently spark outbreaks (Xie et al., 2022). All these factors, generally speaking, not only aid in clinical diagnosis but also facilitate the development of better prevention and response plans, underscoring the crucial role of this toxin in forensic investigations (Figure 7.4).

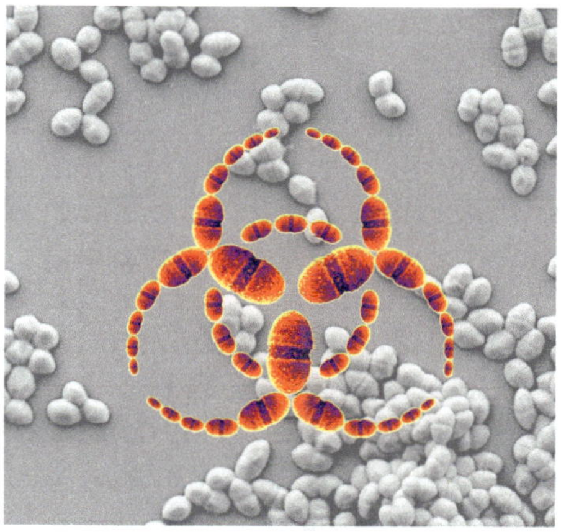

Figure 7.4. Botulinum toxin.

Source: Genetic Engineering and Biotechnology News. (2018). Enterococcus Bacteria (Photo Credit: Francois Lebreton). https://www.genengnews. com/wp- content/uploads/2018/08/ Enterococcus credit Francois Lebretoncopy 7411517610.jpg.

7.1.4. Cyanide

Toxicology and forensic work often mix in odd ways, especially when substances like cyanide are involved. Cyanide, a toxin that works fast and fatally, throws a wrench into postmortem analysis with its sudden effects. Forensic experts, trying to pin down the cause of death, lean on detailed toxicology data and autopsy reports to catch hints of cyanide poisoning. In many autopsy reviews, researchers have, in most cases, highlighted the pressing need for clearer toxicology training – particularly in areas where this expertise is scarce, such as developing countries (Marks et al., 2020). Some findings even suggest that digging into socio-economic factors could boost preventative measures against suicides involving these neurotoxic agents (Albano et al., 2022). All in all, getting a handle on how cyanide messes with the nervous system is not just a lab exercise; it quietly shapes public health moves and forensic procedures aimed at lessening the harm from such dangerous substances.

7.1.5. Strychnine

Forensic cases involving neurotoxins are not a walk in the park—they require a solid understanding of both the composition of these chemicals and their impact on the human body. Strychnine, for example, really catches your eye; it attacks the central nervous system, causing violent convulsions that, in many cases, lead to death. Detecting even a hint of it in bodily samples is crucial when trying to determine if poisoning has occurred. Nowadays, labs often borrow ideas from plant research—techniques like phytochemical fingerprinting (which may sound highfalutin but actually helps pinpoint uncommon markers) add a surprising boost to investigations (Zakaria et al., 2025). Research on other similar toxins generally shows that it is not just about finding the main compound; you also have to look for its breakdown products in forensic samples (Lehner et al., 2018). All in all, mixing clever lab tricks with a flexible, sometimes messy, approach really helps piece together the toxic puzzle (Figure 7.5).

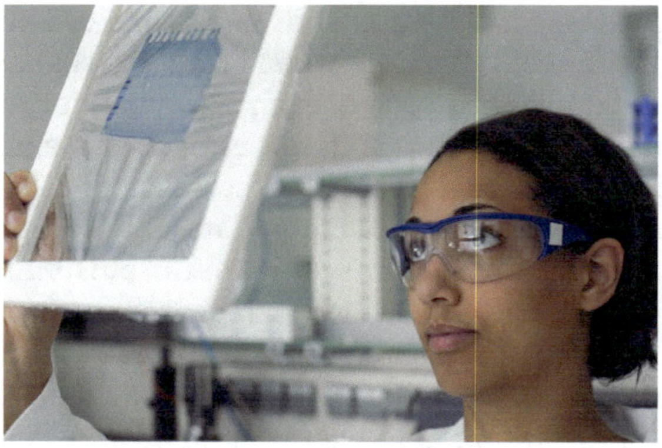

Figure 7.5. Strychnine.

Source: ExploreHealthCareers.org. (2016). *Forensic Chemist at Work in a Laboratory*. https://explorehealthcareers.org/wp-content/uploads/2016/11/forensic_chemist.jpg.

7.1.6. Carbon Monoxide

Environmental toxins and our health often mix in unexpected ways—take carbon monoxide, for example. This gas, which has no color or odor, is dangerous because it binds to hemoglobin much more avidly than oxygen, effectively cutting off the oxygen that our cells need. People can then start showing a host of neurological symptoms; think confusion, gnawing headaches, and in awful cases, even losing consciousness or dying. In forensic work, figuring out a case of carbon monoxide poisoning can be tricky—especially when bodies are decomposed and the usual clues do not show up. Research (Blain et al., 2024) suggests that detecting these neurotoxic effects early, in most cases, can lead to better outcomes in both treatment and investigation. It is also important to note that accurately coding health data is key to understanding the broader impact of these toxins on populations, particularly when several organs end up failing due to a mix of exposures.

7.1.7. Methanol

Neurotoxic substances affect lots of areas, and methanol is one prime example—it is known as a toxic alcohol yet still sees widespread industrial use (Figure 7.6). When accidentally ingested, the body typically converts methanol into chemicals like formaldehyde and formic acid, a process that, in most cases, seriously disrupts metabolism and causes neurological damage. You might start off feeling dizzy, with a headache or even odd visual glitches; then, sometimes, the condition can suddenly escalate to seizures or even coma. Forensic teams investigating such poisoning often struggle to figure out whether the exposure was merely accidental or intentional. Since methanol's harmful effects can overlap with those of other neurotoxins, meticulous documentation and diagnosis—albeit sometimes a bit messy—are essential. In most cases, as ongoing research slowly uncovers more details, the need for accurate detection and regular monitoring continues to rise, echoing similar efforts in studying toxins like phycotoxins that impact marine life and, potentially, human health (Opravil et al., 2023; Sinno-Tellier et al., 2023).

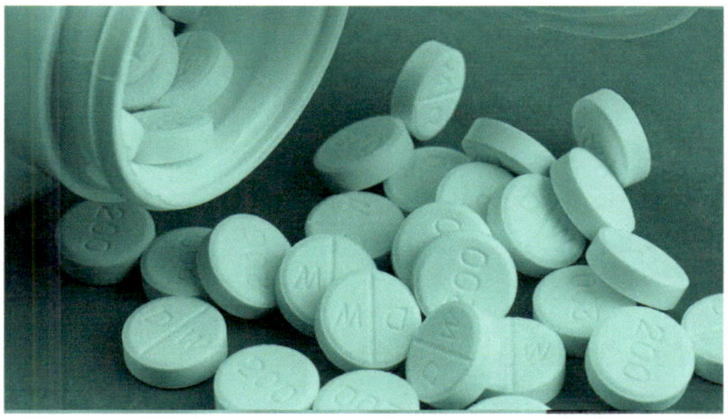

Figure 7.6. Neurotoxic substances affect lots of areas, and methanol is one prime example.

Source: American College of Medical Toxicology. (2022). *Photograph of Cyan-Colored Pills.* https://www.acmt.net/wp-content/uploads/2022/05/1920-x-1080-2022-Pills-Cyan.jpg.

7.1.8. Pesticides

Neurotoxic pesticides are showing up more frequently these days, and that is causing quite a stir in forensic circles, especially with poisoning cases. Take Pyridaben, for example—a pesticide known to mess with the brain in pretty harsh ways—which was involved in a particularly tragic incident with a young girl. She ended up with symptoms like getting unusually drowsy and suffering from stomach pain soon after exposure; lab tests using gas chromatography-mass spectrometry (GC-MS) confirmed it was all due to Pyridaben, underscoring, in most cases, why we need to be extra cautious about how these substances are used (Gautam et al., 2023). And then there's Rotenone—a naturally occurring toxin that, despite its origins, can trigger Parkinson-like symptoms. One fatality even revealed its presence in postmortem samples that were analyzed in a pretty meticulous way to nail down the toxic levels (Rhee et al., 2016). When you consider all this together, it really highlights the urgent need for stricter pesticide regulations.

7.1.9. Fentanyl and Synthetic Opioids

Fentanyl and its synthetic counterparts have recently become a big headache for those in forensic science (Figure 7.7). Generally speaking, the growing use of these drugs is not just a numbers game—it brings along tricky challenges in figuring out how exactly they mess with the brain. People who abuse drugs tend to show some unusual changes in the central nervous system, and while forensic pathologists often look for these clues during autopsies, the way fentanyl uniquely alters brain tissue still is not clear-cut. It turns out that those specific lesions linked to fentanyl toxicity are not very well described, which makes it hard to nail down the exact cause of death in suspected overdose cases. Fentanyl's sheer potency—and its rapid triggering of breathing problems—really pushes the need for more refined forensic methods. By matching what we already know about CNS alterations with drug abuse patterns, experts can slowly piece together how these neurotoxic effects lead to fatal outcomes, as shown in recent studies (Montana et al., 2024). This ongoing, sometimes messy research remains essential for stepping up the reliability of forensic investigations into opioid-related fatalities.

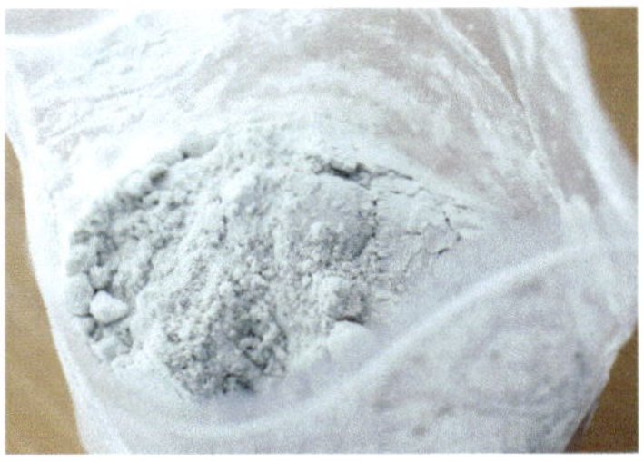

Figure 7.7. Fentanyl and synthetic opioids.

Source: Brookings Institution. (2024). *Former President Donald Trump at a Press Event Related to U.S.-China Tariffs.* https://www.brookings.edu/wp-content/uploads/2024/11/2024-11-28T091149Z_1792799355_RC2UL3AUBB4O_RTRMADP_3_USA-TRUMP-TARIFFS-CHINA.jpg?quality=75&w=1500.

Test Your Knowledge

1. What is a neurotoxic poison?
2. Name three common neurotoxic substances.

7.2. Mechanisms of Action

Learning Outcome

1. Describe oxidative stress
2. Discuss cellular apoptosis
3. Explain blood-brain barrier penetration
4. Explain enzyme inhibition
5. Focus on receptor binding
6. Identify long-term neurological effects
7. Know acute vs. chronic exposure
8. Learn variability in individual responses
9. Understand neurotransmitter disruption

Understanding how neurotoxic poisons really work matters a lot in forensic work—even when you are just trying to tell one substance from another. Take synthetic cannabinoids: they get all tangled up with the body's endocannabinoid system by latching onto cannabinoid receptors, which usually produces effects way stronger than what natural cannabis does. In most cases, this intense action ends up sparking sudden intoxications and, sometimes, even fatalities (Alves et al., 2020). Then there are agents like GHB and mephedrone; often seen in chemsex settings, they come with their own odd methods of ramping up intoxication, which makes forensic analysis even trickier (Giorgetti et al., 2017). All in all, these poisons vary widely in strength and metabolism, so gaining a clear understanding of their drug-like properties is crucial for guiding both legal measures and health responses—a fact that highlights the significant challenges they pose to forensic science.

7.2.1. Neurotransmitter Disruption

Neurotransmitters – essentially the brain's own messengers – and toxins share a surprisingly close bond that sheds light on how our bodies behave both under normal conditions and when things go off course (Figure 7.8). When heavy metals or organic pollutants appear, they can significantly disrupt the smooth flow of these signals, disrupting the usual neuron-to-neuron communication.

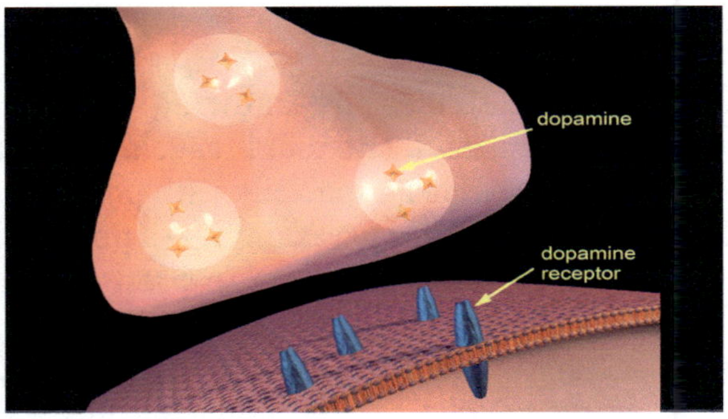

Figure 7.8. Neurotransmitters – essentially the brain's own messengers – and toxins share a surprisingly close bond that sheds light on how our bodies behave both under normal conditions and when things go off course.

Source: Science News Explores. (2019). *Illustration Explaining How Neurotransmitters Work.* https://www.snexplores.org/wp-content/uploads/2019/11/860_main_neurotransmitterexplainer_0.png.

Sometimes, a hiccup in producing these chemicals or getting them to bind to their proper receptors can cause everything from minor memory lapses to severe movement disorders. Often, toxins tend to latch onto cell parts in a way that creates dangerous complexes which eventually push cells toward programmed death and, in turn, trigger brain tissue loss, as seen with heavy metal exposure (de Machado and Dinis-Oliveira, 2023). Toxic nerve issues typically follow an axonal, length-based pattern—sensory neurons are affected first, while motor pathways tend to be spared early on (Smyth et al., 2023). All in all, this kind of disruption not only throws a wrench into forensic checks but also clearly underlines the need to spot and address any suspected poisoning quickly.

7.2.2. Enzyme Inhibition

Neurotoxic agents and enzyme inhibition become entangled in a way that triggers a complex series of biochemical events. Many of these toxins—such as certain mushroom compounds—target enzymes vital for nerve signaling and basic metabolism. For example, amatoxins from the notorious death cap mushroom inhibit RNA polymerase II, which not only halts protein production but also leads to cellular disruptions and ultimately cell death (Wennig et al., 2020). At the same time, synthetic cannabinoids, commonly linked to sudden episodes of intoxication, tend to interfere with how enzymes work, upsetting the endocannabinoid system and boosting neurotoxic effects (Alves et al., 2020). In most cases, understanding exactly which routes these toxins take is essential for forensic work, as it not only helps pinpoint the toxic agent but also lays the groundwork for designing more effective antidotes and treatment strategies. All in all, this biochemical focus deepens our discussion of neurotoxins while firmly establishing their importance in forensic science.

7.2.3. Receptor Binding

Neurotoxic poisons latching onto receptor sites play a significant role in forensic investigations—it really shows how these substances manage to wreak havoc on both the body and mind (Figure 7.9). Certain receptor spots in the central and peripheral nervous systems tend to get targeted by a mix of toxic agents, and this often leads to noticeable shifts in how people feel physically and mentally. Synthetic cannabinoids and other new psychoactive substances (NPS), for example, sometimes display odd binding behaviors that can either speed up or slow down nerve signals; the results can be anything from a quick burst of euphoria to pretty severe toxicity (Berry et al., 2025). Laboratory and clinical work, in most cases, support the idea that the strength of these toxic effects hinges significantly on how receptors are engaged (Costa et al., 2020). In short, examining the details of receptor binding not only helps pinpoint which toxins might be involved in a case but also provides a clearer picture of the overall health risks these substances pose.

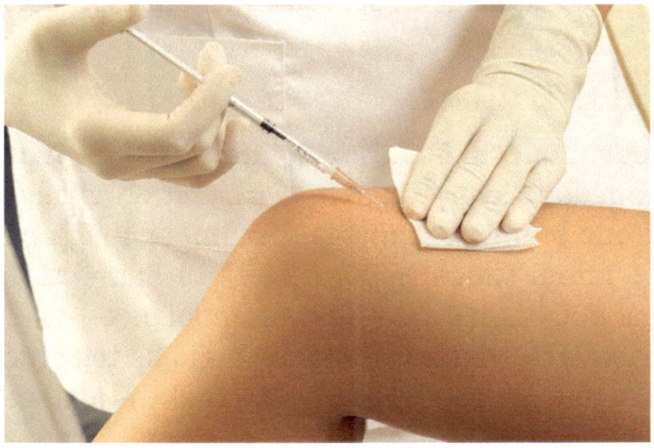

Figure 7.9. Neurotoxic poisons latching onto receptor sites play a big role in forensic investigations—it really shows how these substances manage to wreak havoc on both the body and mind.

Source: Point Performance. (2018). *Close-Up of a Knee Injection Procedure.* https://www.pointperformance.com/wp-content/uploads/2018/11/injection-knee-cropped-1024x689.jpeg.

7.2.4. Cellular Apoptosis

Cell death plays a key role in forensic cases, especially when trying to figure out how neurotoxic substances cause harm. Cells in the process of self-destruction often undergo changes in their biochemistry that suggest they have encountered toxic chemicals. Neurotoxins, for instance, can speed up this demise along several routes, sometimes triggering nerve damage or even leading to death. Extracellular vesicles (EVs) emerge as small messengers, providing insights into how cells respond to these toxins (Bala et al., 2025). You might also notice that agents like hydrogen sulfide (H2S) really shake things up; this compound disrupts everyday mitochondrial work and kicks off the cell's death signals, which ends up harming tissues and causing low oxygen levels throughout the body. All in all, understanding how and why cells opt for this programmed end is crucial in linking toxic exposures to the types of damage observed in forensic studies.

7.2.5. Oxidative Stress

Neurotoxic exposures do not just hit with immediate symptoms; they can set off changes in our brain's chemistry that linger long after the initial shock (Figure 7.10). In many cases, this boils down to a kind of imbalance—when reactive oxygen species (ROS) build up too much and outnumber the body's usual antioxidant defenses. That mismatch, often referred to as oxidative stress, tends to damage cellular structures, and brain tissues are particularly vulnerable to this type of harm. Take synthetic cannabinoid receptor agonists (SCRAs) as an example; chronic use of these substances has been linked to a surge in oxidative stress, which, over time, appears to disrupt normal mitochondrial function and trigger various cellular stress responses (AL-Banaa et al., 2020). You can see that many neurotoxic agents rely on these same mechanisms, making it crucial in forensic work to recognize these oxidative shifts as clues when assessing exposure and planning treatment for suspected poisoning cases (Agelidis et al., 2022).

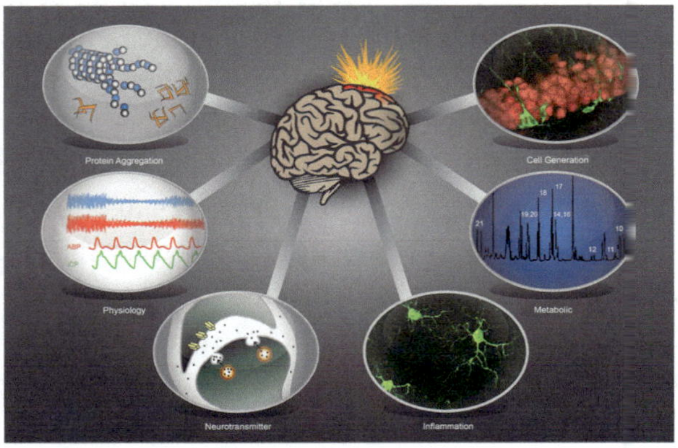

Figure 7.10. Neurotoxic exposures do not just hit with immediate symptoms; they can set off changes in our brain's chemistry that linger long after the initial shock.

Source: Nature Publishing Group. (2018). *Brain Imaging Figure From Study on Neuropsychiatric Disorders.* https://media.springernature.com/full/springer-static/image/art%3A10.1038%2Fs41380-018-0239-6/MediaObjects/41380_2018_239_Fig1_HTML.png.

7.2.6. Blood-Brain Barrier (BBB) Penetration

Neurotoxic poisons make figuring out their impact a real headache, especially when they can slip past the blood-brain barrier (BBB)—that selective shield which usually guards the central nervous system. The BBB acts like a bouncer for chemicals, yet its very function often muddies the waters of forensic analysis. Take ethanol, for example—it can seep into the brain, exposing neural tissues to harm that may later manifest as lingering illnesses or even sudden neurological issues that disrupt behavior and thinking (Herdiana, 2025). Pharmaceutical products are becoming increasingly complex, and in most cases, this means we need stricter checks on how substances interact with this natural defense. Understanding these interactions generally helps craft strategies to identify neurotoxic exposure in forensic work (Committee, 2023). Ongoing research into exactly how these toxins enter the body remains key for protecting public health and refining forensic methods, even if it sometimes feels like trying to catch a moving target.

7.2.7. Long-Term Neurological Effects

Neurotoxic substances messing with the brain have significant implications in forensic science (Figure 7.11). Generally speaking, new studies hint that synthetic cannabinoid receptor agonists—SCRAs, in short—can cause real harm, especially when someone encounters them over a long stretch of time. Even modest, repeated exposure to compounds like MDMB-CHMICA and 5F-ADB appears to alter the functioning of genes and proteins—particularly affecting how cells respond to stress and how mitochondria function—which in turn increases the risk to neurons (AL-Banaa et al., 2020). It is also worth noting that identifying the overall threat posed by these agents is not straightforward; our regulations often lag behind the latest discoveries, leaving gaps that complicate public health responses (Knudsen et al., 2017). All this suggests that more ongoing research and an update of current rules are needed to tackle these lingering neurological issues in forensic investigations.

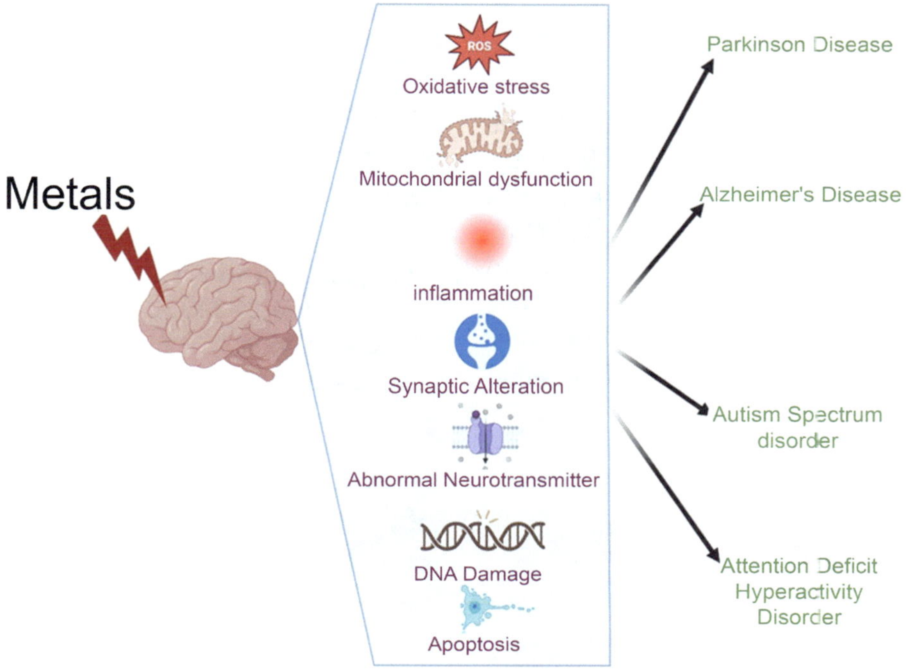

Figure 7.11. Neurotoxic substances messing with the brain have big implications in forensic science.

Source: MDPI. (2024). *Neuroglia Study Figure Showing Glial Cells and Brain Structure.*

7.2.8. Acute vs. Chronic Exposure

Deciding whether exposure to a neurotoxic substance happens in a sudden burst or drips over time really shapes forensic exams, since each path tends to lead to different kinds of health issues. A quick, heavy dose of poison can prompt rapid problems like trouble breathing or jumbled nerve signals—what we generally refer to as an acute event. Then there is the case when someone encounters a low-level toxin repeatedly, letting damage sneak in slowly by muddying organ function or sparking widespread inflammation. Research, in most cases, indicates that an abrupt encounter with organophosphate pesticides (OPs) often results in what is known as cholinergic poisoning; however, prolonged exposure risks such as heightened inflammatory responses and even the onset of cancer appear to increase (Sandilya et al., 2025). Similarly, mycotoxins like aflatoxin B1 behave quite differently depending on how long they persist, which underlines the need for thorough toxicology checks in forensic work (Sacco et al., 2024).

7.2.9. Variability in Individual Responses

Not everyone reacts to toxic chemicals in the same way. Bodies can respond very differently, with factors such as genetics, preexisting health issues, and environmental influences all playing a role (Figure 7.12). Take synthetic cannabinoid receptor agonists (SCRAs) as an example – often, younger, less-developed cells seem to be more sensitive than mature ones, which, in most cases, can lead to serious neurological issues for those already at risk (AL-Banaa et al., 2020). Then there is the case of chemical pesticides in the marine world; even slight differences in exposure can lead to significant differences in outcome, as seen in the example of brown shrimp being more susceptible to fipronil than white shrimp (Al-Badran et al., 2020). All of these observations suggest that forensic evaluations need to be tailored, as the interplay of factors varies for each affected individual.

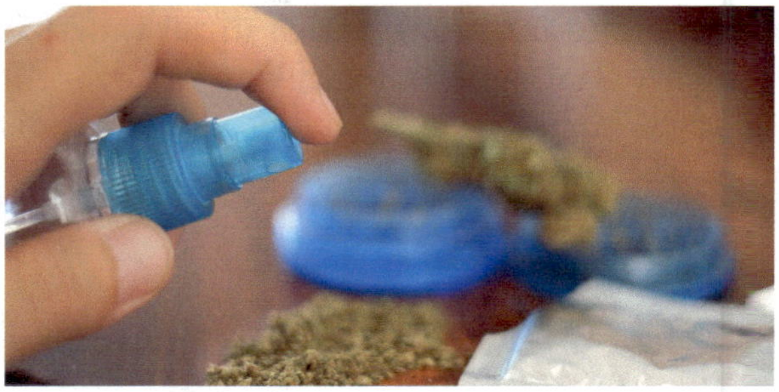

Figure 7.12. Synthetic cannabinoid receptor agonists (SCRAs).

Source: The Conversation. (2024). *Photograph Illustrating Climate Change Impact.* https://images.theconversation.com/files/575640/original/file-20240214-30-1pca5f.jpg?ixlib=rb-4.1.0&rect=7%2C396%2C4977%2C2485&q=45&auto=format&w=1356&h=668&fit=crop.

Test Your Knowledge

1. How do organophosphates cause overstimulation of nerves?
2. What is the mechanism by which botulinum toxin induces flaccid paralysis?
3. How do heavy metals like lead and mercury disrupt neuronal function?

7.3. Detection and Analysis in Forensics

Learning Outcome

1. Discuss immunoassays
2. Explain toxicological screening techniques
3. Focus on gas chromatography-mass spectrometry (GC-MS)
4. Focus on post-mortem analysis
5. Identify challenges in detection
6. Interpretation of results
7. Learn case studies of successful detection
8. Learn liquid chromatography-tandem mass spectrometry (LC-MS/MS)
9. Understand sample collection methods

Forensic science and toxicology converge in unexpected ways when it comes to identifying hazardous neurotoxins in criminal cases. Lately, labs have begun using cutting-edge methods—such as nanoparticle-based sensor technology—that have significantly changed how these poisons are detected, offering, in most cases, sharper sensitivity and precision. Platinum nanoparticles (PtNPs) are a good case in point; they are not only used in conventional chemical setups but also help measure and detect neurotoxins in biological samples, which in turn speeds up and improves the accuracy of forensic analyses (Jeyaraj et al., 2019). Herbal toxins—aconitine being a notable example—are showing up more often, and this trend pushes forensic experts to conduct more detailed toxicology reviews since, frankly, diagnosing these poisoning cases can be tricky (Gao et al., 2018). Forensic methods continue to evolve in unpredictable ways, generally speaking, and this shift provides us with a broader, albeit sometimes messy, insight into neurotoxic agents while bolstering the overall integrity and effectiveness of criminal investigations.

7.3.1. Sample Collection Methods

Neurotoxic investigations are not handled with a one-size-fits-all approach; they require meticulous, sometimes even tedious, sample collection to ensure the integrity of forensic work (Figure 7.13). Instead of sticking to one formula, experts mix things up—grabbing everything from bodily fluids to bits of tissue—to spot traces of toxins scattered across all kinds of surfaces. Touch DNA, for instance, serves as a clever trick by gathering stray genetic clues left behind at crime scenes, which often helps link individuals to toxic exposure (Devika et al., 2024). The National Forensic Laboratory Information System (NFLIS) adds another layer by providing a wealth of data that tracks these harmful chemicals over time; however, it also highlights pitfalls that researchers need to be aware of to prevent misinterpreting the results (Pitts et al., 2023). All in all, these varied sampling methods work together to enhance the accuracy of forensic investigations and generally facilitate solid prosecutions when neurotoxic agents are involved.

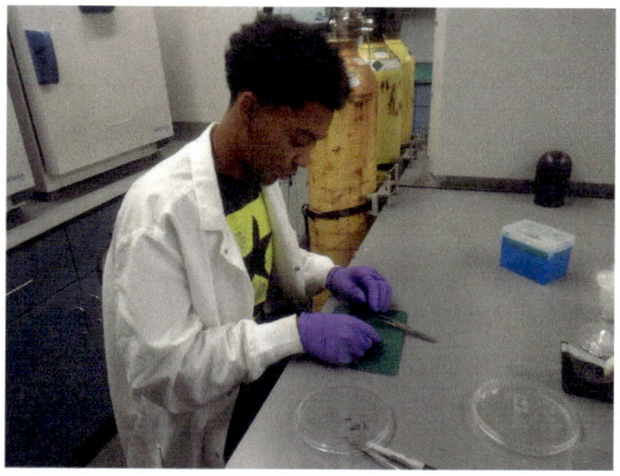

Figure 7.13. Sample collection to keep forensic work solid.

Source: TOPLAB®. (n.d.). *Photograph of Vials of Blood with Evidence Bag and Other Lab Equipment*. https://lh6.googleusercontent.com/KJQ8u5bW4G66bNqg_wttnx5cAhF4U4zTDbBp3PgdlmP3489evFLSHvri79xL-Irx-0VZZ8-5hG1T12FEnjBkLXQjGNUhsN0BKIuGRMWklph_hRS1V2MUXUR6eIl3dRsuChHK0O9c.

7.3.2. Toxicological Screening Techniques

Diagnosing poisoning from neurotoxins is not straightforward—it calls for a screening process that mixes basic tests with sharper, more detailed techniques. Generally speaking, labs start with simple tests for substances like alcohol and carbon monoxide, but then they widen the scope using methods that, for example, employ inductively coupled plasma to detect toxic metals (Pragst, 2025). Sometimes, the approach is not linear at all; initial tests can blur into more refined steps, where headspace GC or a combination of liquid chromatography and mass spectrometry is used to identify nonvolatile organic compounds, which are a significant part of the neurotoxin problem (Pragst, 2025). Recent studies have, in most cases, flagged neurotoxins such as sodium nitrite as a growing concern. This, of course, means that screening methods need to catch up to the challenges in forensic work and public health responses.

7.3.3. Gas Chromatography-Mass Spectrometry (GC-MS)

Detecting neurotoxic poisons in forensic cases is a challenging task that requires methods that are both highly sensitive and precise (Figure 7.14). One tool that has made a mark is GC-MS; it skillfully separates complex mixtures to single out harmful neuroactive compounds. The process kicks off with GC, which breaks down the compound mix before mass spectrometry steps in to lock onto each molecule's signature—generally speaking, this combo proves a real asset in forensic toxicology. Recent investigations have, in most cases, underscored GC-MS's ability to detect emerging contaminants that may be present in everyday items, such as personal care products, as well as in illicit drugs (F-Pereira et al., 2020). Equally, it has been quite helpful when dealing with substances like diquat, an herbicide known for its neurotoxic effects; its ability to trace toxicokinetic and unravel the underlying toxicity mechanisms really sets it apart (Magalhaes et al., 2018). All in all, integrating GC-MS into forensic work gives experts a significantly better chance of understanding and identifying hazardous neurotoxins.

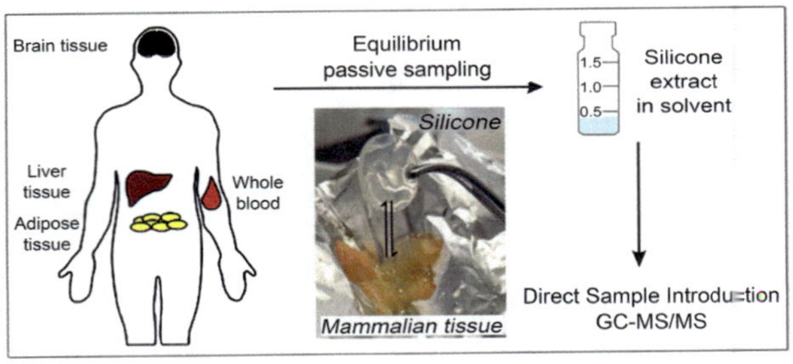

Figure 7.14. Detecting neurotoxic poisons in forensic cases is a challenging task that requires methods that are both highly sensitive and precise.

Source: Baumer, A., Escher, B. I., Landmann, J., & Ulrich, N. (2020). Direct sample introduction GC-MS/MS for quantification of organic chemicals in mammalian tissues and blood extracted with polymers without clean-up. *Analytical and Bioanalytical Chemistry*, *412*, 7295–7305.

7.3.4. Liquid Chromatography-Tandem Mass Spectrometry (LC-MS/MS)

New synthetic opioids and a mix of other neurotoxic compounds keep showing up in forensic toxicology, making it clear that we need better, more advanced testing methods. Take LC-MS/MS—short for liquid chromatography-tandem mass spectrometry (LC-MS/MS)—as an example; it is rapidly becoming the go-to approach for detecting and quantifying these substances in complex biological samples. Its sensitivity is quite impressive – it can detect even the tiniest traces of toxins like flualprazolam and isotonitazene in serum, sometimes down to 0.192 ng/mL (Akbaba et al., 2025). They have even pushed this method into hair analysis, which offers a window into long-term substance use; in most cases, tests with Swiss opioid users have shown only a low rate of these new synthetic opioids (Polke et al., 2024). All in all, LC-MS/MS not only enhances accuracy in forensic work but also provides a better understanding of how these neurotoxic substances spread and impact different groups.

7.3.5. Immunoassays

Forensic toxicology these days relies heavily on advanced techniques to identify and track down neurotoxic poisons. Immunoassays—tools that have really come into their own thanks to their knack for spotting protein toxins—offer a quick way to screen for all sorts of neurotoxins. You can see this in action when tests flag toxins from mushrooms that might be mistaken for edible ones, which can sometimes lead to serious health risks. In most cases, amatoxins found in mushrooms like the infamous death cap trigger life-threatening conditions and call for rapid diagnostic steps (Wennig et al., 2020). It is also interesting that immunoassays can pick up a broad array of biological toxins, including some identified by the Centers for Disease Control and Prevention (Ďuráčová et al., 2018). All in all, incorporating these assays into forensic work generally enhances our ability to address neurotoxic threats and ultimately helps protect public health.

7.3.6. Post-Mortem Analysis

Figuring out why someone died is not a neat, step-by-step process—especially when dangerous toxins might be involved (Figure 7.15). Instead of following a rigid checklist, forensic experts dive into every bit of evidence, examining things like tissue samples and autopsy reports while keeping an eye out for recurring hints about how the poison worked. One case, for instance, involves a heartbreaking three-month-old infant where odd clues—like milk found in unexpected places—hinted that the death might not have been a simple accident but possibly the result of neglect (Tavone et al., 2025). History shows us a similar kind of messy pursuit; back in the Joseon Dynasty, officials dug into perplexing deaths with methods that, although not as advanced as today is, still aimed to uncover hidden truths (Hong et al., 2024). All in all, these deep dives remind us that careful post-mortem checks combine medical insight with forensic expertise, laying the groundwork for sound legal conclusions.

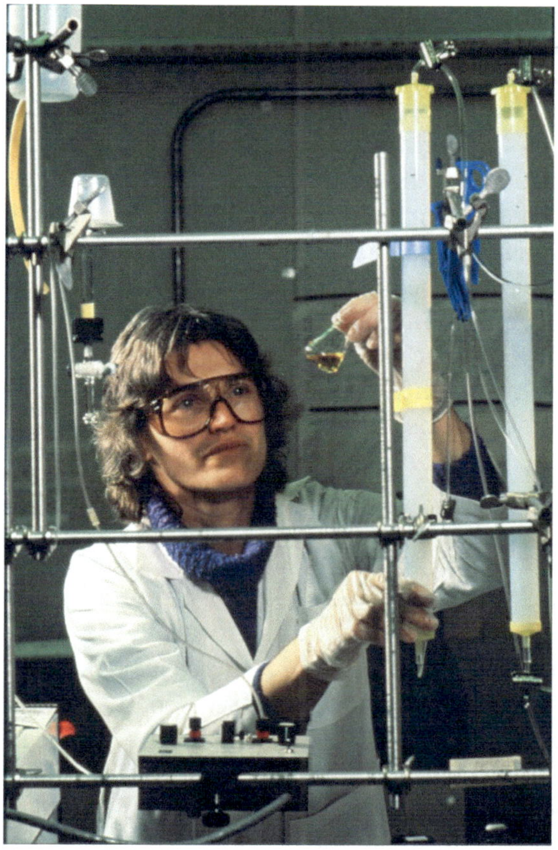

Figure 7.15. Figuring out why someone died is not a neat, step-by-step process—especially when dangerous toxins might be involved.

Source: CENODS. (n.d.). *KW Laboratory Cover Image.* https://s7d1.scene7.com/is/image/CENODS/10021-cover-kwlab?$responsive$&wid=700&qlt=90,0&resMode=sharp2.

7.3.7. Challenges in Detection

Neurotoxic compounds are becoming increasingly complex—this twist poses a significant challenge for forensic tests. Newer poisons, like synthetic cathinones, come in so many unpredictable shapes that the old, routine ways of spotting them just do not cut it anymore. In most cases, this kind of variation forces us to think outside the box. Research, for example, has shown that techniques such as differential pulse voltammetry on boron-doped diamond electrodes can detect unique electrochemical fingerprints (Lima et al., 2024). At the same time, the need for quick and portable detection tools highlights the urgent need for improved biosensors that can handle a wide range of toxins in samples (Gao, 2024). Honestly, keeping up with these twists and turns means that forensic experts must continually refine and reinvent their methods. Ultimately, mastering these advanced approaches is essential if we are to maintain the credibility of forensic investigations.

7.3.8. Interpretation of Results

Neurotoxic poison analysis is a tough nut to crack, meaning that digging into the results is essential if one wants to really nail down a cause of death in forensic cases. One study, for example, showed that in many cases of acute methadone poisoning, lung and brain swelling—pulmonary and cerebral edema—seem to be the main culprits, which generally indicates that metabolic mishaps play a big part in these fatal outcomes (Batotsyrenov et al., 2024). Advanced methods like metabolomics have also proven useful; they can tease apart different intoxication states by revealing unique metabolic changes linked to deadly results from drugs such as chlorpromazine and olanzapine (Bai et al., 2022). These observations, quite plainly, underscore that a keen grasp of metabolic profiles can help identify neurotoxic agents and even enhance forensic evaluations. In the end, carefully reading the results not only ups the accuracy of determining death causes but also highlights how vital metabolic factors are in the whole process leading to death from neurotoxic poisoning.

7.3.9. Case Studies of Successful Detection

Detecting neurotoxins quickly is a real lifesaver in forensic work—especially in remote areas where resources can be scarce. Snakebite cases, for example, demonstrate that when someone is bitten, simple, on-the-spot diagnostic tools are necessary to initiate treatment; this, in most cases, reveals significant disparities in healthcare support that ultimately impact patient outcomes (Knudsen et al., 2021). Then there is the whole issue with synthetic cannabinoids. Their effects can be all over the place, and their chemical makeup is so varied that they often dodge the usual detection techniques, which means law enforcement is forced to keep adjusting its approach to drug policies (Alves et al., 2020). Altogether, these different examples really drive home the point that constantly coming up with new detection methods is key to tackling the messy challenge of neurotoxic poisonings in forensic settings (Figure 7.16).

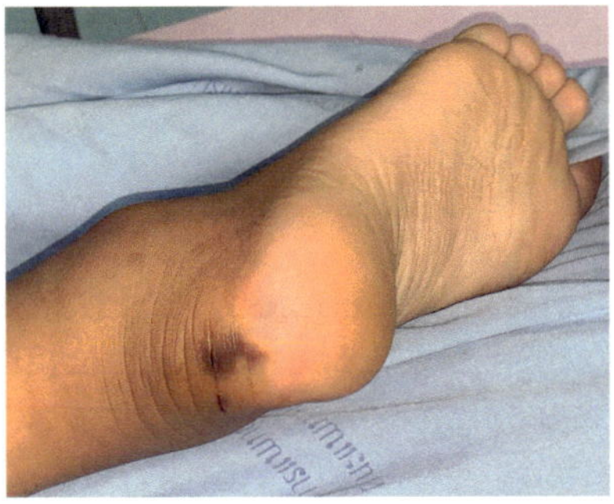

Figure 7.16. Snakebite cases, for example, show us that when someone is bitten, you need simple, on-the-spot diagnostic tools to jump-start treatment.

Source: Chainwit. (2023). Cobra bite in Thailand. *Wikimedia Commons.*

Test Your Knowledge

1. What forensic techniques are commonly used to detect organophosphate poisoning?
2. How does gas chromatography-mass spectrometry (GC-MS) help identify neurotoxic substances in biological samples?

7.4. Legal and Ethical Considerations

Learning Outcome

1. Advocacy for stricter regulations
2. Describe regulatory frameworks for neurotoxic substances
3. Discuss case law related to neurotoxic poisoning
4. Discuss the impact on sentencing and legal outcomes
5. Explain the admissibility of toxicology reports in court
6. Focus on public health implications
7. Know the role of expert witnesses
8. Learn the ethical implications of neurotoxic poisoning
9. Understand the chain of custody in forensic evidence

Forensic science and neurotoxic poisons intersect in ways that raise a multitude of legal and ethical questions that warrant closer examination. In many low- and middle-income countries, traditional lab methods stumble—animal testing debates and hit-or-miss infrastructure keep things murky. One growing workaround is the use of zebrafish; their nearly transparent larvae allow researchers to peek inside without invasive procedures, thereby reducing the harm often seen in larger vertebrates (Mukherjee et al., 2024). This shift is not just about cutting costs and speeding up tests—it also highlights the need for established protocols to ensure that lab data remains reliable, regardless of where it is gathered. All in all, as forensic toxicology ventures into increasingly complex territory, blending innovative ideas with a prudent dose of legal and ethical caution is more than just smart—it is essential.

7.4.1. Chain of Custody in Forensic Evidence

Forensic work depends on a solid chain of custody—it is really the backbone that makes evidence trustworthy, especially when neurotoxic poisons are involved. When you collect specimens from places like toxic plants or algae, you have got to note every person who touches the sample; this careful record-keeping is key to stopping any possible contamination or tampering. Research generally indicates that the distinct chemical signatures present in these plants can serve as important markers in investigations (Zakaria et al., 2025). In a similar vein, collecting and processing algal material requires strict adherence to custody principles to maintain the integrity of all biological matter and prevent contamination throughout the process (Hardy et al., 2012). Ultimately, a rigorously maintained chain of custody validates forensic analyses—even in cases dealing with dangerous neurotoxins.

7.4.2. Admissibility of Toxicology Reports in Court

Forensic work and courtroom cases often pivot on toxicology reports—even more so when neurotoxic poisons are involved. In many instances, the impact of these reports hinges on whether they adhere to strict laboratory methods and employ techniques that people can truly trust. Lately, fresh approaches from recent studies have been providing a boost to the precision with which toxic substances can be pinpointed, which in turn makes the evidence in court much more persuasive. Take, for example, phytochemical fingerprinting; this method can identify unique markers in biological samples that indicate specific neurotoxins, thereby reinforcing the argument against those held responsible for poisoning. Generally speaking, the subtle influence of trace elements on human health, as noted in several pieces of literature (Joseph et al., 2023; Zakaria et al., 2025), adds another layer of complexity to the forensic scene. All in all, these new advances not only strengthen the credibility of toxicology evidence but also keep the conversation going between legal experts and scientists. This dialogue is as important as it is ongoing (Figure 7.17).

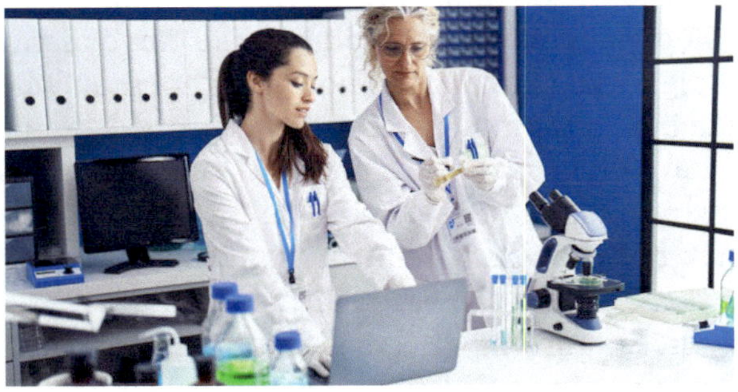

Figure 7.17. Admissibility of toxicology reports in court.

Source: DatoCMS. (n.d.). *Photograph of a Laboratory Setting*. https://www.datocms-assets.com/148522/1740080029-thl_jan_blog_3.jpg?auto=format,compress&w=800.

7.4.3. Ethical Implications of Neurotoxic Poisoning

Neurotoxic poisoning is not just a scientific puzzle—it digs into deep moral territory. Dealing with these toxic exposures means knowing how they can disrupt lives and even tear communities apart, whether the harm is done on purpose or through careless actions. Sometimes, when forensic evidence about these toxins is misused, it can lead to wrongful convictions or misguided public health decisions; generally speaking, this serves as a reminder of why adhering to solid scientific methods and a cautious ethical approach is so crucial.

Forensic experts often find themselves grappling with moral dilemmas as they deliver results that may influence legal decisions, balancing the pursuit of truth against the risk of causing societal harm. This complex interplay between forensic science and ethical duty highlights the need for ongoing, open discussions among practitioners, ethicists, and legal officials, ensuring that our insights support justice rather than perpetuate existing inequalities (Sessa, 2022; Saucedo, 2024).

7.4.4. Role of Expert Witnesses

Expert witnesses play a crucial role in forensic investigations involving neurotoxic poisons—they help clarify complex scientific details for the legal system (Figure 7.18). Their expertise in areas such as toxicology, botany, and forensic science, in most cases, bridges the stubborn gap between complex scientific concepts and the courtroom's needs. They break down how specific neurotoxins affect our bodies and behavior, which often shifts a court's understanding of what really caused harm.

Take, for example, methods such as phytochemical fingerprinting; even advanced procedures like Ultra-High-Performance Liquid Chromatography (UHPLC) (Zakaria et al., 2025) show why experts must carefully interpret detailed data. All in all, these specialists not only support prosecutorial arguments but also serve as essential resources—helping to secure fairness and accuracy in legal decisions involving neurotoxic substances (Saucedo, 2024).

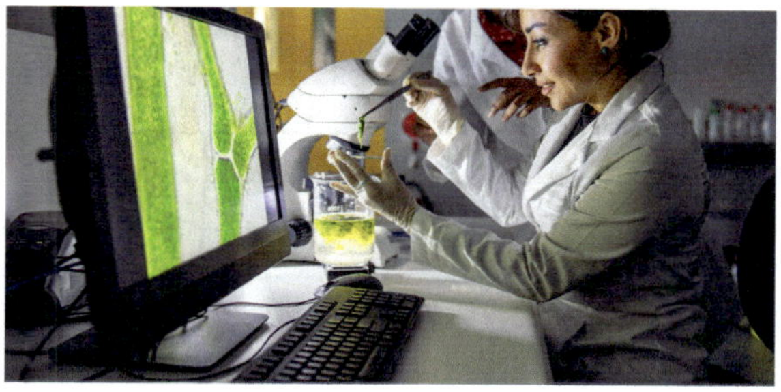

Figure 7.18. Expert witnesses play a crucial part in forensic investigations that involve neurotoxic poisons—they help sort out messy scientific details for the legal system.

Source: Forensis. (n.d.). *Photograph of a Microbiology Laboratory.* https://forensis-website-assets.s3.amazonaws.com/microbiology_57b6f3f770.jpg.

7.4.5. Impact on Sentencing and Legal Outcomes

Neurotoxic poisons really shake up forensic cases, often flipping the whole legal outcome. They trigger unusual shifts in behavior and bodily responses that sometimes make it challenging to determine someone's intent. You get these plant toxins with odd chemical profiles uncovered by tools like Ultra-HPLC, which can serve as key evidence and might even lower blame if it turns out the person was not fully aware or in control (Zakaria et al., 2025). Drugs such as phencyclidine (PCP) add another twist by muddying the link between mental health and legal responsibility, so figuring out if a crime was premeditated gets even more complicated (Bertron et al., 2018). All in all, understanding these neurotoxic effects not only shapes courtroom decisions but also ripples out to broader views on mental health and drug-related issues.

7.4.6. Public Health Implications

Neurotoxic pollutants infiltrate our everyday surroundings, and their impact extends far beyond immediate harm to individuals. Heavy metals, for example, disrupt the natural balance by degrading both soil and water quality; once they enter the environment, these trace elements accumulate in the food chain, affecting what ends up on our plates (Joseph et al., 2023). In rural areas, the situation can be even trickier. Consider how snakebites can sometimes carry neurotoxins; in low-resource regions where a quick diagnosis or proper treatment is not always possible, these exposures exacerbate healthcare gaps (Knudsen et al., 2021). Generally speaking, all these issues mean we need public health strategies that not only prevent these toxic exposures before they spread but also respond promptly when they do occur. Making healthcare accessible and making sure people get the word out seem like significant parts of protecting those who are most at risk.

7.4.7. Regulatory Frameworks for Neurotoxic Substances

Ensuring community safety means we have to keep a close eye on neurotoxic substances—there has been a noticeable uptick in poisoning cases that just cannot be ignored. These toxic compounds, which sometimes appear in both clinical and forensic settings, compel us to reassess our approach; we are now developing less predictable, more hands-on frameworks that not only pinpoint hazards but also attempt to quantify the uncertainties that underlie every assessment. Take, for example, the European Food Safety Authority's initiative on developmental neurotoxicity (DNT)—a move that generally shows how leaning on solid evidence can reshape how we manage these risks. It is not just about identifying dangers immediately; it is also about incorporating systematic reviews and even incorporating probabilistic studies to gain a better understanding of what might happen. And when people are urged to learn about quirky—and sometimes misunderstood—compounds like toad toxin, it reaffirms the need for proactive steps, a point that, in most cases, underscores why our regulatory measures need to be as strict as they are Hernandez-Jerez et al. (2021) and Liu et al. (2025) (Figure 7.19).

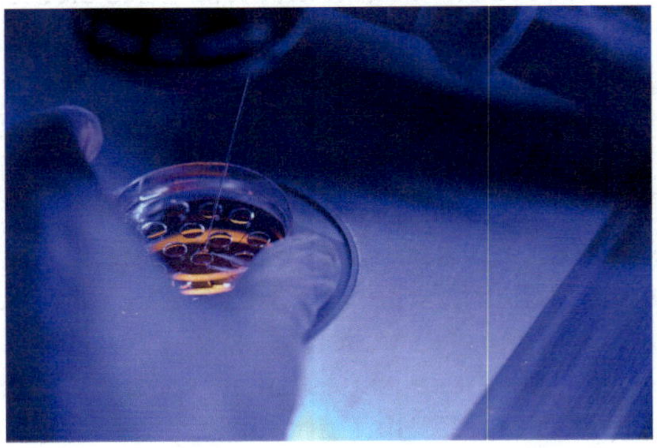

Figure 7.19. Regulatory frameworks for neurotoxic substances.

Source: Organization for Economic Co-operation and Development (OECD). (n.d.). *Photograph of Chemical Testing in a Laboratory.* https://www.oecd.org/content/dam/oecd/en/topics/policy-sub-issues/testing-of-chemicals/shutterstock_2314704833%20(1).jpg.

7.4.8. Case Law Related to Neurotoxic Poisoning

Neurotoxic poisoning and case law often mix in unexpected ways, creating a pretty tangled scene where even small bits of toxic evidence can tip legal decisions. Take, for instance, incidents with phycotoxins – those nasty chemicals from shellfish that sometimes trigger serious nerve problems – which really point to a need for clear-cut legal rules in forensic work. In many cases, linking clinical tests to environmental hazards proves trickier than one might think, as Sinno-Tellier et al. (2023) hint. Then there is the twist of synthetic cannabinoids, which have stirred up new kinds of legal puzzles, especially when it comes to figuring out how they should be classed and controlled across different regions. These substances, all too often sold under names that mislead more than inform, end up muddling court proceedings because their effects are unpredictable and regulations are always a step behind, as noted in Alves et al. (2020). Overall, the blend of neurotoxic cases in the law suggests—generally speaking—that a tighter, ongoing collaboration between scientists and legal experts is needed to effectively address the challenges of toxic exposure.

7.4.9. Advocacy for Stricter Regulations

Neurotoxic poisoning incidents have been on the rise lately, sparking urgent calls for stronger oversight. Field reports reveal sudden poisoning cases often linked to precarious chemicals like Pyridaben—which is well known for its harsh impact on the nervous system—and these exposures have led to severe health crises, particularly among vulnerable communities. In many respects, these episodes point not just to personal tragedies but also to broader lapses in preventing accidental exposure and misuse of dangerous pesticides and similar toxins (Gautam et al., 2023). One study in Bihar, for instance, found that poisoning accounted for roughly 17.6% of unnatural deaths, a figure that in most cases signals a broader public health issue which might be eased by stricter laws and more careful oversight on agrochemical sales (Deepmala et al., 2022). Addressing these challenges appears to require a multifaceted approach: a combination of community awareness, legislative adjustments, and ongoing scientific research – a strategy that may help mitigate the devastating effects of neurotoxins in forensic contexts.

Test Your Knowledge

1. What ethical responsibilities do employers have in preventing neurotoxic exposure in the workplace?
2. How should informed consent be handled in research involving potential neurotoxic substances?

SUMMARY

Neurotoxic substances in forensic work can really complicate how we view toxicology in both hospital labs and court cases. Look at the venom from something like the tiger snake—evidence from (Balmer et al., 2011) shows that these poisons can hit organs in precise ways, often leading to messy clotting issues that make diagnosis and treatment trickier than they should be. Toxic plants such as Datura add another twist; generally speaking, while they sometimes appear to be used for healing, in other cases they are misused in crimes, as Sharma et al. (2020) somewhat point out. This kind of double-edged nature forces forensic experts to stay extra vigilant because pinpointing and understanding where these toxins act is absolutely key to untangling the web of poisoning cases. In most cases, with ongoing research and a bit of teamwork, the forensic community can steadily sharpen its detection methods—thereby supporting both justice and public safety.

Neurotoxic poisons in forensic cases reveal a tangled mix between chemical exposures and brain function issues. Several studies point out that a substance like hydrogen sulfide (H2S) can really mess with the way we think while stirring up our brain's chemistry. In most cases, acute exposure to H2S not only tweaks the brain's metabolome but also shuffles key neurotransmitters such as aspartate, glutamate, and serotonin—a change that might be linked to seizures or even early signs of neurodegeneration (Kim et al., 2024). Even more curiously, prolonged exposure to levels often considered safe by occupational guidelines can unexpectedly lower serotonin and glucose levels (Kim et al., 2024). This sort of split effect suggests – and indeed underscores – that when investigating poisoning, a detailed, sometimes messy, forensic examination is vital; early detection and thorough analysis often bring hidden health risks into view. All things considered, these insights combine to reaffirm just how important the role of neurotoxic poisons is in the realm of forensic science.

KEY TERMS FROM THIS CHAPTER

- Acetylcholinesterase
- Agrochemicals
- Blood
- Botulinum toxin
- carbon monoxide
- Clostridium botulinum
- Cyanide
- Fentanyl
- Food chains
- Formaldehyde
- Formic acid
- Heavy metals
- Lead
- Mercury

CRITICAL THINKING QUESTIONS

1. **Which of the following is a well-known neurotoxin that inhibits acetylcholinesterase?**
   a. Cyanide
   b. Organophosphates
   c. Lead
   d. Ethanol
2. **Botulinum toxin causes paralysis by:**
   a. Enhancing acetylcholine release
   b. Blocking dopamine synthesis
   c. Inhibiting acetylcholine release at neuromuscular junctions
   d. Increasing serotonin activity
3. **Chronic exposure to which metal is associated with tremors, memory loss, and personality changes?**
   a. Mercury
   b. Arsenic
   c. Barium
   d. Aluminum
4. **"Mad Hatter's disease" is a form of neurotoxicity due to exposure to:**
   a. Lead
   b. Mercury
   c. Arsenic
   d. Thallium
5. **Which marine toxin blocks sodium channels, causing rapid-onset neurotoxicity?**
   a. Saxitoxin
   b. Curare
   c. Lead
   d. Carbon monoxide

Short Answer Questions

1. How do organophosphates cause neurotoxicity?
2. What are the clinical signs of acute neurotoxic poisoning?
3. How does botulinum toxin affect the nervous system?
4. What type of paralysis is caused by curare and similar toxins?
5. How does lead affect the developing nervous system in children?
6. What are the neurological effects of chronic mercury exposure?
7. How can neurotoxic effects be assessed in a clinical setting?

Answers to Critical Thinking Questions

1. (b); 2. (c); 3. (a); 4. (b); 5. (a)

REFERENCES

1. Abrosimova, O. L. (2024). *On an Integrated Approach to the Formation of Competencies in Teaching Russian as a Foreign Language at a Russian University*. https://doi.org/10.34660/inf.2020.25.23.006.
2. Akbaba, M., & Isir, A. B. (2025). The development of a highly sensitive liquid chromatography–tandem mass spectrometry (LC-MS/MS) method for the validation of flualprazolam and isotonitazene in serum. *Applied Sciences*. https://www.semanticscholar.org/paper/f6a986b306ada0d39d9ca03172f9aa78910cdcc3 (accessed on 9th May 2025).
3. Al-Badran, A. A. K. (2020). Investigation of lethal and sub-lethal effects of common insecticides, fipronil and imidacloprid, on juvenile brown shrimp, *Farfantepenaeus aztecus*, and white shrimp, *Litopenaeus setiferus*. https://core.ac.uk/download/333659321.pdf (accessed on 9th May 2025).
4. Al-Banaa, I. M. J. (2020). *Epidemiological, Pharmacological and Toxicological Investigation of New Psychoactive Substances.* https://core.ac.uk/download/482028653.pdf (accessed on 9th May 2025).
5. Albano, G. D., Argo, A., Bertol, E., La Spina, C., Malta, G., Provenzano, V., Rifiorito, A., et al. (2022). *Toxicological Findings of Self-Poisoning Suicidal Deaths: A Systematic Review by Countries.* https://core.ac.uk/download/558778364.pdf (accessed on 9th May 2025).
6. Albano, G. D., La Spina, C., Buscemi, R., Palmeri, M., Malandrino, G., Licciardello, F., Midiri, M., et al. (2024). RETRACTED: Systematic review of fatal sodium nitrite ingestion cases: Toxicological and forensic implications. *Toxics, 12*. https://www.semanticscholar.org/paper/0596c7e6e43fe4155aadc5a2d4fd27e757a626a6 (accessed on 9th May 2025).
7. Aleksić, A. A., Aleksić, R. J., Davidov, I., Ivanović, et al. (2022). *The Most Common Intentional Poisoning of Dogs and Cats on the Territory of the Republic of Serbia.* https://core.ac.uk/download/560400642.pdf (accessed on 9th May 2025).
8. Alves, V. L., Gonçalves, J., Aguiar, J., Teixeira, H. M., & Câmara, J. S. (2020). The synthetic cannabinoids phenomenon: From structure to toxicological properties. A review. *Critical Reviews in Toxicology, 50*, 359–382. https://doi.org/10.1080/10408444.2020.1762539.
9. Ambareen, K., & Venkateshwarlu, M., (2023). Sub-lethal effects of chlorpyrifos on Geno-neurotoxic profiles in freshwater fish *Cyprinus carpio* (L.). *Journal of Pharmaceutical Negative Results*. https://www.semanticscholar.org/paper/03bb45c6b1708e2d50bd3107199ad73f54246986 (accessed on 9th May 2025).
10. Bai, R., Dai, X., Miao, X., Xie, B., Yu, F., Cong, B., Wen, D., et al. (2022). Dynamic changes in plasma metabolic profiles reveal a potential metabolite panel for interpretation of fatal intoxication by chlorpromazine or olanzapine in mice. *Metabolites, 12*. https://www.semanticscholar.org/paper/fdde5e9906d4817d73ad275061d549af761a6d6c (accessed on 9th May 2025).
11. Bala, A. A., Oukkache, N., Sánchez, E. E., Suntravat, M., & Galán, J. A. (2025). Venoms and extracellular vesicles: A new frontier in venom biology. *Toxins, 17*, 36. https://doi.org/10.3390/toxins17010036.
12. Balmer, L., Brown, S. G. A., Davern, K. M., Jacoby-Alner, et al. (2011). *Histopathological Analysis and in Situ Localization of Australian Tiger Snake Venom in Two Clinically Envenomed Domestic Animals*. https://core.ac.uk/download/11235854.pdf (accessed on 9th May 2025).

13. Basarslan, S. K., & Basarslan, F., (2023). Intralipid and caffeic acid phenethyl ester reverse the neurotoxic effects of organophosphate poisoning in rats. *Nigerian Journal of Clinical Practice, 26*(6), 686–693. https://www.semanticscholar.org/paper/ab2b333e35e7299728b1e5296c8f1899d346b207 (accessed on 9th May 2025).

14. Batotsyrenov, C. B., Kuznetsov, S., Lodyagin, A. H., Reinuk, V. L., Molin, Y. A., Litvincev, B. S., Klimanov, D. V., et al. (2024). Thanatogenesis and forensic assessment of severe acute methadone poisoning. *Russian Journal of Forensic Medicine.* https://www.semanticscholar.org/paper/9f67cd402bfc269831d4119b28d72243a551ea43 (accessed on 9th May 2025).

15. Berry, A., Shafi, A., Sumnall, H., Tracy, et al. (2025). *New Psychoactive Substances – A Review And Updates.* https://core.ac.uk/download/337612492.pdf (accessed on 9th May 2025)

16. Bertron, J. L., Seto, M., & Lindsley, C. W. (2018). DARK classics in chemical neuroscience: Phencyclidine (PCP). *ACS Chemical Neuroscience, 9*, 2459–2474. https://doi.org/10.1021/acschemneuro.8b00266.

17. Blain, P. G., & Vonberg, F. W. (2024). *Neurotoxicology: A Clinical Systems-Based Review.* https://core.ac.uk/download/613849271.pdf (accessed on 9th May 2025).

18. Brzozowski, K., Daoust-Maleval, I., Geypens, B., Goulart de Medeiros, M., Iatan, A. E., Lequarre, A. S., & Santopolo, D., (2022). *EU CBRNe Glossary*. https://core.ac.uk/download/642865393.pdf (accessed on 9th May 2025).

19. Costa, G., De Luca, M. A., Fattore, L., Marongiu, et al. (2020). *Neuronal and Peripheral Damages Induced by Synthetic Psychoactive Substances: An Update of Recent Findings from Human and Animal Studies.* https://core.ac.uk/download/268908564.pdf (accessed on 9th May 2025).

20. Deepmala, D., Singh, R., Das, R., & Bhushan, V., (2022). The socio-demographic profile of unnatural death in Bihar. *International Journal of Medical Reviews and Case Reports.* https://www.semanticscholar.org/paper/b28019b69e466a792878d02c3d00f1582a8f41c4 (accessed on 9th May 2025).

21. Devers, K. G., & Nine, J., (2010). Autopsy findings in botulinum toxin poisoning. *Journal of Forensic Sciences, 55*. https://www.semanticscholar.org/paper/7f008535e3d440a3435cafa15d2ecbcb03005e8f (accessed on 9th May 2025).

22. Devika, G., Vaishnavi, S., & Mane, M., (2024). Forensic significance of touch deoxyribonucleic acid. *Journal of Forensic Science and Medicine*. https://www.semanticscholar.org/paper/[illegible]f939b95224481fa3b276090d2bf302f85fe5d84 (accessed on 9th May 2025).

23. Ďuráčová, M., Klimentová, J., Fučíková, A., & Dresler, J., (2018). Proteomic methods of detection and quantification of protein toxins. *Toxins, 10*, 99. https://doi.org/10.3390/toxins10030099.

24. Gao, A., (2024). Advances in biosensors for poison detection applications. *E3S Web of Conferences.* https://www.semanticscholar.org/paper/936186f7c381c230226f330e91ce1a15f983463d (accessed on 9th May 2025).

25. Gao, X., Hu, J., Zhang, X., Zuo, Y., Wang, Y., & Zhu, S., (2018). Research progress of aconitine toxicity and forensic analysis of aconitine poisoning. *Forensic Sciences Research, 5*, 25–31. https://doi.org/10.1080/20961790.2018.1452346.

26. Gautam, A. K., Paul, S. K., & Verma, D., (2023). A case report on the toxicological evaluation of pyridaben from a human cadaver. *Austin Journal of Forensic Science and Criminology*. https://www.semanticscholar.org/paper/ebc4ce40d79f4ae5dbdd5f4982a80feb63358c55 (accessed on 9th May 2025).

27. Giorgetti, R., Tagliabracci, A., Schifano, F., Zaami, S., Marinelli, E., & Busardò, F. P. (2017). When "Chems" meet sex: A rising phenomenon called "ChemSex." *Current Neuropharmacology, 15.* https://doi.org/10.2174/1570159x15666161117151148.

28. Hardy, C. R., & Wallace, J. R. (2012). *Algae in Forensic Investigations.* https://doi.org/10.1002/9781119945734.ch9.

29. Herdiana, Y., (2025). Alcohol in daily products: Health risks, cultural considerations, and economic impacts. *Risk Management and Healthcare Policy, 18,* 217–237. https://doi.org/10.2147/rmhp.s495493.

30. Hernandez-Jerez, A., Adriaanse, P., Aldrich, A., Berny, P., Čoja, T., Duquesne, S., Focks, A., et al. (2021). Development of integrated approaches to testing and assessment (IATA) case studies on developmental neurotoxicity (DNT) risk assessment. *EFSA Journal.* https://www.semanticscholar.org/paper/4afe5cf178a461914a5a7338a7ddeedf33317268 (accessed on 9th May 2025).

31. Hong, S., Lee, S. D., & Shin, D. H. (2024). Forensic anthropological analysis of the Korean Empire's post-mortem examination report on Park Bong-Un of Unbong County. *Korean Journal of Legal Medicine.* https://www.semanticscholar.org/paper/b05799c5fe4ba4b222da43e0fe184c20d82b4e9b (accessed on 9th May 2025).

32 Jeyaraj, M., Gurunathan, S., Qasim, M., Kang, M. H., & Kim, J. H. (2019). A comprehensive review on the synthesis, characterization, and biomedical application of platinum nanoparticles. *Nanomaterials, 9,* 1719. https://doi.org/10.3390/nano9121719.

33. Joseph, D., Ahuja, P., Dockrell, M. E. C., Purchase, D., Price, R., Krishna, S., García-Muñoz, J., et al. (2023). *Trace Metals in the Environment.* IntechOpen eBooks. https://doi.org/10.5772/intechopen.1001530.

34. Kharmate, S. A., & Yadav, P. N. (2024). Determine the various types of fungi found on corpse – A review. *International Journal of Scientific Research in Science and Technology*. https://www.semanticscholar.org/paper/66191968296009c56c01437f1f4ae16fdd9f3ad0 (accessed on 9th May 2025).

35. Kim, D. S., Santana, M. C. M., Giulivi, C., & Rumbeiha, W. K. (2024). Metabolomic signatures of brainstem in mice following acute and subchronic hydrogen sulfide exposure. *Metabolites, 14,* 53–53. https://doi.org/10.3390/metabo14010053.

36. Knudsen, C., Jürgensen, J. A., Føns, S., Haack, A. M., Friis, R. U. W., Dam, S. H., Bush, S. P., et al. (2021). Snakebite envenoming diagnosis and diagnostics. *Frontiers in Immunology, 12.* https://doi.org/10.3389/fimmu.2021.661457.

37. Knudsen, S. H. (2017). *Regulating Cumulative Risk.* https://core.ac.uk/download/267973167.pdf (accessed on 9th May 2025).

38. Lehner, A. F., Bokhart, M. T., Johnson, M., & Buchweitz, J. P. (2018). Characterization of bromethalin and its degradation products in veterinary toxicology samples by GC–MS-MS. *Journal of Analytical Toxicology, 43,* 112–125. https://doi.org/10.1093/jat/bky072.

39. Lima, C. D., Arantes, L. C., Machado, L. L., Paixão, T., & Dos Santos, W. T. P. (2024). Synthetic cathinones' comprehensive screening and classification by voltametric and chemometric analyses: A powerful method for on-site forensic applications. *Analytical Chemistry, 96,* 17746–17753. https://www.semanticscholar.org/paper/f842a4ec8590008a15d2db499e4866fa1280dad0 (accessed on 9th May 2025).

40. Liu, Y., Zhang, J., Wang, B., Zheng, F., & Yan, J., (2025). Epidemiological patterns and therapeutic approaches of toad toxin poisoning in a retrospective case study. *Scientific Reports, 15*. https://www.semanticscholar.org/paper/6dbb347e000126d867d45969e9a126d380b8a336 (accessed on 9th May 2025).

41. Machado, C. de C., & Dinis-Oliveira, R. J. (2023). Clinical and forensic signs resulting from exposure to heavy metals and other chemical elements of the periodic table. *Journal of Clinical Medicine, 12*, 2591. https://doi.org/10.3390/jcm12072591.

42. Magalhaes, N. P., Carvalho, F., & Dinis-Oliveira, R. J. (2018). Human and experimental toxicology of diquat poisoning: Toxicokinetics, mechanisms of toxicity, clinical features, and treatment. *Human & Experimental Toxicology, 37*, 1131–1160. https://doi.org/10.1177/0960327118765330.

43. Marks, C. J. (2020). *The Core Competencies Required by Toxicology Students in Order to Function Effectively in a Poisons Information Center: A Delphi Study*. https://core.ac.uk/download/328346641.pdf (accessed on 9th May 2025).

44. Marsico, F. L., & Egeland, T., (2024). Likelihood ratios for physical traits in forensic investigations. *bioRxiv*. https://www.semanticscholar.org/paper/56eccb5263af905f0ae79413284c4a6b06baf23c (accessed on 9th May 2025).

45. Miliano, C., Serpelloni, G., Rimondo, C., Mereu, M., Marti, M., & De Luca, M. A. (2016). Neuropharmacology of new psychoactive substances (NPS): Focus on the rewarding and reinforcing properties of cannabimimetics and amphetamine-like stimulants. *Frontiers in Neuroscience, 10*. https://doi.org/10.3389/fnins.2016.00153.

46. Montana, A., Alfieri, L., Neri, M., Piano, D., Renier, E., Marti, M., Palpacelli, M., et al. (2024). Macroscopic and microscopic cerebral findings in drug and alcohol abusers: The point of view of the forensic pathologist. *Biomedicines, 12*, 681. https://doi.org/10.3390/biomedicines12030681.

47. Mukherjee, S., Mohanty, A., Chinnadurai, R. K., Deb Barman, D., & Poddar, A., (2024). Zebrafish: A cost-effective model for enhanced forensic toxicology capabilities in low- and middle-income countries. *Cureus*. https://doi.org/10.7759/cureus.76223.

48. Opravil, J., Pejchal, J., Finger, V., Korábečný, J., Rozsypal, T., Hrabinová, M., Múčková, L., et al. (2023). A-agents, misleadingly known as "Novichoks": A narrative review. *Archives of Toxicology, 97*, 2587–2607. https://doi.org/10.1007/s00204-023-03571-8.

49. Pena-Pereira, F., Bendicho, C., Mutavdžić, P. D., Martín-Esteban, A., Díaz-Álvarez, M., Pan, Y., Cooper, J. M., et al. (2020). Miniaturized analytical methods for determination of environmental contaminants of emerging concern – A review. *Analytica Chimica Acta, 1158*, 238108–238108. https://doi.org/10.1016/j.aca.2020.11.040.

50. Pitts, W. J., Heller, D., Smiley-McDonald, H., Weimer, B., Grabenauer, M., Bollinger, K., Ropero-Miller, J., et al. (2023). Understanding research methods, limitations, and applications of drug data collected by the National Forensic Laboratory Information System (NFLIS-Drug). *Journal of Forensic Sciences, 68*, 1335–1342. https://www.semanticscholar.org/paper/bccea6744dcce483dea8faf459e4dbe3c35fabf9 (accessed on 9th May 2025).

51. Polke, M., Concheiro, M., Cooper, G., Bogdal, C., Baumgartner, M., Kraemer, T., & Binz, T., (2024). Development and validation of a liquid chromatography-tandem mass spectrometry (LC-MS/MS) method including 25 novel synthetic opioids in hair and subsequent analysis of a Swiss opioid consumer cohort. *Drug Testing and Analysis*. https://www.semanticscholar.

org/paper/508e4b9dbbb99af0821b1884de84398ed949dc25 (accessed on 9th May 2025).

52. Pragst, F., (2025). Systematic toxicological analysis in forensic and clinical laboratories: A challenging task of analytical chemistry. *ChemTexts*. https://www.semanticscholar.org/paper/9ea88b3c70dafdaff6c1dfe3569b42da439bc82f (accessed on 9th May 2025).

53. Rhee, J., Yum, H., Moon, S., In, S., Lee, S., & Seo, J., (2016). Rotenone analysis by liquid chromatography-tandem mass spectrometry with information-dependent acquisition in a fatal case of rotenone poisoning with a commercial organic insecticide being sold in Korea. *Journal of Analytical Toxicology, 40*(6), 460–465. https://www.semanticscholar.org/paper/512fe6af54288d6691c96af4893a4f617a68f1da (accessed on 9th May 2025).

54. Sacco, M. A., Gualtieri, S., Tarallo, A. P., Verrina, M. C., Carbone, A., Mazzuca, W., Gratteri, S., et al. (2024). The role of AFB1, OTA, TCNs, and patulin in forensic sciences: Applications in autopsy, criminal investigations, and public health prevention. *Toxins, 16*. https://www.semanticscholar.org/paper/a8458b432d71236b27dea352d34b3e6d13e9a285 (accessed on 9th May 2025).

55. Sandilya, V., El-Gameel, D., Atashi, M., Nguyen, T., Fowowe, M., Bhuiyan, M. M. A., Daramola, O., et al. (2025). LC-MS/MS-profiling of human serum unveils significant increase in neuroinflammation and carcinogenesis following chronic organophosphate exposure. *Journal of Proteome Research*. https://www.semanticscholar.org/paper/fe76045a0bab4e2c233524e31b37b6f14574abe1 (accessed on 9th May 2025).

56. Saucedo, C., (2024). NUBE abstract issue. *Western Journal of Emergency Medicine, 25*. https://doi.org/10.5811/westjem.19410.

57. Sessa, F., (2022). *Forensic Science and Legal Medicine.* MDPI eBooks. https://doi.org/10.3390/books978-3-0365-4193-8.

58. Sharma, A., & Yadav, S., (2020). *A Toxicological Review of Dhatura.* https://core.ac.uk/download/478521846.pdf (accessed on 9th May 2025).

59. Singh, R. R., Tripathi, S. K., Bharti, A., & Yadav, P. K. (2025). Analyzing the efficacy of artificial intelligence in facilitating medico-legal investigations and enhancing forensic processes for emergency trauma patients: A systematic review. *Journal of Forensic Science and Medicine*. https://www.semanticscholar.org/paper/43b6e94c4f01224ec121d449ebc50f605a5e1d66 (accessed on 9th May 2025).

60. Sinno-Tellier, S., Abadie, É., Guillotin, S., Bossée, A., Nicolas, M., & Delcourt, N., (2023). Human shellfish poisoning: Implementation of a national surveillance program in France. *Frontiers in Marine Science, 9*. https://doi.org/10.3389/fmars.2022.1089585.

61. Smyth, D., Kramarz, C., Carr, A., Rossor, A. M., & Lunn, M. P. (2023). Toxic neuropathies: A practical approach. *Practical Neurology, 23*, 120–130. https://doi.org/10.1136/pn-2022-003444.

62. Tavone, A., Servadei, F., Cazzato, F., Giacobbi, E., Bonfiglio, R., Oliva, A., & Marella, G., (2025). Diagnosing milk aspiration as a cause of death in sudden unexpected infant death: Forensic insights from post-mortem analysis impacting criminal investigations. *Forensic Science, Medicine, and Pathology*. https://www.semanticscholar.org/paper/5ca5a328591258e02ca6f3f7a29dd479ca03a385 (accessed on 9th May 2025).

63. The Scientific Committee. (2023). Proceedings of the workshop NANO23@uniVR – 8–9 June 2023, University of Verona, Italy. *European Journal of Histochemistry, 67*. https://doi.org/10.4081/ejh.2023.3778.

64. Ulloa, M., Rivero, M. A., & Fernández, A., (2024). Contribution to the knowledge of cetacean strandings in Chile between 2015 and 2020. *Oceans, 5*, 1–20. https://doi.org/10.3390/oceans5010001.

65. Wankhede, A., (2024). The role of fingernails in death investigation. *The American Journal of Forensic Medicine and Pathology*. https://www.semanticscholar.org/paper/6227214027f81c3295a7a1a7f4e32fbda8955da9 (accessed on 9th May 2025).

66. Wennig, R., Eyer, F., Schaper, A., Zilker, T., & Andresen-Streichert, H., (2020). Mushroom poisoning. *Deutsches Ärzteblatt International*. https://doi.org/10.3238/arztebl.2020.0701.

67. Xie, X., Li, B., Fan, Y. H., Duan, R., Gao, C., Zheng, Y., & Tian, E., (2022). Identification of *Gyromitra infula*: A rapid and visual method based on loop-mediated isothermal amplification. *Frontiers in Microbiology, 13*. https://www.semanticscholar.org/paper/7e78cb9d194a81f4a944b1b637b3cca00c8bbfed (accessed on 9th May 2025).

68. Zakaria, N., El-Sayed, A. S. A., & Ali, M. G. (2025). Phytochemical fingerprinting of phytotoxins as a cutting-edge approach for unveiling nature's secrets in forensic science. *Natural Products and Bioprospecting, 15*. https://doi.org/10.1007/s13659-024-00484-6.

CARDIOTOXIC AND MISCELLANEOUS POISONS

8

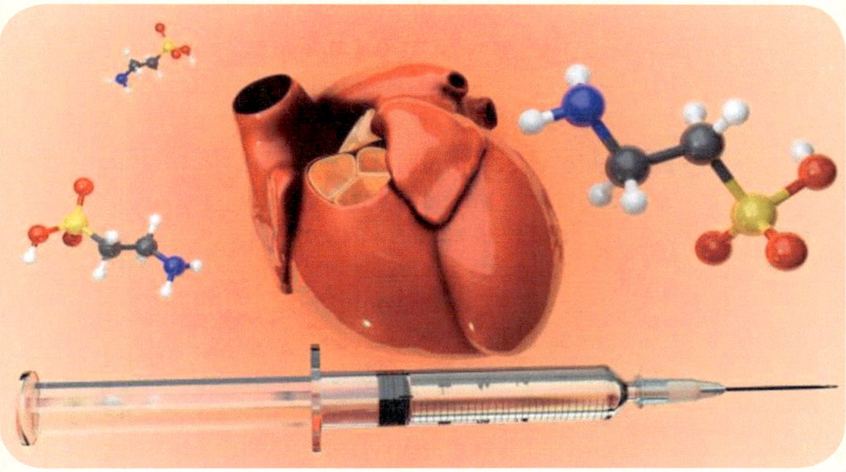

LEARNING OBJECTIVES

After studying this chapter, you will be able to:

1. Understand cardiotoxic poisons
2. Identify miscellaneous poisons in forensic science
3. Explain forensic toxicology techniques
4. Focus on legal and ethical considerations.

Introduction

Chemicals interact with our bodies in surprisingly complex ways, and in forensic work, this is not a straightforward, step-by-step process. Poisonous substances—whether they target the heart or are of a more miscellaneous nature—can really throw off the assessment of how and why someone died; in many cases, investigators stumble through these challenges because the lines blur between apparent toxic effects and subtle physiological changes. To figure this out, one must look closely at how these compounds act inside the body—studying not just their chemical properties but also the intricate metabolic pathways they follow. For example, Prothipendyl and cannabinoids, when measured at their usual blood levels along with specific markers hinting at recent use, point to the need for rock-solid forensic data. Meanwhile, the constant arrival of new psychoactive substances (NPS) keeps shaking things up, as these ever-changing chemicals make detection and interpretation even more unpredictable (Guirguis et al., 2017). In most cases, blending tried-and-true methods with newer, innovative techniques seems the only way to untangle the complex reality of poison-related investigations; a flexible, integrated approach is key for forensic toxicology to capture every nuance, however messy the process may be.

Definition of Cardiotoxic and Miscellaneous Poisons

Forensic toxicology is not as cut-and-dry as it may seem; you really have to get a grip on how various substances can damage health. Cardiotoxic agents, for instance, tend to be particularly sneaky—they zero in on the heart, often messing up its rhythm and structure so badly that arrhythmias, heart attacks, or even death can result. In many cases, substances such as certain pharmaceuticals, heavy metals, and even natural toxins can disrupt a heart's normal rhythm by interfering with its electrical signals and muscular function.

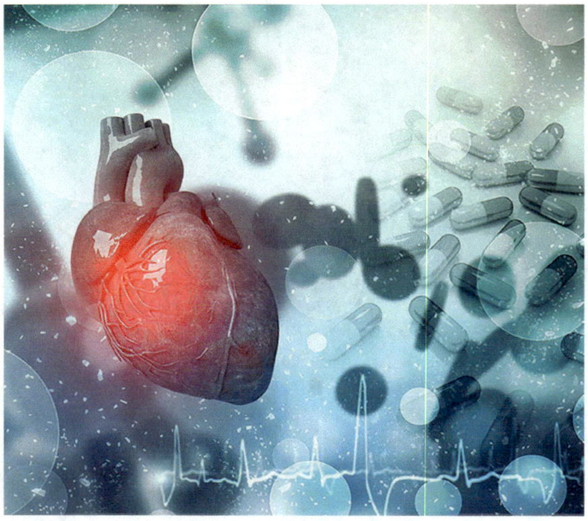

Figure 8.1. Cardiotoxic agents.

Source: Enzo Life Sciences. (2023). *Cardiotoxic Drugs and Mechanisms of Cardiotoxicity.* https://www.enzo.com/wp-content/uploads/2024/05/2023-02-TN-Cardiotoxic-drugs-and-mechanisms-of-cardiotoxicity.jpg.

Then again, there is a whole mix of other poisons that do not fit into one neat box—industrial chemicals, everyday household products, and environmental toxins that accumulate over time all fall under this jumbled category (Payne-James et al., 2011). Their different ways of wreaking havoc only make investigations tougher since each one calls for its own testing method to figure out whether it is present and how it is affecting the body. Overall, obtaining a clear picture of these differences is crucial for forensic specialists attempting to investigate poisoning cases (Figure 8.1).

Importance of Studying Poisons in Forensics

Forensic cases involving poison tend to be unexpectedly messy. Often, a case's complex details force us to delve deeply into the range of harmful substances around us. Take yellow oleander—this plant might look harmless at a glance. Still, it carries dangerous cardiac glycosides that, in recent studies (Professor, 2018), have been linked with life-threatening heart rhythm issues after people ingest it. Then there's carbon monoxide poisoning, which in most cases does not receive the attention it deserves, underscoring the vital importance of forensic expertise in detecting even the faintest signs of trouble and avoiding a misdiagnosis. Examining these diverse poisons closely, forensic teams can gradually refine their detection methods and analytical techniques, thereby generally enhancing the success of criminal casework. Knowledge about both cardiotoxic substances and other toxins not only helps in figuring out the cause and manner of death but also plays a vital role in public health tracking and in taking preventive measures against toxic exposures.

Overview of the Impact of Poisons on Human Health

Poisoning hits human health in ways that are not always straightforward. A strong dose of a toxin—especially one that messes with the heart—can cause a crisis, like the body struggling to breathe, organs failing, or even death. Yet sometimes the damage is slow and sneaks up over time; continuous exposure may lead to nerve problems, reproductive issues, and an increased risk of certain cancers. Not everyone is affected the same way, either—factors such as age, gender, and pre-existing conditions mix in, complicating the picture and keeping forensic experts on their toes. Generally speaking, knowing these little nuances really helps in weighing the risks and is key to setting up effective treatment and prevention plans (Casarett et al., 2001) (Figure 8.2).

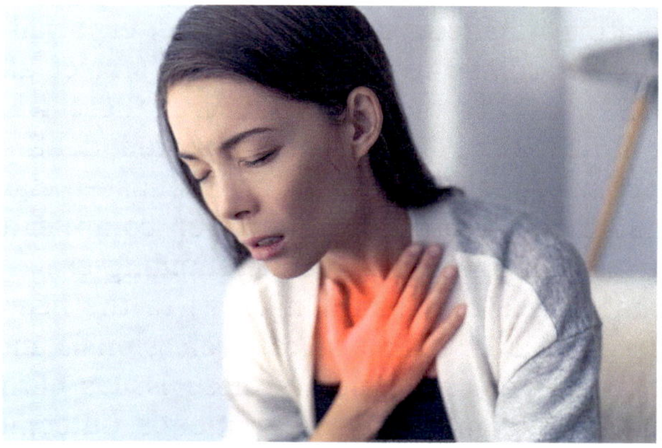

Figure 8.2. A strong dose of a toxin—especially one that messes with the heart—can cause a crisis, like the body struggling to breathe, organs failing, or even death.

Source: PatientPop. (n.d.). *Photograph of a Medical Professional.* https://sa1s3optim.patientpop.com/assets/images/provider/photos/2252940.jpeg.

Historical Context of Poison Use in Criminal Cases

Poison has a strange pull that has woven itself through the history of crime for centuries. In Ancient Rome, the powerful sometimes slipped it into political schemes—quiet kills done under the radar; one well-known case is that of Emperor Claudius, who, it is said, was taken out with poison by his wife Agrippina. Over time, the way people used poison got more nuanced; during the Victorian era, stuff like arsenic and strychnine—often passed off as everyday medicine—became infamous.

That era also saw a growing curiosity about how these toxins affected the body, which generally nudged forensic science into new territory (it is interesting to consider how things evolved). Even now, echoes of those old poisoning cases still show up in modern forensic investigations, reminding us that the dark allure and danger of poison remains ever present (Mozayani et al., 2003).

Methodology for Researching Poisons

Investigating toxic substances in forensic contexts is not a neat, step-by-step process—it is more of a spontaneous mix of different methods. Researchers often combine chemical assays with toxicological screens, sometimes incorporating tools like mass spectrometry and chromatography to unravel puzzles in compounds like the toad toxin, which can serve both as a remedy and a deadly agent in surprising ways.

New studies, in most cases, indicate that understanding the drug-like behavior and the effects on the heart of these substances is just as critical as the careful techniques used to pinpoint issues like ARP Spoofing in network security. By merging time-tested forensic practices with fresh, innovative tech, scientists have, in many instances, fine-tuned their approaches to not only manage and treat poison cases better but also to deepen our grasp of how these compounds really work, as highlighted in Herman et al. (2025) and Liu et al. (2025).

8.1. Understanding Cardiotoxic Poisons

Learning Outcome

1. Describe treatment and management of cardiotoxicity
2. Discuss diagnostic methods for detecting cardiotoxicity
3. Explain mechanisms of action on the cardiovascular system
4. Identify common types of cardiotoxic substances
5. Know the legal implications of cardiotoxic poisoning
6. Learn case studies involving cardiotoxic poisons
7. Learn the symptoms and signs of cardiotoxicity
8. Understand the definition and characteristics of cardiotoxic poisons
9. Understand future research directions in cardiotoxicity

Digging into how various substances meddle with the heart's workings is pretty much a cornerstone in forensic toxicology. In most cases, determining the effects of certain heart-harming toxins reveals their breakdown pathways and the risks they pose. Sometimes, checking how a substance behaves in the blood—where its usual levels pop up during tests—really helps crack the mystery behind an incident. Studies that detail metabolites and biomarkers (and, yes, they do repeat these patterns) can assist in distinguishing between poison-induced deaths and those caused by other issues. A good example lies with cannabinoids; these chemicals often stick around in the body longer than you would expect, hinting at a rather complex metabolic behavior. Meanwhile, the emergence of new toxicants, such as novel psychoactive compounds, underscores the need for researchers to delve deeper to establish a baseline for potential cardiotoxicity (Akindahunsi et al., 2013). All this information, albeit a bit messy at times, proves critical for shaping forensic assessments and guiding public health actions.

8.1.1. Definition and Characteristics of Cardiotoxic Poisons

Toxins can really disrupt how our heart and blood vessels function—this is one big reason to take a closer look at those poisons that can harm the cardiovascular system (Figure 8.3). They may disrupt the natural rhythm of the heart, damage the heart muscle, or alter blood flow conditions. Take xylazine, for example: its unpredictable symptoms make spotting and treating its effects a real headache, especially when it comes to forensic work (Mai et al., 2023). During the COVID-19 era, there was a noticeable boost in heart-related deaths, particularly among vulnerable groups—a sign that extra stressors can further complicate matters. In most cases, understanding exactly what makes a poison dangerous to the heart is essential for both medical professionals and legal experts, as detecting these issues early can significantly impact a patient's outcome and affect legal decisions.

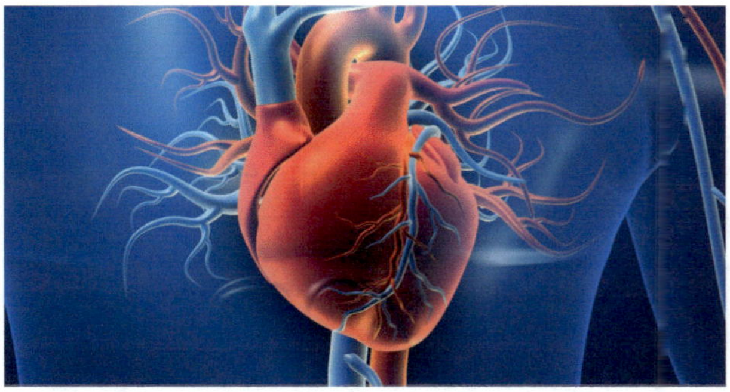

Figure 8.3. Toxins can really disrupt how our heart and blood vessels function—this is one big reason to take a closer look at those poisons that can harm the cardiovascular system.

Source: Bhadramani, R. (2020). *Human Heart with Blood Vessels.*

8.1.2. Common Types of Cardiotoxic Substances

Determining which substances harm the heart is crucial in forensic toxicology. Take aconitine—it is well known for triggering dangerous arrhythmias and causing neurological issues, and accidentally ingesting Aconitum products with this alkaloid can have serious consequences. In many cases, reports of aconitine poisoning show that forensic experts struggle to pinpoint its effects in autopsies because its signs often mirror other cardiovascular problems, which really muddies the investigation (Gao et al., 2018). Similarly, methadone—a drug used for both pain management and opioid dependence—has been linked to a notable increase in death rates, especially among groups that tend to mix multiple substances. In Tehran, for instance, there has been an apparent rise in methadone-related fatalities; this, generally speaking, underscores the urgent need for tighter regulations to curb its misuse (Akhgari et al., 2017). All in all, knowing these harmful substances inside and out is key to both improving forensic analyses and shaping effective public health strategies.

8.1.3. Mechanisms of Action on the Cardiovascular System

Poisons can impact heart function in ways we might not immediately expect, so it is essential to really understand how they work (Figure 8.4). Take oleandrin, for example - it is derived from the oleander plant and is generally known to be extremely toxic to the heart. This substance's fat-friendly nature allows it to easily enter cell membranes; by blocking the Na+/K+ ATPase pump, it disrupts the ion balance inside heart cells, which can lead to irregular rhythms and elevated calcium levels (Zhai et al., 2022). On a similar note, researchers looking into MDMA—formally known as 3,4 methylenedioxymethamphetamine—have discovered that even though it is mainly talked about for its drug interactions, its own toxic effects can seriously unsettle cardiovascular stability. Elevated MDMA levels in the bloodstream, generally speaking, are linked to increased mortality, mainly because its stimulant properties push the heart into tachycardia and may even provoke a near-collapse of heart function (Roxburgh et al., 2021). Overall, knowing how these mechanisms operate is not just academic; it plays a critical role in forensic investigations into poisoning cases.

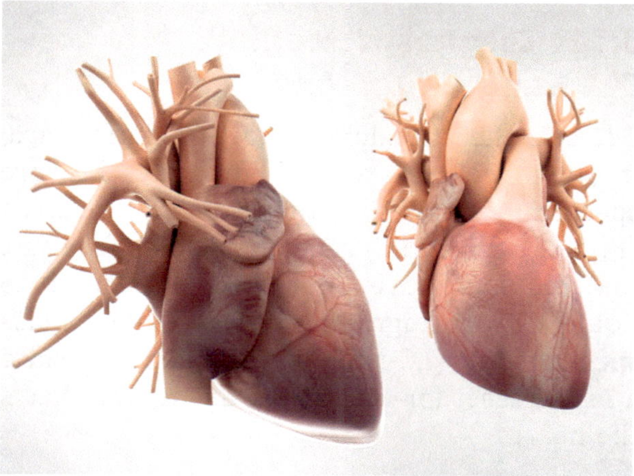

Figure 8.4. Poisons can impact heart function in ways we might not immediately expect, so it is important to really understand how they work.

Source: American Heart Association. (2019). *Heart health.* https://www.heart.org/-/media/Images/News/2019/January-2019/0201HeartHealth_SC.jpg?sc_lang=en.

8.1.4. Symptoms and Signs of Cardiotoxicity

Detecting heart damage in forensic cases really matters - catching it early can make all the difference in treatment. You may notice signs such as irregular heartbeats, chest discomfort, or sudden shortness of breath that indicate more serious issues with the heart. Sometimes, low blood pressure or subtle features of heart failure show up and are misread as something else, which muddies the diagnostic waters. Different toxins can trigger these signals, so a careful, step-by-step toxicology check is essential. Forensic toxicologists, using pretty advanced techniques, dig into these clues to reveal the presence of dangerous agents, helping figure out why someone died or if poisoning is to blame. All in all, the messy overlap of these symptoms really underscores why detailed exams are a must, especially when heart toxicity often mixes with other urgent health issues (Pragst 2025; Viktor et al., 2025).

8.1.5. Diagnostic Methods for Detecting Cardiotoxicity

Detecting heart toxicity is not straightforward; it often requires testing methods that are specifically tailored to the chemicals involved (Figure 8.5). In recent times, forensic toxicologists have increasingly turned to liquid chromatography coupled with mass spectrometry (LC-MS) – a tool many consider a major asset for identifying agents that harm the heart.

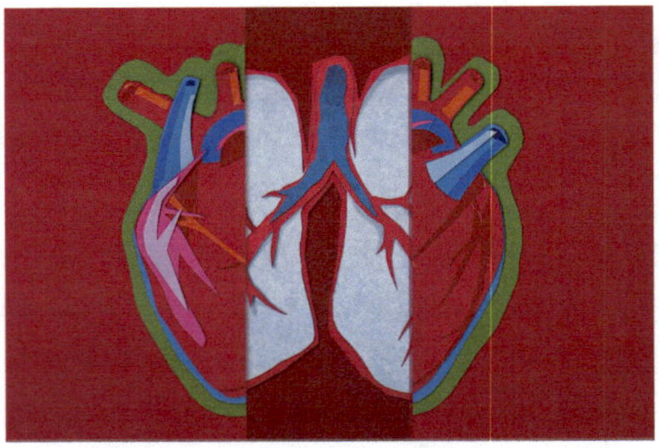

Figure 8.5. Detecting heart toxicity is not straightforward; it often calls for testing methods that are fine-tuned to the specific chemicals involved.

Source: Getty Images. (n.d.). *Getty Images sJEE4J4ZIrA Unsplash.* https://townsendletter.com/wp-content/uploads/2023/07/getty-images-sJEE4J4ZIrA-unsplash.jpg.

This approach generally does well at spotting both familiar compounds and newer ones like α-PVP, a substance known to trigger rapid heartbeats and high blood pressure, which—since it muddles clinical assessments—is especially challenging (Nóbrega et al., 2018). Also, while conventional toxic screenings sometimes miss certain toxins, techniques such as ion mobility spectrometry are gaining favor for their knack for sorting through complex biological samples, particularly in cases involving substances like kratom that can display a range of dangerous heart effects (Fluyau et al., 2017). Ultimately, precise detection remains key for prompt medical intervention and for deepening our understanding of cardiotoxicity's broader impact in forensic investigations.

8.1.6. Case Studies Involving Cardiotoxic Poisons

Exploring case studies about poisons that mess with the heart paints a vivid, if sometimes chaotic, picture of forensic toxicology—especially when you consider how exposure to different compounds plays out. Take Prothipendyl, for example; it demonstrates that understanding not only what a substance does in the body but also how it alters and changes over time is crucial.

This kind of insight keeps popping up when trying to decode toxicology reports in cases that might involve an overdose or poisoning. And honestly, things get even trickier with the surge of New Psychoactive Substances (NPS)—their varied makeup makes it a real challenge to pin them down. In most cases, new tools like Raman spectroscopy (*as noted in* Guirguis et al., 2017) are stepping in to help identify and detect these compounds more quickly, which in turn sheds light on their heart-related effects. All in all, these developments not only help us identify which substances are involved but also inform our understanding of their role in acute poisoning situations.

8.1.7. Legal Implications of Cardiotoxic Poisoning

Sometimes charges of involuntary manslaughter pop up when it turns out that a poison affecting the heart was involved—often with signs of carelessness or even a clear intent to hurt. The way the toxin is administered - whether it is done with negligence or with malicious intent - can significantly escalate legal consequences into a more severe zone. Forensic work, like that carried out by Forensic Science Laboratories (FSL), basically rests on toxicology reports for nailing down the cause of death; generally speaking, these reports are critical since the process can be pretty tricky.

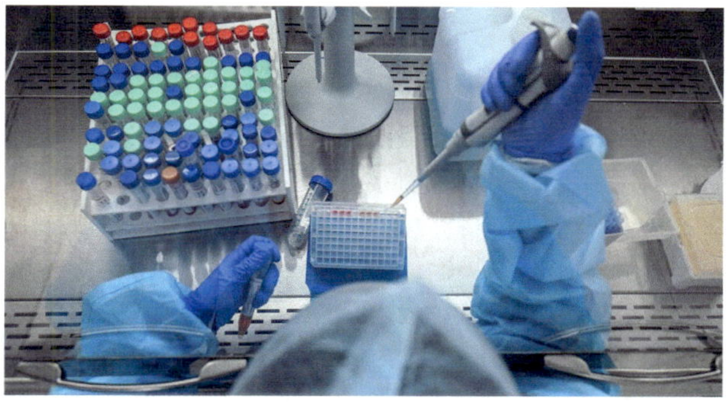

Figure 8.6. The way the toxin is administered - whether it is done with negligence or with harmful intent - can really push legal consequences into a tougher zone.

Source: Carnegie Endowment for International Peace. (n.d.). *Getty Images Photo of U.S.-China Trade Negotiations.* https://carnegieendowment.org/static/media/images/GettyImages-1228545815edit-1-2400x1301.jpg.

In many instances, viscera samples are examined after death to detect any traces of these heart toxins; however, if the tests run negative, complications can arise, potentially undermining the prosecution's case and delaying justice (Dixit et al., 2024). With forensic technology continuously shifting, legal guidelines need to keep pace too - ensuring that police methods stay both compelling and answerable (Vashisth et al., 2024). All in all, this highlights the importance of continually refining our legal standards to address the complex challenges posed by cardiotoxic poisoning in forensic investigations (Figure 8.6).

8.1.8. Treatment and Management of Cardiotoxicity

Treating heart toxicity is not a one-size-fits-all deal—it is about juggling a bunch of approaches, especially when you are in a forensic scene where pinning down the exact poison really matters. Identifying issues early and minimizing exposure as soon as possible is vital; consider carbon monoxide poisoning, for example—administering oxygen quickly can significantly reduce heart damage and accelerate recovery (Agoro, 2020). It also helps to keep an eye on any quirky changes on an ECG, since drugs like opiates and stimulants can trigger unexpected heart rhythm shifts that then steer treatment options aimed at lowering the risk of serious issues. Mixing in some extra supportive care, such as using antidotes when necessary, naturally complements the medications used to bring the heart back to normal. And, generally speaking, with NPS popping up these days, it is not only about spotting the poison anymore—it is also about swiftly tweaking treatment plans to handle the ever-shifting challenges of heart toxicity in emergencies.

8.1.9. Future Research Directions in Cardiotoxicity

Cardiotoxicity is a complex subject that requires multiple approaches in future studies, particularly when considering forensic applications. As we continue to learn about the various substances that can harm the heart, it is clear that we need reliable methods to determine both how these chemicals function and what long-term effects they may have. Research that digs into how a person's genetic quirks mix with these harmful agents might actually offer clues for predicting toxic outcomes. Additionally, exploring new methods to detect subtle biomarkers may help identify heart damage much sooner, potentially guiding treatment in the right direction. In some cases, combining various techniques—such as incorporating isotopic analysis into classic methods—can reveal hidden metabolic pathways triggered by these agents, which in turn enriches forensic studies on chemical exposure. Delving into these angles will not only boost forensic results but also back broader public health efforts against heart-related risks (Coster et al., 2024; Nishchal, 2024).

Test Your Knowledge

1. What is a cardiotoxic poison?
2. Name two common cardiotoxic drugs or substances.

8.2. Miscellaneous Poisons in Forensic Science

Learning Outcome

1. Explain the definition and classification of miscellaneous poisons
2. Give examples of commonly encountered miscellaneous poisons
3. Identify routes of exposure and absorption
4. Know the toxicological effects of miscellaneous poisons
5. Focus on detection methods in forensic toxicology
6. Discuss challenges in identifying miscellaneous poisons
7. Learn case studies highlighting miscellaneous poisons
8. Describe prevention and public health implications

Forensic work sometimes forces us to dig into substances that might seem unimportant at first glance—but they can be key when figuring out what led to a death. You find that a jumble of poisons, each with its own story of origin and action, can really complicate an investigation. Take cobalt, for example; it is common in industrial settings and, over time, builds up in the body, causing heart issues, a classic case of toxins affecting cardiac function. In most cases, there is also the matter of setting limits for harmful agents, such as the spacecraft maximum allowable concentrations (SMACs) for contaminants—a practice detailed by the National Research Council—that demonstrates how toxicology is applied even in closed-off environments, where seemingly random poisons become a serious threat. Knowing these agents, generally speaking, enriches forensic analysis; it offers a broader view of their potential impact on health and helps in piecing together those complex cases, even if the details occasionally seem somewhat disorganized.

8.2.1. Definition and Classification of Miscellaneous Poisons

Toxicology looks into a whole mix of harmful substances that come from all sorts of sources and work in different ways. You might notice that not every poison fits neatly into the usual boxes—say, heavy metals or toxins from plants. Often, these hazardous compounds pop up from industrial byproducts, everyday household items, or even drugs when they are taken in the wrong way.

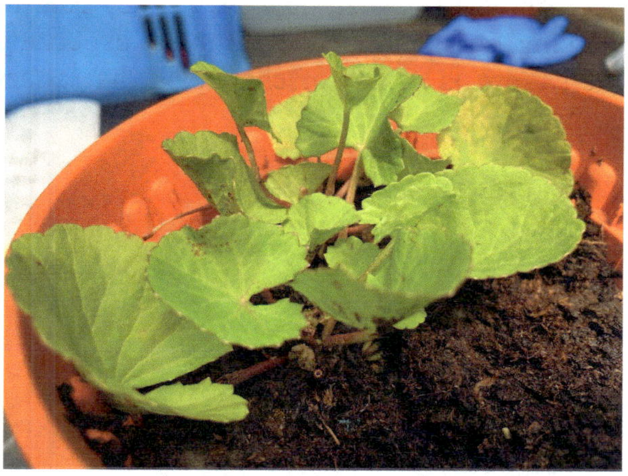

Figure 8.7. Heavy metals or toxins from plants.

Source: Science X. (2022). *Tropical Plants in a Natural Environment.*

In many cases, trying to pin them down is no simple task; sometimes a single substance can behave a bit like a neurotoxin at one moment and then act like a cytotoxin under other conditions, depending on how much you are exposed to and how it enters the body. People often focus on the immediate, acute effects, yet generally speaking, uncovering the long-term outcomes and subtle interactions with other chemicals is a research puzzle that forensic experts are keen to solve. Identifying and understanding these poisons is crucial for both medical response and legal work, especially since individual reactions can vary significantly (Vale et al., 2012) (Figure 8.7).

8.2.2. Examples of Commonly Encountered Miscellaneous Poisons

Forensic work often hinges on spotting an array of poisons, which can really help figure out how someone died or what exactly went on. Heavy metals—like lead and arsenic that you would typically encounter in industrial settings—can slowly build up in a person, leading to poisoning over time. Then there's carbon monoxide; coming from incomplete combustion, it turns dangerous especially in tight, enclosed spaces, sometimes causing not just asphyxiation but even subtle nerve damage. Oddly enough, you also find poisons like ethylene glycol, commonly found in antifreeze, mixed in with plant toxins such as oleander and yew that can affect the heart; these substances seem to appear in various scenarios. It is generally clear that a comprehensive toxicology check is crucial in forensic science, helping to determine the cause and clarify legal responsibilities. In most cases, understanding how these different agents function—and their origins—is crucial for both clinical assessments and legal interpretations in toxicology (Aggrawal, 2025).

8.2.3. Routes of Exposure and Absorption

Grasping how toxins sneak into our bodies matters a lot, especially when you are dealing with poisons that hit the heart or cause other kinds of harm. Toxins usually get in by being breathed in, swallowed, or even absorbed through the skin – and each path carries its own type of risk, depending on what the substance is like (Figure 8.8). Consider certain airborne pollutants that can lead to sudden toxic effects simply from inhaling them; this clearly calls for strict limits on exposure—NASA, for instance, has established SMACs guidelines for the air inside spacecraft. Then there's cobalt, which frequently appears in toxicology reports; its effects depend largely on how it enters the body and how long it remains there. In a nutshell, understanding the various ways toxins can reach you is crucial for conducting thorough forensic investigations and maintaining public health.

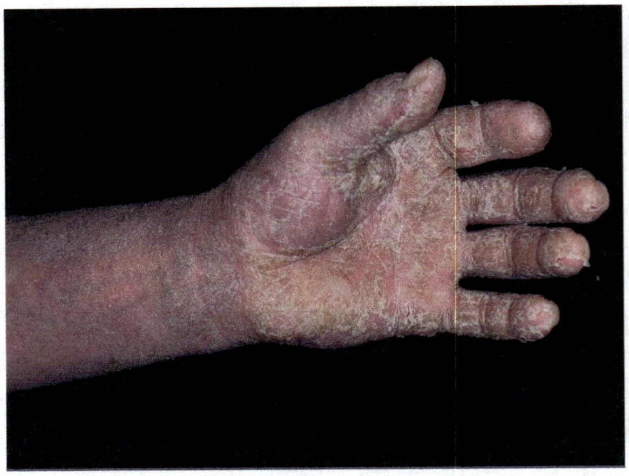

Figure 8.8. Toxins usually get in by being breathed in, swallowed, or even absorbed through the skin – and each path carries its own kind of risk, depending on what the substance is like.

Source: NOSA. (2017). *Cover Image for the NOSA Safety Blog.* https://blog.nosa.co.za/hubfs/Cover%20image%2023%20November%202017.jpg.

8.2.4. Toxicological Effects of Miscellaneous Poisons

Exploring how different toxins impact the body often reveals unexpected insights into heart health. Take yellow oleander—a plant you might see in southern India—which packs compounds that really upset the heart's steady rhythm. One study found that approximately 64% of individuals who ingested it developed abnormal ECG readings. Then there's carbon monoxide poisoning, which works in its own strange way; it is frequently misdiagnosed and can suddenly lead to neurological, cardiac, and other bodily issues. In many cases, forensic toxicology acts like a detective, piecing together clues about these hidden dangers—even if the process is not always perfectly linear. Overall, these examples serve as a gentle reminder that substances we may encounter in everyday settings can harbor risks that are not immediately apparent.

8.2.5. Detection Methods in Forensic Toxicology

Forensic toxicology is not a simple field—figuring out poisons is often a real challenge that calls for more than just basic tests. Advanced tools like gas chromatography-mass spectrometry (GC-MS) and liquid chromatography-mass spectrometry (LC-MS) now play a key role in breaking down biological samples, especially when there is a hint of chemicals that affect the heart.

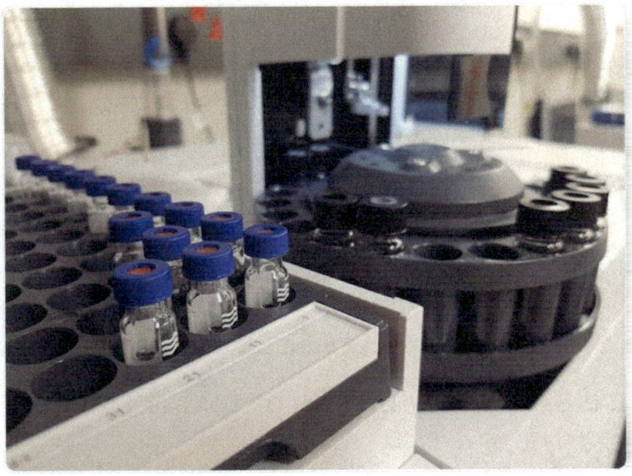

Figure 8.9. Advanced tools like gas chromatography-mass spectrometry (GC-MS) and liquid chromatography-mass spectrometry (LC-MS) now play a key role in breaking down biological samples, especially when there is a hint of chemicals that affect the heart.

Source: Shutterstock. (2020). *Image Depicting a Laboratory Setting with Toxic Substances.* https://d1g9yur4m4naub.cloudfront.net/image-handler/picture/2020/4/shutterstock_1216853737.jpg.

These tests help labs separate and identify various toxins, even when they appear in only tiny traces. Generally speaking, some new protocols even lean on ideas borrowed from frameworks used initially for other contaminants;

take, for instance, how NASA set up SMACs to keep controlled habitats safe. When you mix in environmental and workplace exposure issues, knowing a bit about the toxic profiles of elements like cobalt shows just how vast the net of forensic toxicology's relevance to public health really is. Overall, as detection methods continue to improve, they not only deepen our understanding of poisons but also give forensic investigations a much-needed boost—role of miscellaneous poisons in criminal investigations (Figure 8.9).

Poison plays a crucial role in solving complex criminal cases. Toxic substances—in all kinds of chemical forms—can really hide what truly caused a death or left someone incapacitated. Experts use methods such as mass spectrometry and gas chromatography (GC) to detect these toxins; each one often exhibits a unique pattern that distinguishes it from the usual suspects. In many cases, a close look at the toxicology results can hint at underlying motives or sketch out shady methods, which then feeds into the legal process. Understanding how these poisons work in the body—essentially, their pharmacodynamics—further helps piece together the timeline and determine if the exposure was accidental or intentional. All in all, combining deep chemical insights with hands-on detective work provides law enforcement with a significant boost in building cases that advance justice (Casarett et al., 2001).

8.2.6. Challenges in Identifying Miscellaneous Poisons

Forensic toxicology gets even messier when you throw in all these assorted poisons that do not give themselves away easily. Often, these substances show off varying levels of toxicity and sometimes copy symptoms of other conditions, which tends to throw off a precise diagnosis. Take cobalt and toluene, for example; you find them popping up everywhere in industrial settings, yet each one has its own baffling biological quirks that make them hard to pin down. In many cases, studies have noted that exposure to cobalt tends to be linked with heart problems, kind of a blend of cardiotoxicity mixing with toxicology. On the other hand, toluene is well known for its potential to disrupt nerve function, thereby making forensic identification even more challenging. When these substances exhibit overlapping symptoms, it typically forces investigators to delve into case histories and employ advanced analytical techniques, all in an effort to determine the underlying cause (Figure 8.10).

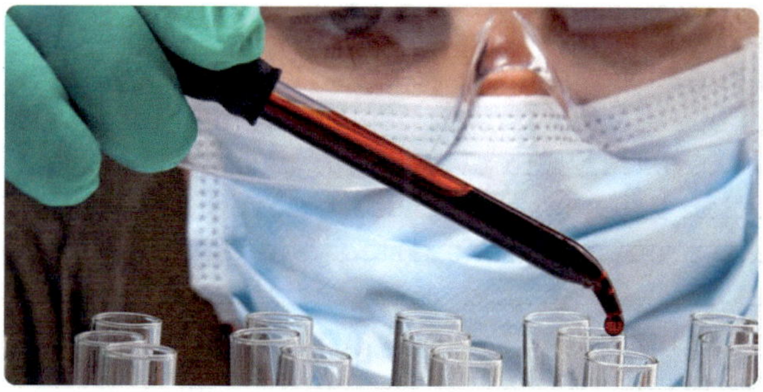

Figure 8.10. Identifying miscellaneous poisons is sometimes challenging.

Source: IKA. (2017). *Forensic Laboratory Equipment in Use.*

8.2.7. Case Studies Highlighting Miscellaneous Poisons

Poisons can be a real mess since cases keep proving just how dangerous they might be, mixing up severity with tricky forensic puzzles. Yellow oleander serves as a clear example—a plant that is visually appealing yet conceals some seriously toxic seeds. At the Karuna Institute of Medical Sciences & Hospital, a study found that among 25 patients who ingested parts of yellow oleander, approximately 64% exhibited ECG abnormalities, indicating arrhythmias caused by the plant's cardiac glycosides. These findings, in most cases, remind us that understanding how different poisons behave is vital, and they highlight why constant, careful monitoring in forensics is crucial. Additionally, tools like capillary electrophoresis—an approach that provides in-depth detection and characterization of these toxins—add another layer of insight to help manage a variety of poisoning cases (Issaq, 1997).

8.2.8. Prevention and Public Health Implications

Toxic substances and public health mix in ways that are not simple at all. When you consider heart-harming chemicals along with a range of other poisons that pop up in forensic reviews, it is clear that a broad prevention plan is needed right away. Getting people informed about the dangers that lurk around—in homes, workplaces, and even in fun spots—is a must. Strict rules on how these hazardous materials are produced, transported, and disposed of go a long way in mitigating their harmful effects on communities. Health groups, environmental advocates, and law enforcement teams can work together to make it easier to spot and track these threats, which often prevent poisoning cases from escalating. Quick, easy-to-find information on symptoms and the right steps to take gives both regular people and healthcare workers a better chance to react quickly. In most cases, jumping on prevention not only addresses issues in the moment but also builds a stronger shield for public health over the long term (Frank, 2001) (Figure 8.11).

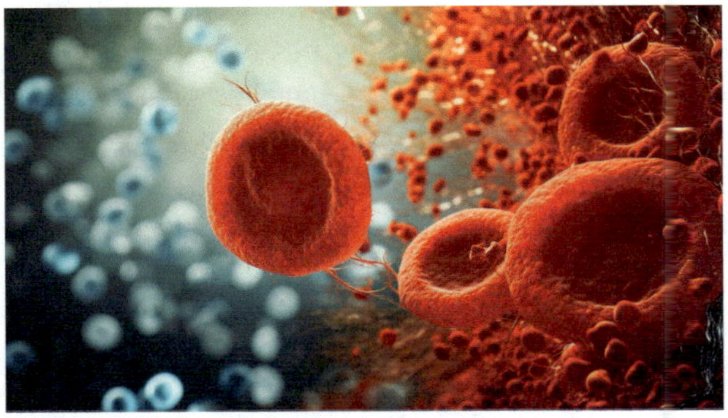

Figure 8.11. When you consider heart-harming chemicals along with a range of other poisons that pop up in forensic reviews, it is clear that a broad prevention plan is needed right away.

Source: Sponaugle Wellness. (n.d.). *Mold Toxicity and Its Potential Link to Pernicious Anemia.* https://sponauglewellness.com/wp-content/uploads/can-mold-toxicity-cause-pernicious-anemia.jpg.

Test Your Knowledge

1. What are the toxic effects of ethylene glycol ingestion?
2. How can solvents like toluene cause systemic toxicity?

8.3. Legal and Ethical Considerations

Learning Outcome

1. Understand the legal framework surrounding poison-related cases
2. Explains ethical dilemmas in forensic toxicology
3. Know future legal trends in forensic toxicology
4. Identify challenges in proving intent in poisoning cases
5. Know the impact of forensic findings on legal outcomes
6. Focus on privacy concerns in toxicological investigations
7. Discuss the role of forensic toxicologists in the justice system
8. Learn case law examples involving poisons
8. Know the role of expert witnesses in court

Forensic work in poisoning cases is not simply about lab tests on toxins—it is a messy blend of legal, ethical, and scientific concerns that often come crashing together. When a poisoning is suspected, investigators go beyond just checking chemicals; they face ethical duties toward the deceased as well as tangled legal questions that can pop up unexpectedly. Experts have recently noted that issues like physician burnout, even if not directly tied to the case at hand, highlight broader struggles in medicine that can subtly affect forensic work (Kentor et al., 2024). The National Association of Medical Examiners, for instance, recommends conducting thorough autopsies and paying close attention to the scene—steps that are crucial for maintaining accurate legal records and ensuring the accuracy of public health data (Davis et al., 2019). In short, adhering to ethical guidelines is crucial when navigating a legal maze, ensuring that both victim rights and overall public safety remain at the forefront.

8.3.1. Legal Framework Surrounding Poison-Related Cases

Forensic work involving poison cases requires a legal framework that balances public safety and individual rights (Figure 8.12). Experts often find themselves lost in a maze of rules, outdated case precedents, and moral guidelines tied to toxicology data, making it difficult to know which path to take. Laws tend to break down toxins—say, those that hurt the heart—by explaining how they should be used, shared, or punished when misused, even if it sometimes feels a bit haphazard. In most cases, proving a poison charge is not just about showing a toxin was involved; it means establishing why it was used and what effect it had, placing a heavy burden on prosecutors who must prove everything beyond a reasonable doubt. Sometimes, not following the correct steps can send a case off track—a reminder that our legal framework must remain flexible enough to keep pace with the ever-changing world of forensic science and toxicology (Vale et al., 2012).

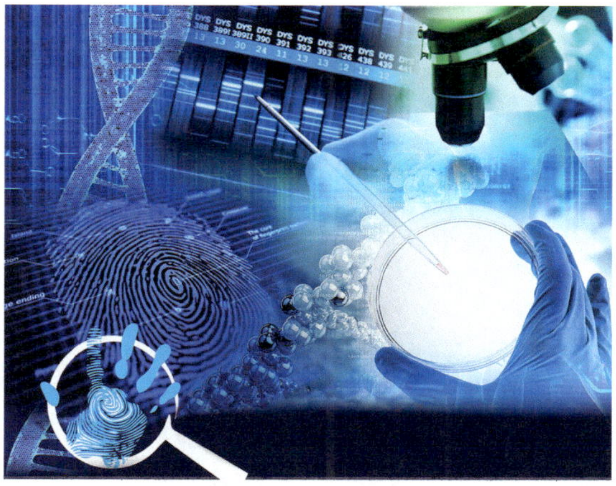

Figure 8.12. Forensic work with poison cases demands a legal setup that juggles public safety and the rights of individuals.

Source: Legal Service India. (n.d.). *3rd-Year Law Student at Presidency University Bangalore.* https://www.legalserviceindia.com/legal/uploads/3rdyearlawstudentpresidencyuniversitybangalore_4764558229.jpg.

8.3.2. Ethical Dilemmas in Forensic Toxicology

Ethics and forensic toxicology frequently intersect in ways that demand more than a straightforward answer. Toxicologists wrestle with issues like getting consent, keeping things confidential, and the risk that their hard-earned data might end up misused. The challenge mounts when they deal with substances that, even in tiny doses, serve as lethal agents or mess with the heart. Consider wheat pills loaded with potent toxins – this not only presses for clear treatment protocols but also sparks stubborn debates about who is really responsible when an overdose turns out to be accidental or intentional (Pervez et al., 2024). Extra pressure from medico-legal probes often fuels the dilemmas over bias in weighing evidence and the broader social impact of toxicology findings (Kenton et al., 2024). All in all, balancing meticulous scientific work with a deep, sometimes messy, sense of moral responsibility remains a challenging yet essential task in the field.

8.3.3. Role of Expert Witnesses in Court

Expert witnesses really matter in forensic cases, especially when you are dealing with odd toxins like those that mess with the heart or other miscellaneous poisons (Figure 8.13). They not only come armed with deep knowledge but can also break down complicated scientific data into plain talk that juries and judges can actually follow. Take wheat pill poisoning, for example – generally speaking, when a case involves these substances, the toxic elements throw up peculiar challenges in medical care because there is simply no well-established treatment protocol (Pervez et al., 2024). In many instances, the National Association of Medical Examiners has pointed out that expert opinions are essential in pinning down the causes and classifications of deaths linked to substance misuse (Davis et al., 2019). All in all, these professionals bridge the sometimes complex gap between deep scientific inquiry and legal accountability, helping ensure the process is as informed as possible.

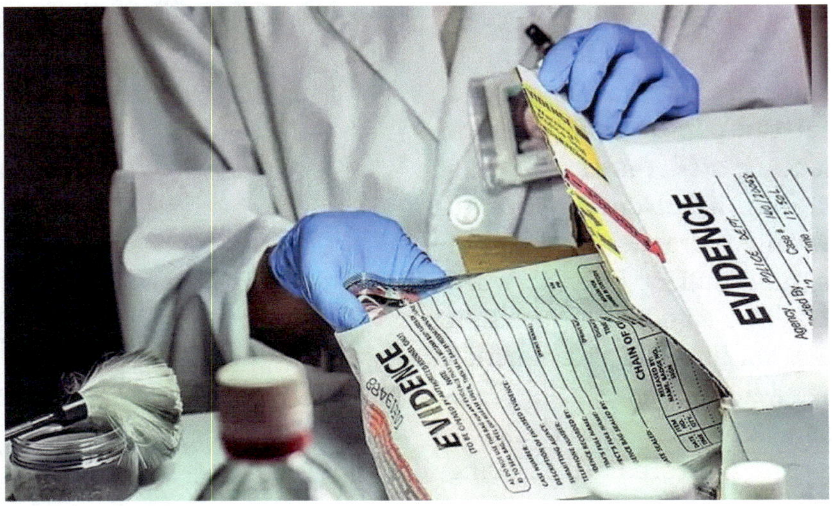

Figure 8.13. Expert witnesses really matter in forensic cases, especially when you are dealing with odd toxins like those that mess with the heart or other miscellaneous poisons.

Source: ET Bureau. (n.d.). *Photograph of a Business Conference.* https://etimg.etb2bimg.com/photo/111549048.cms.

8.3.4. Challenges in Proving Intent in Poisoning Cases

Poisoning cases present a complex web of legal complications, and determining intent is a significant challenge for investigators. Showing that someone meant harm is key when deciding between murder, attempted murder, or manslaughter – generally speaking, it all hinges on whether the act was planned or just a disastrous accident. In many situations, the ease of obtaining a substance and the specific circumstances behind its use only add layers to this puzzle. Take, for instance, areas where everyday poisons like zinc or aluminum phosphide are available over the counter; here, determining whether ingestion was intentional or accidental becomes particularly challenging (Pervez et al., 2024). The plot thickens further when toxic heavy metals are present in various settings, as they can easily obscure the origin and path of exposure, making it challenging to attribute a clear malicious motive to a single individual (Pandey, 2013). Often, these challenges necessitate a thorough examination of forensic work—utilizing toxicology reports and circumstantial evidence—to construct a narrative of intent that withstands courtroom scrutiny.

8.3.5. Impact of Forensic Findings on Legal Outcomes

Forensic evidence can tip the scales in a trial—detailed screens of toxins from blood or tissues often reveal clues about both how and why someone died, and cases dealing with substances that affect the heart or other assorted poisons tend to be no exception. A precise count of these chemicals sometimes hints at wrongdoing, nudging the burden of proof onto the prosecution and, in many cases, paving the way for harsher penalties. At the same time, hazy or ambiguous test results might ultimately benefit the defendant, demonstrating that these investigations can cut both ways. In most situations, courts rely on forensic toxicologists to interpret the data, which highlights the importance of solid, careful methods. Generally speaking, the mix of science and law is not always neat; unexpected findings can suddenly shift a case's trajectory. All in all, the trustworthiness of these forensic results remains a key piece in the puzzle of delivering justice within our legal system (Vale et al., 2012).

8.3.6. Privacy Concerns in Toxicological Investigations

Forensic toxicology and privacy issues have become a real tangle—something investigators now face head-on. Labs are increasingly leaning on toxic assessments to decide cases involving dangerous cardiotoxins and other poisons, and in doing so, they sometimes end up handling loads of sensitive information. Traditional methods typically utilize biological samples that not only indicate the presence of a toxin but also reveal personal health information, which naturally sparks ethical debates about informed consent and the risk of misuse. At the same time, new approaches—such as those that use zebrafish because they are cost-effective and efficient—raise their own set of questions about the security of the generated data. Balancing the need for critical toxic insights with maintaining personal details under wraps proves to be no simple matter, particularly in situations that may lead to public exposure or even legal repercussions (Mukherjee et al., 2024; Rajan et al., 2025). All in all, this ongoing challenge, in most cases, requires solid frameworks that ensure ethical standards remain intact in forensic practices (Figure 8.14).

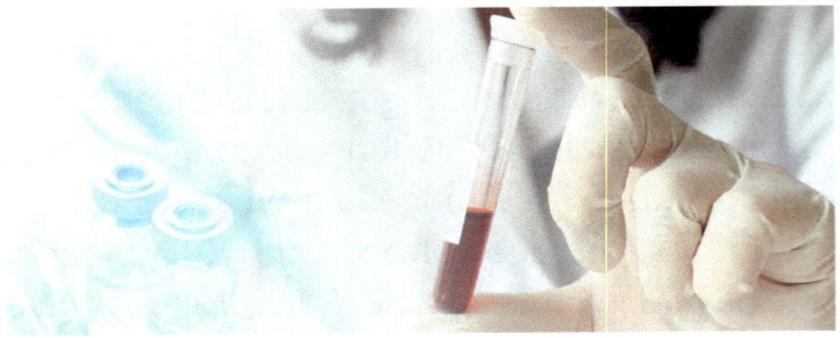

Figure 8.14. Privacy concerns in toxicological investigations.

Source: UCSF Health. (n.d.). *Photograph of a Toxicology Screening Process.* https://www.ucsfhealth.org/-/media/project/ucsf/ucsf-health/medical-tests/hero/toxicology-screen-2x.jpg?rev=ee9b1e590f984ba69075f261e2d9d971.

8.3.7. The Role of Forensic Toxicologists in the Justice System

Forensic chemistry and law often meet in unexpected ways, with forensic toxicologists playing a surprisingly hands-on role. These experts dig into biological samples, checking for drugs, alcohol, and even poisons – sometimes including cardiotoxic substances that might have been tied to criminal acts or baffling deaths. They use techniques like mass spectrometry and GC (yes, the really high-tech ones) to spot and measure toxins that could easily slip by unnoticed. Their findings help pinpoint not just the cause of death, but also shed light on tricky cases where things do not add up. In most cases, the painstaking work of these professionals underpins our judicial system, ensuring that justice is served effectively overall (Vale et al., 2012).

8.3.8. Case Law Examples Involving Poisons

Forensic science truly comes alive in court, and cases involving poisons tend to highlight its more complex aspects. Often, legal battles reveal how science and emotion intersect—juries are left trying to separate hard evidence from dramatic stories. Take *State v. McKee,* for example; experts there examined aconitine, a potent substance known for its heart-harming effects, and in many cases, it was found to be consistent with what the defendant was accused of doing. The prosecution, in most instances, leaned on lab reports and toxicology findings to argue that the poison led directly to the victim's death, stressing the role toxicologists play in the courtroom (Vale et al., 2012). It seems that cases like these remind us that lawyers and scientists really need to work side by side, as the path to justice depends on interpreting such evidence correctly. In the end, these legal decisions not only advance forensic methods but also shape public perceptions of how poisons are involved in criminal acts.

8.3.9. Future Legal Trends in Forensic Toxicology

Forensic science is changing fast, and legal rules are now mixing with toxicology in ways that really grab your attention. Drug profiles are getting trickier these days—especially with synthetic and designer drugs popping up everywhere—which means our legal standards need to keep pace with new toxic findings. This hit is felt hard when we deal with substances that mess with the heart; the public health risks here are huge. Courts need solid, dependable guidelines for toxicology evidence since even a minor misunderstanding might send someone the wrong way, ending up in a wrongful conviction or an odd acquittal. In most cases, legal experts are taking a closer look at fresh research, like studies on drug dependence and its ripple effects on health outcomes; look at the situation in the Netherlands, where harm reduction policies are already reshaping forensic toxicology (Amsterdam et al., 2011; Kentor et al., 2024). All in all, these shifts are bound to change how justice is delivered in cases involving heart-affecting toxins and a mishmash of other poisons (Figure 8.15).

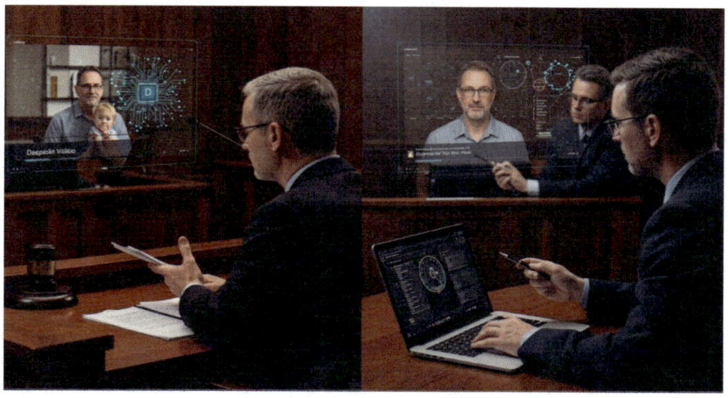

Figure 8.15. Courts need solid, dependable guidelines for toxicology evidence since even a small misunderstanding might send someone the wrong way—ending up in a wrongful conviction or an odd acquittal.

Source: LinkedIn. (n.d.). *Courts Need Solid, Dependable Guidelines for Toxicology Evidence Since Even a Small Misunderstanding Might Send Someone the Wrong Way—Ending Up in a Wrongful Conviction or an Odd Acquittal.* https://media.licdn.com/dms/image/v2/D4E12AQE2VhRs7wJKIw/article-cover_image-shrink_720_1280/B4EZUCQOJUHUAI-/0/1739499561922?e=2147483647&v=beta&t=E 72omLOotI-XQ8md5OiyNhGymoye4gaKMhdLXciUWzQ.

Test Your Knowledge

1. What is the legal definition of poisoning in criminal law?
2. How is chain of custody maintained in poisoning investigations?

SUMMARY

Understanding the impact of certain toxins on the heart in forensic cases is not just about spotting what is poisonous. Obtaining diagnoses and handling cases—especially when dealing with substances like yellow oleander or carbon monoxide—is crucial for a sound forensic review and proper medical care. Research generally indicates that exposure to yellow oleander can trigger a range of cardiovascular issues; one study found that approximately 64% of cases exhibited clear ECG changes, suggesting that patients require careful, ongoing monitoring during treatment. Carbon monoxide, for instance, often muddles things even further, since its symptoms can mimic those of other conditions and sometimes lead to misdiagnoses. In all, deepening our grasp of such poisonings not only sharpens legal proceedings but also boosts healthcare outcomes by bridging toxicology with everyday medical practice.

Investigating toxic substances impacts both legal cases and health care in ways you might not expect. Figuring out how substances that hurt the heart actually work is essential for nailing down the right diagnosis and treatment—even minor missteps can add up. For example, cobalt often proves to be a real troublemaker; its tendency to disrupt normal heart rhythms poses serious public health concerns. Toluene, although primarily known for its effects on the nervous system, also poses risks to cardiac function – a reminder that these compounds can be hazardous on multiple levels. Generally speaking, as toxins mix in increasingly complex ways, forensic experts find themselves untangling these intricate connections to refine toxicology assessments. This blend of insight not only bolsters legal investigations but also deepens our understanding of how chemical exposures can lead to harmful health outcomes, highlighting the broader dangers lurking in our environment and workplaces.

KEY TERMS FROM THIS CHAPTER

- Asphyxiation
- Cardiotoxic substances
- Compounds
- Echoes
- Forensic technology
- Oleandrin
- Reproductive issues
- Biomarkers
- Chemical assays
- Cytotoxin
- Ethylene glycol
- New Psychoactive Substances
- Pain management
- Toxins

CRITICAL THINKING QUESTIONS

1. **Which of the following is a classic cardiotoxic drug that increases intracellular calcium and contractility?**
   a. Lidocaine
   b. Digoxin
   c. Atropine
   d. Propranolol
2. **What is a common electrocardiographic (ECG) finding in digoxin toxicity?**
   a. Prolonged QT interval
   b. ST depression with a "scooped" appearance
   c. Peaked T waves
   d. Sinus tachycardia
3. **Beta-blocker overdose typically leads to which of the following?**
   a. Hypertension and tachycardia
   b. Bradycardia and hypotension
   c. Hypothermia and hyperkalemia
   d. Seizures and fever
4. **Which of the following poisons can lead to cardiac arrest due to inhibition of cytochrome oxidase in mitochondria?**
   a. Cyanide
   b. Lead
   c. Benzene
   d. Iron
5. **What is the specific antidote for digoxin toxicity?**
   a. Atropine
   b. Digibind (digoxin-specific antibody)
   c. Naloxone
   d. Flumazenil

Short Answer Questions

1. Name two common cardiotoxic drugs or substances.
2. What ECG changes are commonly seen in cardiotoxic poisoning?
3. How do beta-blockers and calcium channel blockers cause cardiotoxicity?
4. What are the clinical signs of carbon monoxide-induced myocardial injury?
5. How does cyanide poisoning affect cardiac output?
6. What role does potassium play in cardiac poisoning cases?
7. How is cardiotoxicity managed in poisoning cases in the emergency setting?

Answers to Critical Thinking Questions

1. (b); 2. (b); 3. (b); 4. (a); 5. (b)

REFERENCES

1. Aggrawal, A., (2025). *APC Textbook of Forensic Medicine and Toxicology*. Avichal Publishing Company. https://play.google.com/store/books/details?id=zbjiCQAAQBAJ&source=gbs_api (accessed on 9th May 2025).
2. Agoro, E. Y. S. (2020). *Vitreous Humor Biochemical Indicators of Acute CO Intoxication Associated Deaths: A Review of the Literature*. https://core.ac.uk/download/612900612.pdf (accessed on 9th May 2025).
3. Akhgari, M., Amini-Shirazi, N., & Sardari, I. F., (2017). Forensic toxicology perspectives of methadone-associated deaths in Tehran, Iran, a 7-year overview. *Basic & Clinical Pharmacology & Toxicology, 122*, 436–441. https://doi.org/10.1111/bcpt.12930.
4. Akindahunsi, A. A., Lawa, A. T., Ogunlana, O. O., & Ogunlana, et al. (2013). *Antioxidant and DPPH-Scavenging Activities of Compounds and Ethanolic Extract of the Leaf and Twigs of Caesalpinia Bonduc L. Roxb*. https://core.ac.uk/download/159129373.pdf (accessed on 9th May 2025).
5. Anderson, B., de Peyster, A., Gad, S. C., Hakkinen, P. J. B., Kamrin, M., Locey, B., Mehendale, H. M., et al. (2005). *Encyclopedia of Toxicology*. Elsevier. http://books.google.com/books?id=dEnbcGW44RYC&dq=Emerging+technologies+in+forensic+toxicology+for+cardiotoxic+and+miscellaneous+poisons+analysis&hl=&source=gbs_api (accessed on 9th May 2025).
6. Ashry, S., Khater, A., Wahdan, M., & Eweda, S. A. (2023). The possible role of partial pressure of carbon dioxide level changes in the outcome of acute carbon monoxide poisoning. *Zagazig Journal of Forensic Medicine, 21*, 131–147. https://doi.org/10.21608/zjfm.2023.216580.1151.
7. Casarett, L. J. (1980). *Casarett and Doull's Toxicology*. MacMillan Publishing Company. http://books.google.com/books?id=XlJrAAAAMAAJ&dq=toxicological+interpretation+of+cardiotoxic+and+miscellaneous+poisons+in+forensic+science&hl=&source=gbs_api (accessed on 9th May 2025).
8. Coelho, M. M., Fernandes, C., Remião, F., & Tiritan, M. E. (2021). Enantioselectivity in drug pharmacokinetics and toxicity: Pharmacological relevance and analytical methods. *Molecules, 26*, 3113. https://doi.org/10.3390/molecules26113113.
9. Davis, G. G., Cadwallader, A. B., Fligner, C. L., Gilson, T., Hall, E., Harshbarger, K., Kronstrand, R., et al. (2019). *Recommendations for the Investigation, Diagnosis, and Certification of Deaths Related to Opioid and Other Drugs*. https://docs.gato.txst.edu/666186/Opioid%20position%20paper%20Final%2012-17-2019.pdf (accessed on 9th May 2025).
10. De Coster, M., Ammer, S., Laning, T., & Kootker, L., (2024). The relevance of Sr–O–C isotope analysis on burnt human skeletal remains in archeological and forensic contexts: A review and future directions. *WIREs Forensic Science*. https://www.semanticscholar.org/paper/b3687b6f45225d1872efc72e438e9a8c9b54ed18 (accessed on 9th May 2025).
11. Dildy, G. A. III., Belfort, M. A., Saade, G. R., Phelan, J. P., Hankins, G. D. V., & Clark, S. L. (2004). *Critical Care Obstetrics*. http://ndl.ethernet.edu.et/bitstream/123456789/56617/1/4065.pdf#page=518 (accessed on 9th May 2025).
12. Dixit, P., & Kumari, M., (2024). Challenges in viscera analysis: Addressing errors in forensic reporting and their medico-legal implications. *Indian Internet Journal of Forensic Medicine and Toxicology*. https://www.semanticscholar.org/paper/92f73203c17266faa2ab4cb227dc8516d35bd3d8 (accessed on 9th May 2025).

13. Ekins, S., (2007). *Computational Toxicology: Risk Assessment for Pharmaceutical and Environmental Chemicals*. http://ndl.ethernet.edu.et/bitstream/123456789/49347/1/197.pdf#page=26 (accessed on 9th May 2025).

14. Fakiha, B., (2024). Analysis of forensic toxicology of carbon monoxide cases in Jeddah, Saudi Arabia. *African Journal of Biomedical Research*. https://www.semanticscholar.org/paper/f1c8fad1d1da5c065fb36f0e4c75ecedee36fb65 (accessed on 9th May 2025).

15. Fluyau, D., & Revadigar, N., (2017). Biochemical benefits, diagnosis, and clinical risks evaluation of Kratom. *Frontiers in Psychiatry, 8*. https://doi.org/10.3389/fpsyt.2017.00062.

16. Frank, A. L. (2001). *Taking an Exposure History*. https://play.google.com/store/books/details?id=XabmcKmdNysC&source=gbs_api (accessed on 9th May 2025).

17. Gao, X., Hu, J., Zhang, X., Zuo, Y., Wang, Y., & Zhu, S., (2018). Research progress of aconitine toxicity and forensic analysis of aconitine poisoning. *Forensic Sciences Research, 5*, 25–31. https://doi.org/10.1080/20961790.2018.1452346.

18. Guirguis, A., (2017). *Identification and Classification of New Psychoactive Substances Using Raman Spectroscopy and Chemometrics*. https://core.ac.uk/download/83960858.pdf (accessed on 9th May 2025).

19. Gunawardena, S., Dassanayake, N., Keerawelle, B. I., Kanthasamy, S., Ranganatha, H., & Gunawardana, J. W. (2023). The effect of the COVID-19 pandemic on the trends and characteristics of natural and unnatural deaths in an urban Sri Lankan cohort viewed through retrospective analysis of forensic death investigations from 2019 to 2022. *Osong Public Health and Research Perspectives, 14*, 468–482. https://www.semanticscholar.org/paper/0a4bfcb078d6ff1e0283fd6626b66a4a5989152b (accessed on 9th May 2025).

20. Herman, R. U., & Prasetyo, A., (2025). Analysis of address resolution protocol poisoning attacks on Mikrotik routers using live forensics methods. *International Journal of Engineering Business and Social Science*. https://www.semanticscholar.org/paper/90bbc22aa5d62f70efbff2f23cd138f7bd2bf75a (accessed on 9th May 2025).

21. Issaq, H. J. (1997). Capillary electrophoresis of natural products. *Electrophoresis, 18*, 2438–2452. https://doi.org/10.1002/elps.1150181234.

22. Kentor, M., Daven, M., Greg, C., Andrew, B., (2024). Conversations on burnout: Part two. *ACEP Now, 43*(1). www.acepnow.com (accessed on 9th May 2025).

23. Liu, Y., Zhang, J., Wang, B., Zheng, F., & Yan, J., (2025). Epidemiological patterns and therapeutic approaches of toad toxin poisoning in a retrospective case study. *Scientific Reports, 15*. https://www.semanticscholar.org/paper/6dbb347e000126d867d45969e9a126d380b8a336 (accessed on 9th May 2025).

24. Mai, T., Zhang, Y., & Zhao, S., (2023). Xylazine poisoning in clinical and forensic practice: Analysis method, characteristics, mechanism and future challenges. *Toxics, 11*. https://www.semanticscholar.org/paper/6043a270b541c87e7fa139f48abcb6685b021935 (accessed on 9th May 2025).

25. Malar, K. M., Kavitha, R., & Sonawane, K. S. (2024). Nanomaterials as game changers in forensic toxicology and trace analysis. *South Asian Journal of Engineering and Technology*. https://www.semanticscholar.org/paper/0c2d9248c492284cae543d74070c1c7e3c17afdb (accessed on 9th May 2025).

26. Mozayani, A., & Raymon, L., (2003). *Handbook of Drug Interactions*. Springer Science & Business Media. https://play.google.com/store/books/details?id=dwMyBwAAQBAJ&source=gbs_api (accessed on 9th May 2025).

27. Mukherjee, S., Mohanty, A. K., Chinnadurai, R. K., Deb Barman, D., & Poddar, A., (2024). Zebrafish: A cost-effective model for enhanced forensic toxicology capabilities in low- and middle-income countries. *Cureus, 16*. https://www.semanticscholar.org/paper/512b3900314799a96e8f01a6f71592b32f631aea (accessed on 9th May 2025).

28. Neole, N., & Rajan, S., (2025). Green forensic toxicology: Optimizing chlordiazepoxide detection in milk, whiskey, and whiskey cream matrices. *Indian Journal of Forensic Medicine & Toxicology*. https://www.semanticscholar.org/paper/394699352df614680e98fa8548f44abe468649d (accessed on 9th May 2025).

29. Nishchal, S., (2024). Forensic analysis of WhatsApp: A review of techniques, challenges, and future directions. *Journal of Forensic Science and Research*. https://www.semanticscholar.org/paper/dcc16c19e342f89567252da86bf5fd771b777f50 (accessed on 9th May 2025).

30. Nóbrega, L., & Dinis-Oliveira, R. J. (2018). The synthetic cathinone α-pyrrolidinovalerophenone (α-PVP): Pharmacokinetic and pharmacodynamic clinical and forensic aspects. *Drug Metabolism Reviews, 50*, 125–139. https://doi.org/10.1080/03602532.2018.1448867.

31. Pandey, G., (2013). *Heavy Metals Poisoning in Fish (Manual on Aquatic Toxicology)*. http://www.isca.co.in (accessed on 9th May 2025).

32. Payne-James, J., Jones, R., Karch, S., & Manlove, J., (2011). *Simpson's Forensic Medicine*. CRC Press. http://books.google.com/books?id=UCzSBQAAQBAJ&dq=Definition+of+cardiotoxic+poisons+and+miscellaneous+poisons+in+forensics&hl=&source=gbs_api (accessed on 9th May 2025).

33. Pervez, T., Malik, M., & Khan, N. A. (2024). Therapeutic dilemma of wheat pill poisoning: A narrative review and management proposal. *Medical & Clinical Case Reports Journal, 2*(2), 213–218. https://doi.org/10.51219/MCCRJ/Tamkeen-Pervez/59 (accessed on 9th May 2025).

34. Pragst, F., (2025). Systematic toxicological analysis in forensic and clinical laboratories: A challenging task of analytical chemistry. *ChemTexts*. https://www.semanticscholar.org/paper/9ea88b3c70dafdaff6c1dfe3569b42da439bc82f (accessed on 9th May 2025).

35. Radhika R. H. (2018). Cerebra Thevetia poisoning: A prospective study at a tertiary care hospital, Kerala. *Indian Journal of Forensic and Community Medicine, 5*, 123–126. https://doi.org/10.18231/2394-6776.2018.0028 (accessed on 9th May 2025).

36. Roxburgh, A., Şam, B., Kriikku, P., Mounteney, J., Castañera, A. A., Dias, M., & Giraudon, I., (2021). Trends in MDMA-related mortality across four countries. *Addiction, 116*, 3094–3103. https://doi.org/10.1111/add.15493.

37. Suzuki, O., & Watanabe, K., (2006). *Drugs and Poisons in Humans*. Springer Science & Business Media. https://play.google.com/store/books/details?id=HGWi4MB1qiUC&source=gbs_api (accessed on 9th May 2025).

38. Vale, J. A., & Meredith, T. J. (2012). *Poisoning Diagnosis and Treatment*. Springer Science & Business Media. https://play.google.com/store/books/details?id=ne7qCAAAQBAJ&source=gbs_api (accessed on 9th May 2025).

39. van Amsterdam, J., Pennings, E., Brunt, T., & van den Brink, W., (2011). *Physical Damage*

Due to Drug Dependence (ZonMw Study). https://projecten.zonmw.nl/sites/zonmw/files/typo3-migrated-files/lichamelijke_effecten_van_drugs_01.pdf (accessed on 9th May 2025).

40. Vashisth, S., Singh, N., & Dudi, S. (2024). An in-depth investigation into police operations and their impact on delivering speedy justice in criminal proceedings: Efficiency, challenges, and legal implications. *Library Progress International.* https://www.semanticscholar.org/paper/ed82e101a395a7f3cf6faa2b8735c2137b8e985c (accessed on 9th May 2025).

41. Viktor, P., Kaur, L., Pillai, J. S. H. P., Khalaf, O. M., Mudhafar, M., Hasan, H., Devi, J., et al. (2025). Exposures to poisoning to forensic investigations and public health views – A toxicology tapestry. *Research Journal of Pharmacy and Technology.* https://www.semanticscholar.org/paper/e490d3e8ab4acf56cbeeb7c920e1d500c086ce1f (accessed on 9th May 2025).

42. Zhai, J., Dong, X., Yan, F., Guo, H., & Yang, J., (2022). Oleandrin: A systematic review of its natural sources, structural properties, detection methods, pharmacokinetics and toxicology. *Frontiers in Pharmacology, 13.* https://doi.org/10.3389/fphar.2022.822726.

SUBSTANCE ABUSE

9

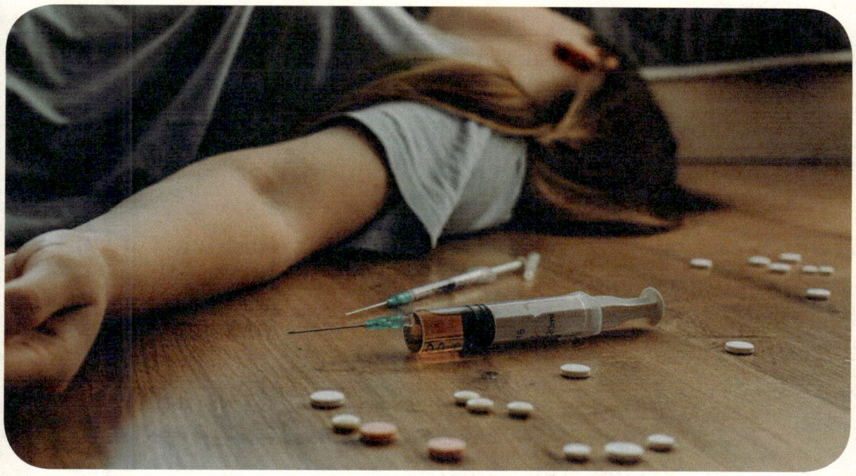

Introduction

Drug misuse is a stubborn problem touching many parts of everyday life—public health and criminal justice included. Lately, stats hint that more young folks are falling into drug use, which in most cases ties into serious issues like strokes, with cocaine, for example, showing its own kind of damaging effects (Patel et al., 2024). It becomes essential to get a good read on how these drugs change the body's functions and behavior—this helps doctors nail down tough cases and even guides investigations by legal authorities. Even the mouth is not spared; substance abuse often messes with oral health, offering both challenges and unexpected clues for forensic work (Nilendu, 2024). When toxicology, medicine, and dental findings are all pulled together, they usually tell a fuller story of someone's history with drugs and might even flag potential criminal ties. Bringing all these elements together really strengthens how cases are handled and reminds us that tackling drug problems means examining a whole range of issues.

LEARNING OBJECTIVES

After studying this chapter, you will be able to:

1. Know the impact of substance abuse on criminal behavior
2. Understand forensic analysis of substances
3. Focus on substance abuse and mental health
4. Explain prevention and intervention strategies.

Definition of Substance Abuse

Mental and behavioral issues can be a real tangled mess, and it really calls for clear-cut definitions – especially when things get messy in forensic settings where legal concerns mix with medical ones over substance abuse. Usually, substance abuse pops up as a noticeable pattern of problematic use, one that messes with everyday life – at home, socially, or at work. You might note, in many cases, that substance abuse is not just one neat definition; instead, it covers a range of behaviors that point to underlying brain or emotional issues, not simply a single, tidy category (Haslam et al., 2011). Generally speaking, our definitions also need to align with global standards, such as those outlined in the World Health Organization's ICD-11 revisions – these emphasize practical use and help keep global health discussions on the same page. All in all, having a consistent method is crucial for forensic evaluations, ensuring that diagnoses and interpretations of substance abuse stay in line across both legal and healthcare settings (Figure 9.1).

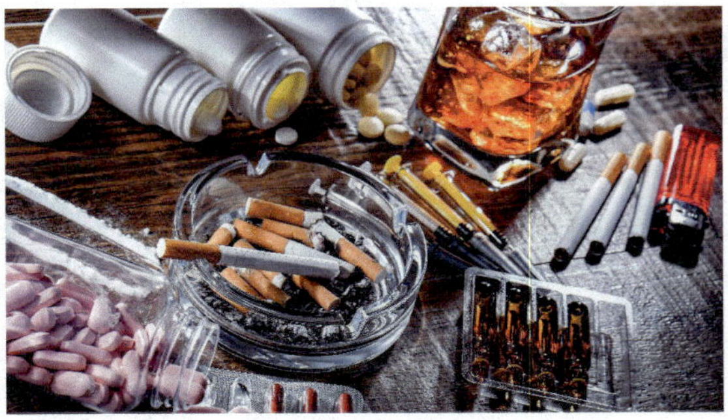

Figure 9.1. Substance abuse.

Source: Getty Images. (n.d.). *Getty Images sJEE4J4ZIrA Unsplash*. https://d35oenyzp35321.cloudfront.net/substance_abuse_in_men_df9c0e2b63.jpg.

Importance of Studying Substance Abuse in Forensics

Illicit substances have shifted in unexpected ways lately, pushing forensic experts to rethink their methods. New drugs—often promoted as legal alternatives—keep popping up and tripping up our old detection tools, which means we are forced to continuously try out fresh research strategies and adaptation (Brandt et al., 2014).

Forensics is not just about identifying these substances anymore; it is also about understanding their effects on the human body—details that ultimately play a role in legal cases and public health responses. Generally speaking, drug abuse tends to tie in with criminal behavior, so getting a grip on these messy connections really matters when evaluating a crime scene. And when you consider that substance abuse sometimes walks hand-in-hand with mental health struggles, like those encountered in adult ADHD cases (Kooij et al., 2018), thorough evaluations need to juggle both psychological and neurological angles. In short, examining the intersection of drug use and forensic science not only sharpens the pursuit of justice but also addresses broader questions about society's overall well-being.

Historical Context of Substance Abuse in Criminal Cases

Substance abuse and crime have tangled together for ages, a topic that is been looked at from many angles. Back in the day, people mostly chalked drug misuse up to a personal moral failing—ignoring how it is really a mix of mental and bodily challenges, which in most cases swayed legal responses. Slowly, psychiatric research nudged us toward seeing these issues as lying on a spectrum rather than as separate, fixed problems (Haslam et al., 2011). This gradual shift in thinking has, in many instances, reshaped criminal cases; forensic experts now often find they can better gauge a defendant's state of mind and how drugs, in fact, played into the crime. Similarly, newer approaches that factor in overlaps with issues like ADHD advocate for more in-depth, nuanced legal evaluations (Kooij et al., 2010). Clearly, weaving clinical insights into forensic work remains a crucial piece of the puzzle when aiming for just outcomes.

Scope of the Discussion

Substance abuse in forensic cases is not just a simple matter—it is tangled up with how people think, their social ties, and the way laws come into play (Figure 9.2). The issue often stretches beyond linking drug use to criminal behavior; it spills into how mental health is gauged during forensic exams and how community programs try to tackle the deeper social causes. In most cases, examining these areas reveals that enhancing mental health through both promotion and prevention strategies requires a broader approach than just addressing individual issues, and instead, it should consider the broader social context (Castillo et al., 2019).

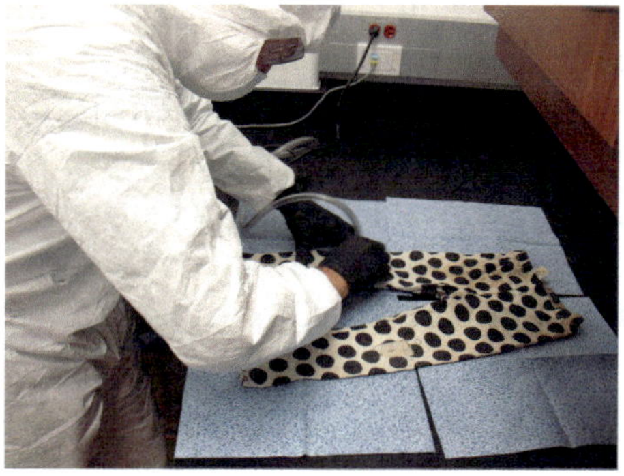

Figure 9.2. Substance abuse in forensic cases is not just a simple matter—it is tangled up with how people think, their social ties, and the way laws come into play.

Source: U.S. Customs and Border Protection. (n.d.). *Description of the Image*. https://www.cbp.gov/sites/default/files/Vacumming%20Baby%20Doe%20pants_0020.JPG.

Generally speaking, new ways of classifying behavioral disorders—as seen in the latest updates, such as those in ICD-11—underscore that updated diagnostic methods play a significant role in shaping how forensic assessments and legal guidelines are developed (Reed et al., 2016). All in all, this view paints a broad, interconnected picture of substance abuse in forensic settings, reminding us that real cases are often complicated and call for a thoughtful, multifaceted approach from legal experts, clinicians, and policymakers alike.

Key Terms and Concepts

Understanding these basic words and concepts in forensic substance abuse analysis is crucial when dealing with legal cases. Consider malingering, performance validity tests (PVTs), and symptom validity tests (SVTs) - they help distinguish between genuine cognitive issues and those that are faked, especially when someone may be motivated to gain an external benefit. In most cases, the Slick, Sherman, and Iverson criteria have long served as a sort of roadmap for detecting feigned neurocognitive problems in clinical work and research; however, these standards could use a modern update to keep pace with current malingering detection methods (Sherman et al., 2020). Also, evolving classification systems like those in the ICD-11 now offer more detailed guidelines for diagnosing mental and behavioral disorders tied to substance abuse, which, in many contexts, improves clinical practice across varied settings (Stein et al., 2020). All in all, truly grasping these key terms and their evolving meanings is crucial for forensic assessments that are both scientifically sound and legally robust.

Relevance to Current Forensic Practices

Forensic science breakthroughs are stepping in to tackle the shifting challenges of substance abuse in sports and other areas. The COVID-19 crisis exposed how traditional doping controls sometimes fell short, prompting labs to adopt remote sample collection and more rigorous testing methods to catch performance enhancers more reliably (Negro et al., 2022). These moves demonstrate that, generally speaking, forensic experts can adapt quickly to unexpected pressures while maintaining the integrity of substance detection. At the same time, forensic toxicology is getting more attention for its work in exploring long-term brain effects from substance use, like the concussions often seen in retired athletes with a drug history (Manley et al., 2017). This mixed approach not only helps in identifying banned substances but also provides insights into their lasting impact on individuals, which in turn informs legal and medical responses. As a result, modern forensics is becoming more dynamic and flexible—melding new techniques with occasional, cross-field teamwork to enhance detection accuracy, uphold fairness, and support public health efforts against substance abuse.

9.1. The Impact of Substance Abuse on Criminal Behavior

Learning Outcome

1. Understand the correlation between substance abuse and crime rate
2. Identify types of substances commonly abused
3. Know the psychological effects of substance abuse
4. Explain the influence of substance abuse on decision-making
5. Learn case studies illustrating substance abuse in criminal acts
6. Describe demographic factors influencing substance abuse and crime
7. Focus on substance abuse as a motive for criminal behavior
8. Discuss recidivism rates among substance abusers
9. Know legal implications of substance abuse in criminal cases

Substance abuse and criminal behavior create a complex mix that really challenges both the justice system and forensic work. Substance use tends to worsen underlying behavior issues, nudging folks toward criminal actions—a fact that is not as clear-cut as it might seem. Often, the best way to untangle these complications is by blending scientific insights with everyday social understanding; many forensic science courses even emphasize this practical mix to prepare students for what they will truly face beyond textbooks (Brockport et al., 2008). Recidivism among former offenders shows time and again that substance abuse and mental health struggles stubbornly stick around, pushing people back into the cycle of crime. In most cases, studies have found that giving focused counselling and mental health support during reentry helps reduce the chances of slipping back into criminal habits (Dadashazar et al., 2017). Addressing substance abuse, then, is not just a side note—it is key to lowering crime and boosting true rehabilitation. Forensic professionals now must go beyond simply examining physical evidence; they also need to consider the human and behavioral aspects of criminal acts. This broader view kind of shapes the strategies used to lower the risks of crimes linked to substance use, and it steers smarter decisions in forensic settings. Generally speaking, keeping an eye on both the hard facts and the messy human elements makes it possible to build plans that work more reliably in real life.

9.1.1. Correlation Between Substance Abuse and Crime Rates

Substance misuse and criminal behavior are not tidy issues—they are tangled up in ways that keep forensic experts busy, probing into both the social factors and the mental struggles involved (Figure 9.3). Research generally shows that when someone misuses drugs, it often makes their existing mental problems even worse, which can sometimes steer them toward violent or unlawful actions. Forensic psychiatry, for instance, puts a lot of weight on risk assessment when dealing with mentally troubled individuals who also struggle with substance abuse, making it really hard to predict or nip violent acts in the bud (Zhu et al., 2014). Additionally, behaviors such as avoiding the problem and shifting blame outward have been identified as early indicators of criminal patterns later in life (Idemudia, 2014). All in all, blending treatment for substance misuse with broader mental health care seems to be a promising way to bring down crime rates. In short, truly understanding how these issues mix is key to developing forensic protocols and risk management tools that are rooted in solid, evidence-based practices.

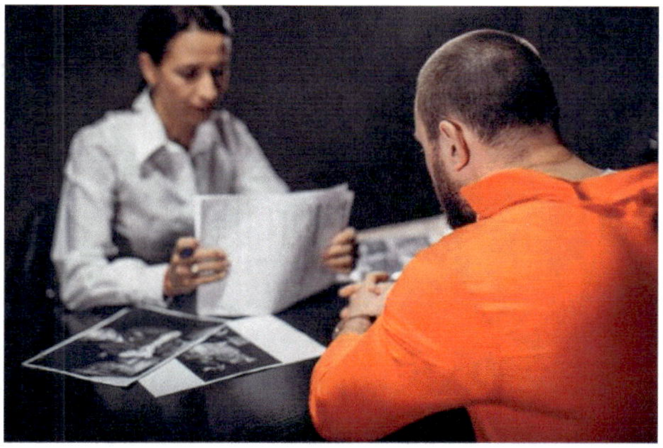

Figure 9.3. Substance misuse and criminal behavior are not tidy issues—they are tangled up in ways that keep forensic experts busy, probing into both the social factors and the mental struggles involved.

Source: American Public University. (n.d.). *What is a Criminal Psychologist?* https://www.apu.apus.edu/images/site/cards/what-is-a-criminal-psychologist.jpg.

9.1.2. Types of Substances Commonly Abused

Pinpointing abused substances is one of the trickier parts of forensic work. Each drug—whether it is alcohol, nicotine, cannabis, opioids, stimulants like cocaine or methamphetamine, or even synthetic types—leaves its own unique traces and affects the body in less predictable ways. In many cases, these substances do not simply blend into the background; they create both physical and chemical clues that often signal different health risks. It is not uncommon to see signs in the mouth—such as dental cavities, gum issues, and even unusual mucosal lesions (Nilendu, 2024)—which, as some experts note, can indicate prolonged misuse. Recent techniques, such as tracking wastewater, have opened up new ways to observe community-level trends in near real-time; this approach monitors not only legal substances, like nicotine and alcohol, but also illicit drugs (Da Nğlıoğlu et al., 2024). Generally speaking, having a good grasp of these varied effects helps sharpen the accuracy of an investigation and also supports public health efforts aimed at mitigating substance-related harm (Figure 9.4).

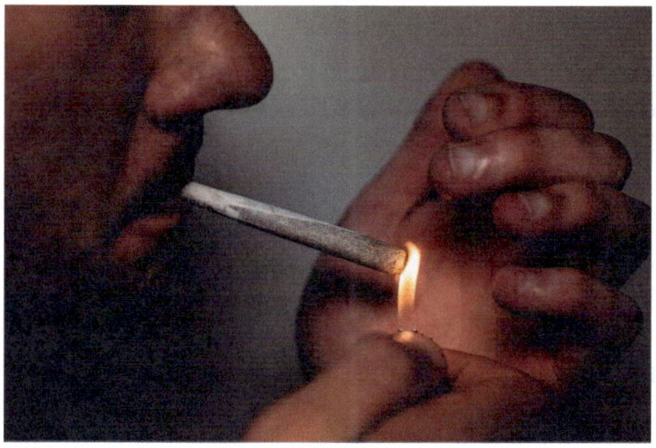

Figure 9.4. Nicotine.

Source: Refocus. (n.d.). *How Does Drug Abuse Affect Society?* https://refocus.com.au/wp-content/uploads/How-Does-Drug-Abuse-Affect-Society.jpg.

9.1.3. Psychological Effects of Substance Abuse

Substance abuse and mental health issues mix in ways that really complicate forensic work

(Figure 9.5). Long-term drug use messes with memory, judgment, and emotional balance, which in turn muddies how behavior or intent is read during investigations. People who suffer from prolonged substance misuse can show signs like anxiety, depression, or even episodes of psychosis – and these symptoms may, in most cases, affect their ability to face trial or engage fully in legal proceedings. At the same time, some substances push individuals toward riskier actions that could lead to criminal acts or self-harm, making legal evaluations even trickier. Take salbutamol, for example – while its toxic profile is generally milder, its mental side effects when misused or taken in overdose still call for careful examination (Kycler et al., 2024). Spotting these psychological changes is key to building a solid forensic profile, helping to tell if actions were voluntary or not (Nilendu, 2024).

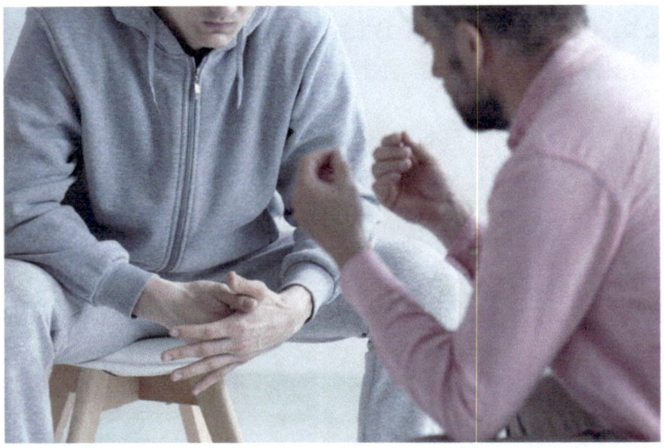

Figure 9.5. Substance abuse and mental health issues mix in ways that really complicate forensic work.

Source: Casa Palmera. (2019). *Optimized AdobeStock_150581294-2.* https://marvel-b1-cdn.bc0a.com/f00000000200278/casapalmera.com/wp-content/uploads/2019/09/Optimized-AdobeStock_150581294-2.jpeg.

9.1.4. Influence of Substance Abuse on Decision-making

Psychoactive substances can really throw off our ability to decide, mainly when they are used as a quick fix during high-stress times. People taking drugs meant to boost brainpower often miss the whole picture—they might not see the legal and health dangers linked to their clouded judgment, sometimes putting not just themselves but others (say, while driving or getting medical care (Dominik et al., 2022)) at risk (Figure 9.6). Studies in forensic samples generally show that repeated drug use can further mess with vital mental skills like planning and decision-making. For example, some forensic inpatients with a history of substance abuse struggled noticeably with tasks that test these abilities; meanwhile, simple targeted strategies like dietary supplements even offered a hint of improvement (Hansen et al., 2015). All in all, it seems that the brain glitches tied to substance abuse are pretty complex but, in most cases, at least partly reversible—an idea that really underlines the need to address these issues in forensic settings to cut down risky behavior and help rehabilitation work better.

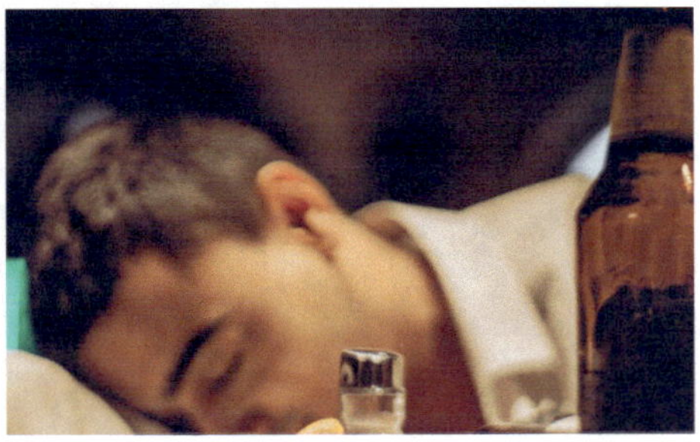

Figure 9.6. People taking drugs meant to boost brainpower often miss the full picture.

Source: Futures Recovery Healthcare. (2023). *Alcohol Effects on Society*. https://i0.wp.com/futuresrecoveryhealthcare.com/wp-content/uploads/2023/03/Alcohol-Effects-on-Society.png?fit=1280%2C791&ssl=1.

9.1.5. Case Studies Illustrating Substance Abuse in Criminal Acts

Grasping how substance misuse ties into criminal behavior often means digging into real-life cases that quietly expose hidden mental and social struggles. Look at forensic studies on autistic adults—here, crimes usually are not driven by drugs but seem more linked to thinking and social snags that dampen motivation and twist behavior (Helverschou et al., 2015). On the other hand, early abuse, measured by tools like MACE, generally sets up long-term paths where initial maltreatment nudges people toward mental issues and substance reliance, which can then spiral into criminal acts (Teicher et al., 2015). These examples remind us that drug-related crimes are not isolated incidents; they are mixed into a wider, sometimes messy, developmental, and social fabric. By melding forensic insights with detailed histories of early abuse and neurodevelopment challenges, researchers and practitioners can—often imperfectly—spot patterns in offending linked to substance use, ultimately refining both preventive and rehabilitative efforts in forensic settings.

9.1.6. Demographic Factors Influencing Substance Abuse and Crime

Age, income, and access to mental health care all seem to play a role in turning substance use into criminal behavior—this mix gives forensic experts plenty to chew on (Figure 9.7). Sometimes it is clear that being young, having limited funds, and not getting enough support nudges folks toward using substances, which can then lead to run-ins with the law. Research shows that among ex-offenders, risk factors measured by tools such as the Level of Service Inventory-Revised (LSI-R) tend to match up with higher recidivism rates, especially when mental health counselling during reentry is patchy or even missing (Dadashazar et al., 2017). This finding generally highlights the need for targeted support for individuals facing demographic challenges. Variations in forensic support and public awareness—seen in different regions—further complicate effective policing and rehabilitation, blurring the lines between background and criminal activity (Quansah et al., 2022). In short, grasping these background influences is pretty essential if we are to build robust forensic strategies to tackle crimes tied to substance abuse.

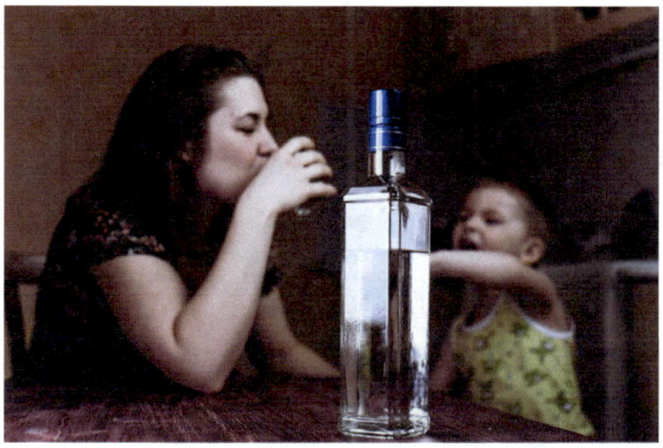

Figure 9.7. Age, income, and access to mental health care all seem to play a role in turning substance use into criminal behavior—this mix gives forensic experts plenty to chew on.

Source: Alcohol Help. (2018). *AdobeStock_106669390.* https://www.alcoholhelp.com/app/uploads/2018/07/AdobeStock_106669390.jpeg.

9.1.7. Substance Abuse as a Motive for Criminal Behavior

Criminal behavior often comes out of a messy mix of inner struggles, social pressures, and even environmental cues—with substance abuse, in many cases, lighting the fuse. When someone has been drinking or using drugs, their decision-making gets fuzzy, and a spark of aggression might unexpectedly flare up, sending them down a path that can range from violent clashes to property offenses. At times, the grip of addiction makes people feel pushed into breaking the law to keep feeding their habit—a loop that keeps reinforcing both the addiction and criminal acts. For instance, research into serial killings generally shows that substance misuse can blend with other risks—like mental health challenges and social disadvantages—thereby raising the odds of dangerous behavior (Brennan et al.,

2019). Domestic disputes, too, remind us that intoxication is often tied to a rapid escalation in personal conflicts, occasionally ending in grim outcomes such as intimate partner homicide-suicide (Salari et al., 2007). All in all, seeing substance abuse as a crucial factor behind criminal acts is key for both forensic digs and in working out better ways to prevent such behavior (Figure 9.8).

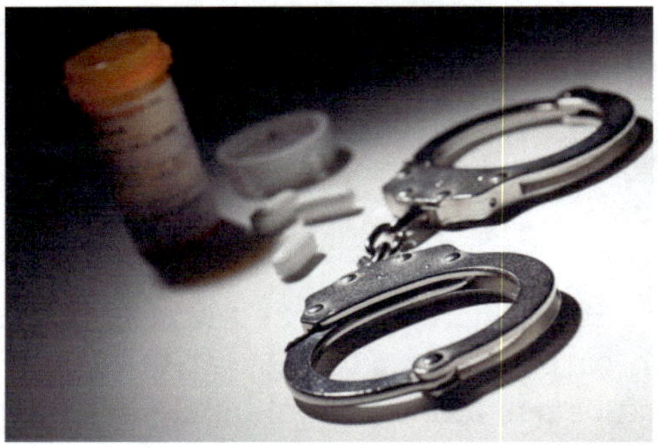

Figure 9.8. Substance abuse as a motive for criminal behavior.

Source: NADA Acudetox UK. (n.d.). *Substance-Abuse.* https://nadaacudetox.co.uk/wp-content/uploads/2016/03/substance-abuse.jpg.

9.1.8. Recidivism Rates Among Substance Abusers

Exploring how mental health issues mix with substance abuse really gets to the heart of why some individuals fall back into criminal patterns. Forensic psychiatric groups, for example, often see a bump in reoffending risks when substance misuse is in play—especially with conditions like schizophrenia spectrum disorders. A Finnish study found that about 63.5% of these patients also deal with substance problems, and, in most cases, this combination leads to more criminal recidivism after they leave psychiatric care. Interestingly, longer treatment spans tend to link with lower general recidivism, suggesting that sustained care addressing both psychiatric symptoms and substance issues is key to rehabilitation. Plus, interventions such as dialectical behavior therapy—which focuses on regulating emotions and building coping skills—have shown promise in cutting down impulsive behaviors and substance use, which might help reduce those reoffending risks tied to addiction and erratic behavior. All in all, these insights emphasize the importance of dedicated substance abuse treatment within forensic settings to prevent a return to criminal activity (Ojansuu et al., 2023; Marshall et al., 2024) (Figure 9.9).

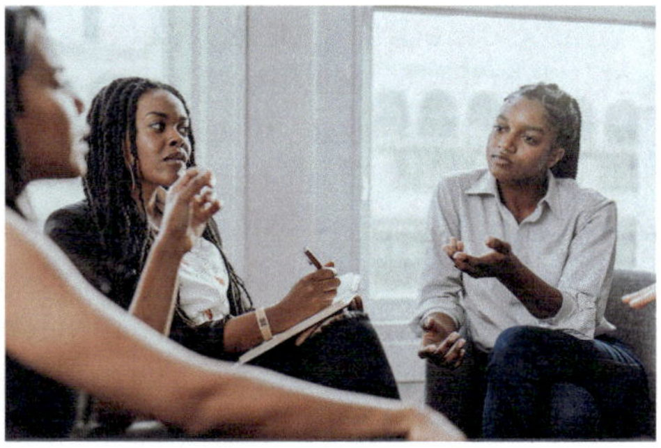

Figure 9.9. Forensic psychiatric groups.

Source: BetterHelp. (n.d.). *What is a Forensic Psychiatrist?* https://advice.cdn.betterhelp.com/md/what-is-a-forensic-psychiatrist-1_.JPG.jpg.

9.1.9. Legal Implications of Substance Abuse in Criminal Cases

Substance abuse mixed with criminal law really creates a tangled set of challenges for legal practitioners and forensic experts. In most cases, figuring out exactly how intoxication or addiction might nudge a defendant's mental state calls for a forensic review that is anything but straightforward – it relies on weighing clinical findings against legal norms in ways that are not always neat. Experts, then, tread a careful line; they avoid blunt claims about guilt to keep ethical limits intact while still hinting at how substance issues might impair behavior or even boost the risk of reoffending (Apodaca et al., 2015). At the same time, cultural factors get thrown into the mix, influencing forensic psychiatric evaluations in ways that can shift how we interpret behavior linked to substance use—and that, in turn, may change perceptions of legal responsibility (Tseng et al., 2004). The legal system, for its part, has to juggle these various aspects to deliver decisions that feel fair, even as it wrestles with the impact addiction can have on criminal actions. Ultimately, blending solid forensic evidence on substance abuse into criminal trials demands not only scientific care but also a touch of cultural sensitivity to keep justice on track.

Test Your Knowledge

1. How does chronic drug use influence an individual's decision-making and impulse control?
2. What is the relationship between alcohol intoxication and violent crimes?

9.2. Forensic Analysis of Substances

Learning Outcome

1. Identify methods of substance identification in forensics
2. Explain the role of toxicology in forensic investigations
3. Know the chain of custody in substance evidence
4. Discuss challenges in analyzing substances
5. Know advances in forensic technology for substance analysi
6. Describe the interpretation of toxicology reports;
7. Learn limitations of current forensic methods
8. Focus on case examples of forensic analysis in substance abuse cases
9. Describe ethical considerations in forensic substance analysis

Substance abuse is on the rise these days, and forensic teams now find themselves needing advanced techniques to track and measure psychoactive drugs in criminal investigations. Recent work has demonstrated that broad toxicology screenings—utilizing methods like high-resolution liquid chromatography-mass spectrometry, along with gas chromatographic techniques—play a crucial role in identifying both well-known substances and newer ones, such as gabapentinoids. In many cases, these tools help forensic experts untangle the messy mix of drugs found among victims and suspects, offering critical clues about how substance use ties in with various criminal acts.

For example, some analyses have pointed out that stimulants and cannabinoids often appear together with gabapentinoids, which not only highlights an evolving drug scene but also suggests that legal guidelines and screening methods might need to be tweaked (Saglam et al., 2025).

Collecting samples on time and in a somewhat organized way boosts the overall value of the toxicology data, thereby supporting both preventive strategies and more informed judicial decisions (Heinsvig et al., 2024). All in all, blending these forensic approaches is pretty crucial for handling the substance abuse challenges within our criminal justice system.

9.2.1. Methods of Substance Identification in Forensics

Forensic science often kicks off with pinpoint techniques that tie substances to both criminal acts and health issues—substance abuse being a prime example (Figure 9.10). Analysts have long relied on classic tests like chromatography and spectrometry; these methods reliably detect drugs and their byproducts in human samples, as well as in environmental ones. Lately, technological improvements have enabled these tests to run faster and with greater sensitivity, generally speaking. One intriguing, newer twist is wastewater-based epidemiology (WBE): by analyzing sewage for traces of substances and their metabolites, investigators can piece together community drug usage patterns almost in real-time (Da Nğlıoğlu et al., 2024). Sometimes, a closer look at oral health offers clues too—this route can be advantageous when the usual direct chemical evidence is not available (Nilendu, 2024). All in all, mixing these varied approaches tends to widen the net and sharpen the overall accuracy of substance identification, ultimately bolstering efforts in both criminal justice and public health arenas.

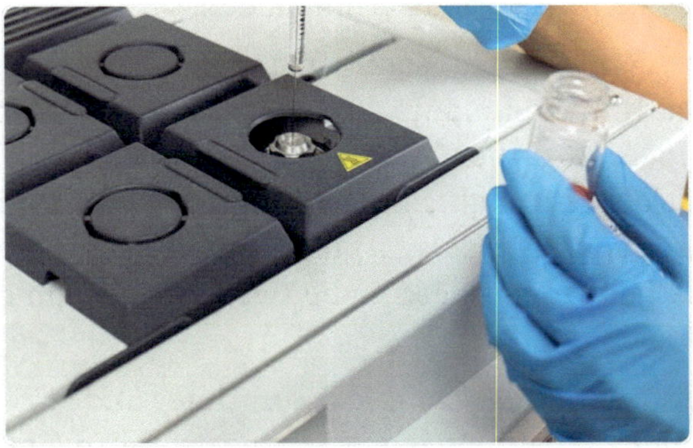

Figure 9.10. Substance identification methods in forensics.

Source: Lerner, V. (2019). *By Lerner Vadim-1.* https://d2jx2rerrg6sh3.cloudfront.net/image-handler/picture/2019/5/By_Lerner_Vadim-1.jpg.

9.2.2. Role of Toxicology in Forensic Investigations

Investigating substance abuse in forensic settings is not just about running tests—it demands a nuanced feel for how drugs mingle with the body and subtly shape behavior, sometimes swaying legal decisions.

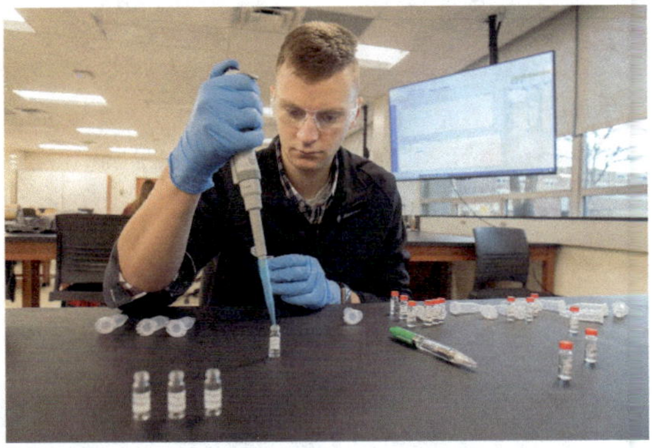

Figure 9.11. Role of toxicology in forensic investigations.

Source: Bowling Green State University. (n.d.). *Student in Forensics Lab.* https://www.bgsu.edu/content/dam/BGSU/academics/forensic-science/Student-in-Forensics-Lab.jpgs.

Forensic toxicology, in this context, acts as a key bridge between scientific inquiry and the law; its advanced analytical techniques help detect and measure compounds in a range of biological samples, shedding light on why someone might be impaired or, tragically, why death occurred. Generally speaking, reading toxicology reports is no walk in the park: differences in drug metabolism between genders and the unique ways drugs affect the body often complicate postmortem examinations (Giorgetti et al., 2025). Plus, as synthetic and novel psychoactive substances pop up more frequently, labs are pushed to keep their detection methods on their toes—with instruments like gas chromatography (GC)-mass spectrometry (MS) and liquid chromatography-tandem mass spectrometry now playing a significant role in spotting these tricky chemicals (Sacco et al., 2025). At the end of the day, these approaches not only help clarify the messy details of substance-related incidents but also inform public health strategies and shape judicial decisions. Clearly, forensic toxicology remains essential, quietly bridging the gap between rigorous scientific analysis and the pragmatic demands of the courtroom (Figure 9.11).

9.2.3. Chain of Custody in Substance Evidence

In substance abuse cases, keeping evidence intact is crucial—even a small slip might throw the whole legal process off track. A chain of custody that is carefully recorded at every turn, ensuring each item is gathered, stored, and handed off without any unwanted tampering or contamination, serves as a critical safeguard. Lately, technology has made significant strides: blockchain and smart contracts now offer ways to create unalterable digital records that tend to reduce human error and even help prevent tampering (Imrankhan et al., 2024). This setup, which generally enhances transparency and accountability, still relies heavily on hands-on expertise; for example, forensic veterinarians handling animal poisoning cases emphasize the importance of getting every detail right in the records (Kulnides et al., 2023). As forensic science advances, a solid chain of custody remains the backbone for meeting the strict standards of admissible, reliable evidence in court.

9.2.4. Challenges in Analyzing Substances

Forensic work is not simple—substance analysis itself presents a multitude of unexpected challenges. In many cases, the chemicals in materials vary significantly, especially with illicit drugs that are often cut or blended with substances we are unaware of, which makes it extremely challenging to obtain exact identifications and measurements. Substances may break down over time or under different environmental conditions, too, further muddying attempts at reliable detection. Often, these issues overlap with problems in the criminal justice system, where mental health challenges and substance dependencies mix, calling for careful, layered approaches (Forsythe, 2013). Furthermore, factors such as prison overcrowding ultimately limit resources and disrupt procedural timelines, leading many to advocate for improved policies and new testing methods (Wootton et al., 2016). All in all, these stumbling blocks underscore the ongoing need to develop more refined, sensitive, and specific techniques in forensic toxicology to support just and effective legal outcomes (Figure 9.12).

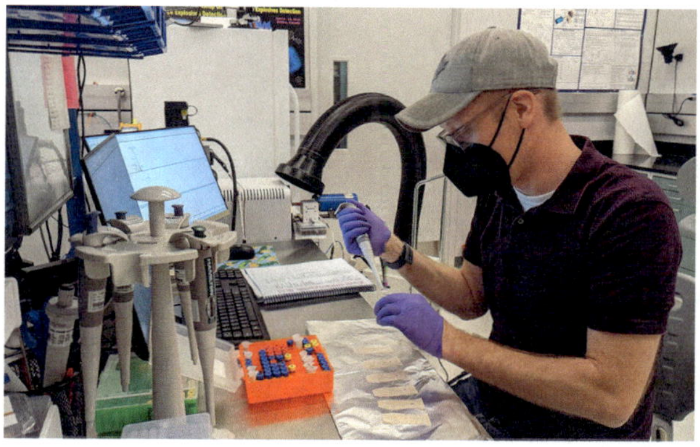

Figure 9.12. Substances may break down over time or under different environmental conditions, too, further complicating attempts at reliable detection.

Source: Sisco, E. (2021). *Ed Sisco Analyzing Wipe Samples of Suspected Drug Packaging Using TD-DART-MS.*

9.2.5. Advances in Forensic Technology for Substance Analysis

Forensic substance testing has really taken an unexpected turn lately—new tech is not just upgrading methods but reshuffling everything about how we spot drug use patterns. High-resolution instruments, such as liquid chromatography-mass spectrometry, now enable experts to detect multiple substances simultaneously, including newer ones like gabapentinoids, often at levels that are barely detectable (Figure 9.13). In most cases, this improvement matters a lot; studies (Saglam et al., 2025) have hinted that drugs like methamphetamine and THC often appear alongside these emerging compounds, which generally call for a rethink in our screening routines. Sometimes, practitioners even mix these lab techniques with a bit of an oral health check, naturally linking visible symptoms to a person's drug history (Nilendu, 2024). Overall, these fresh approaches not only stretch the limits of detection but also back legal proceedings by offering richer toxic profiles, paving the way for more informed court decisions in drug-related cases.

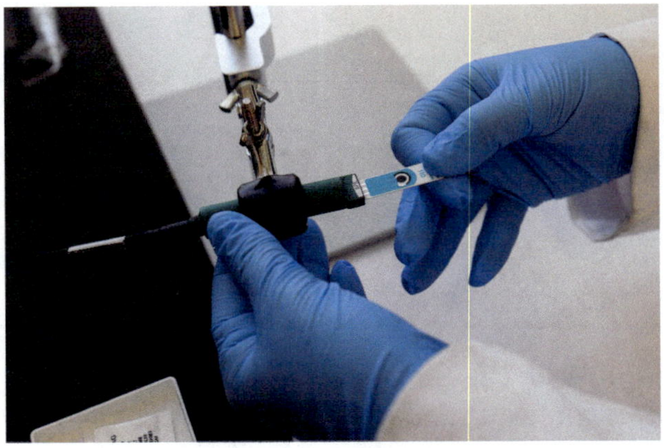

Figure 9.13. High-resolution instruments, such as liquid chromatography-mass spectrometry, enable experts to detect multiple substances simultaneously, including newer ones like gabapentinoids, often at barely detectable levels.

Source: National Institute of Justice. (2024). *Drug Identification Using a Screen-Printed Carbon Electrode.* https://nij.ojp.gov/sites/g/files/xyckuh171/files/images/2024-08/figure1-drug-identification-using-a-screen-printed-carbon-electrode_0.jpg.

9.2.6. Interpretation of Toxicology Reports

Interpreting toxicology reports well is not just a routine task—it is really central to forensic work (Figure 9.14). It calls for a solid, even if sometimes winding, grasp of both pharmacology and what we might call toxicokinetics so that experts can tell therapeutic use apart from abuse or a mere accidental contact. Lately, you see more cases where substances like gabapentinoids are present. Generally, speaking, their appearance alongside other illicit chemicals such as methamphetamine and THC complicates things a bit, making it challenging to pin down cause and effect (Saglam et al., 2025).

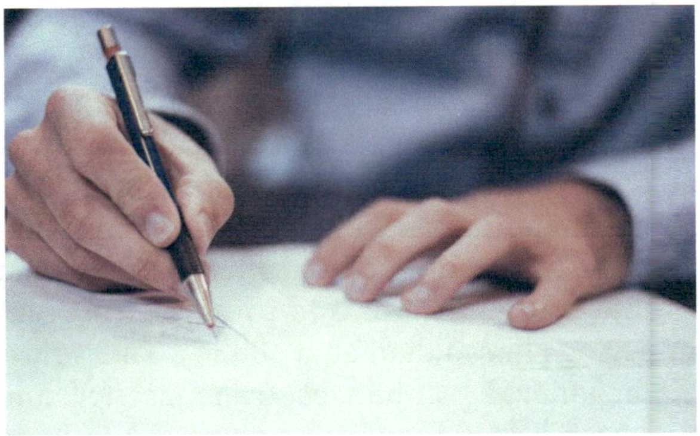

Figure 9.14. Interpreting toxicology reports.

Source: Graham, S. (n.d.). Photograph of a person writing on paper. *Unsplash*. https://www.dnalegal.com/sites/default/files/styles/content_image/public/blog-images/scott-graham-OQMZwNd3ThU-unsplash_0.jpg?itok=CCxTOC0t.

Sometimes, it is not only about noticing what substances are there; one also has to look at the patterns when multiple drugs mix and how every individual processes them. Forensic specialists, as they often say, need to work hand in hand with clinicians to put lab results into a wider, almost conversational picture that takes into account possible abuse, trauma, and related clinical symptoms—especially when vulnerable groups are part of the picture. A small slip in how the data is read can, in most cases, lead to an underdiagnosis or even to really off-track conclusions that might ripple seriously through legal and healthcare settings (Focardi et al., 2025). In the end, merging a full spectrum of toxicological details with clear clinical and circumstantial clues remains pretty much the cornerstone for drawing sound conclusions about substance misuse.

9.2.7. Limitations of Current Forensic Methods

Analyzing psychoactive substances is no simple task—it puts a severe strain on the methods used in forensics today. Imagine trying to spot drugs that have been altered or blended, like when codeine gets mixed with ephedrine; such cases demand top-notch techniques that are not always handy, so investigators sometimes end up with the wrong picture.

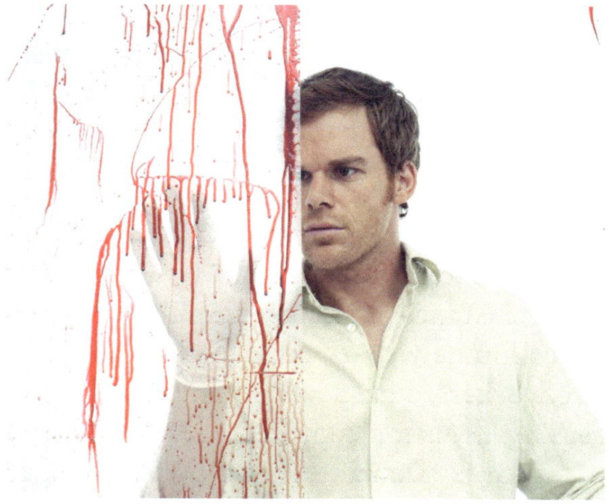

Figure 9.15. Prisoners with a background of childhood abuse tend to show cycles of drug use combined with criminal activity.

Source: Weber, C. (n.d.). *Photograph of the TV Character Dexter Looking at Blood Splatter on a Wall*. https://opentextbc.ca/introductiontosociology/wp-content/uploads/sites/12/2013/12/Dexter.jpg.

In many instances, substance abuse itself shifts unpredictably, often fueled by early-life trauma, which only complicates the effort to link behavior with drug use. Take, for example, prisoners with a background of childhood abuse; they tend to show cycles of drug use combined with criminal activity, yet many forensic methods do not capture these intertwined social and psychological details fully (Ali et al., 2024). Meanwhile, as the world of narcotics continues to evolve, forensic protocols are also forced to keep pace—though technical and logistical issues still arise (Titova, 2024). All of these challenges, in most cases, seriously restrict how wholly and accurately substance abuse can be evaluated in forensic settings (Figure 9.15).

9.2.8. Case Examples of Forensic Analysis in Substance Abuse Cases

Forensic analysis is crucial when attempting to unravel complex substance abuse cases, as it provides solid evidence to support legal inquiries. Toxicology tests, for one, have been flagging a growing misuse of gabapentinoids – think pregabalin and gabapentin – among younger people caught up in judicial issues. In one study that looked at over 10,000 urine samples, about 21.6% came out positive; often these positives showed up alongside methamphetamine or THC-COOH, suggesting a trend that is on the rise even with current regulatory checks (Saglam et al., 2025). These results, in general, support the case for updating routine forensic screenings to include emerging substances. Forensic pathology, on its part, has wedded advanced methods, such as scanning electron microscopy with energy-dispersive X-ray spectrometry (SEM/EDX), to identify unique chemical markers—such as those found in cigarette burns linked to abuse situations (Tambuzzi et al., 2024). Altogether, these mixed analytical approaches enhance the accuracy of forensic readings, thereby supporting legal outcomes and, in most cases, informing public health responses to address substance abuse.

9.2.9. Ethical Considerations in Forensic Substance Analysis

Forensic substance analysis plays a crucial role in maintaining the fairness of our justice system—if evidence is mishandled, it can significantly impact legal outcomes and affect real lives. Usually, the process begins with careful sample storage and accurate identification, ensuring that, in most cases, contamination or decay does not alter the substance's true nature. Analysts, trying to be as objective as possible, need to avoid any bias or outside pressure that might sneak in, and, frankly, that is easier said than done.

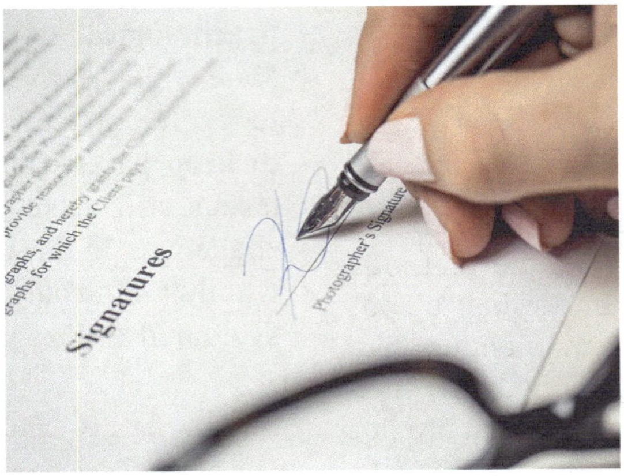

Figure 9.16. Confidentiality is also key; keeping sensitive case details under wraps protects privacy and legal rights, even if the lines sometimes get a bit blurred.

Source: energepic.com. (n.d.). *Person Holding Silver Pen Signing Photographer's Signature*. https://www.zoppi.co.uk/_next/image?url=https%3A%2F%2Fcms.gaffneyzoppi.com%2Fwp-content%2Fuploads%2F2023%2F11%2FFree-Person-Holding-Silver-Pen-Signing-Photographers-Signature-Stock-Photo.jpg&w=1920&q=75.

Confidentiality is also key; keeping sensitive case details under wraps protects privacy and legal rights, even if the lines sometimes get a bit blurred. Occasionally ethical issues occur in environments like prisons or clinical settings, where, for instance, Buddhist-inspired programs may show promise—though they still need a strong moral framework to back them up (Griffiths et al., 2013). Furthermore, the fact that many healthcare workers, such as emergency nurses, lack sufficient forensic knowledge only reinforces the pressing need for comprehensive training to maintain evidentiary integrity and meet medicolegal standards (Donaldson et al., 2020) (Figure 9.16).

Test Your Knowledge

1. What is the purpose of forensic analysis in substance-related cases?
2. Which biological samples are commonly used for substance detection?

9.3. Substance Abuse and Mental Health

Learning Outcome

1. Understand the relationship between mental health and substance abuse
2. Identify common mental health disorders associated with substance abuse
3. Know the impact of substance abuse on forensic evaluations
4. Explain the role of mental health professionals in forensic settings
5. Discuss treatment options for substance abuse in offenders
6. Focus on recidivism and mental health treatment outcomes
7. Describe legal defenses based on mental health and substance abuse
8. Know the importance of interdisciplinary approaches in forensics
9. Understand future directions for research on mental health and substance abuse

Mental health issues and substance misuse often show up tangled in forensic environments nowadays, which calls for a close look and flexible approaches. Daily strains from social and personal factors—and even some brain-based quirks—can combine to exacerbate these problems, making it challenging to determine the right diagnosis and treatment. In most cases, the COVID-19 pandemic has made matters even more complicated, exacerbating neuropsychiatric symptoms and substance use; factors such as increased brain inflammation and heightened daily stress appear to play a role (Munipalli et al., 2024). Early rough experiences, like childhood neglect or abuse, also tend to kick off a chain reaction leading to increased substance misuse and sometimes more aggressive criminal acts—a recurring loop in many forensic settings (Ali et al., 2024). All in all, getting a grip on these mixed influences is really key when crafting mental health interventions that tackle both the lingering scars of trauma and the ongoing challenges of substance dependence among vulnerable folks.

9.3.1. Relationship Between Mental Health and Substance Abuse

In forensic settings, mental health issues and substance abuse get tangled up in ways that often muddy both diagnosis and treatment. Many people in the criminal justice system show overlapping symptoms—say, signs of posttraumatic stress or personality problems mixed in with drug dependency—which tends to make clear clinical assessments pretty tricky. Going into the depth, you see that underlying problems, issues like trauma and shaky attachment bonds, generally feed into both the mental struggles and the substance use, further complicating the picture.

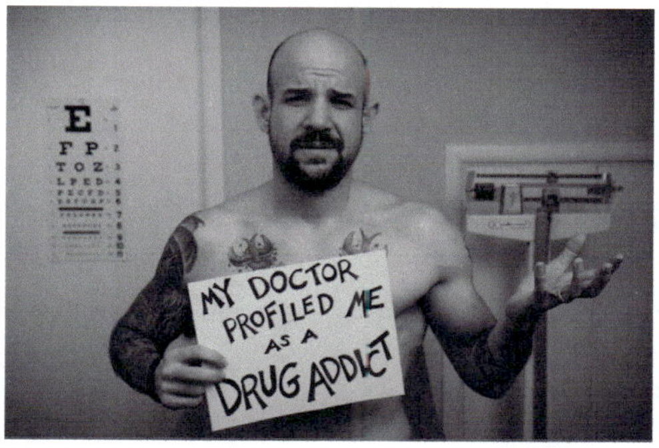

Figure 9.17. Many people in the criminal justice system show overlapping symptoms—say, signs of posttraumatic stress or personality problems mixed in with drug dependency—which tends to make clear clinical assessments pretty tricky.

Source: Ideal Medical Care. (2014). *Double_-51*. https://www.idealmedicalcare.org/blog/wp-content/uploads/2014/01/Double_-51-1024x678.jpg.

Dual diagnoses pop up a lot, especially among incarcerated women, and when their psychological signals are misinterpreted, it can lead to care that is either off-target or even biased. Effective forensic interventions, then, really must be trauma-aware and gender-sensitive, paving the way for more accurate assessments and smoother rehabilitation within correctional settings (Gillette et al., 2011). Public health frameworks also emphasize the crucial role that state services play in addressing these interconnected issues in forensic contexts (Figure 9.17).

9.3.2. Common Mental Health Disorders Associated with Substance Abuse

Substance abuse is not just about a physical dependency—it often gets mixed up with mental health struggles that make both spotting the problem and treating it a real challenge. In forensic settings, many individuals show signs of anxiety, depression, and even post-traumatic stress disorder; these issues can get even worse when substance misuse is in the picture.

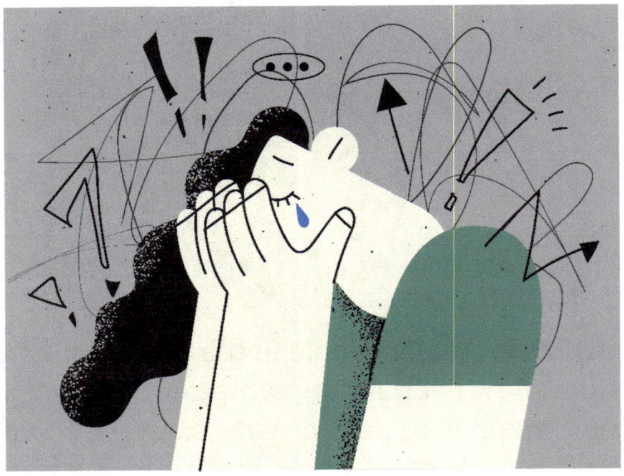

Figure 9.18. In forensic settings, many individuals show signs of anxiety, depression, and even post-traumatic stress disorder; these issues can get even worse when substance misuse is in the picture.

Source: Self. (n.d.). Physical symptoms of anxiety. *Condé Nast.* https://media.self.com/photos/6201544646024e0a717b9306/4:3/w_6664,h_4998,c_limit/physical-symptoms-of-anxiety.jpg.

When mental health problems and substance abuse feed off each other, they create a cycle that is tough for forensic professionals to break. Research, in most cases, shows that forensic scientists who have been exposed to trauma tend to have higher rates of anxiety paired with PTSD (Sistrunk et al., 2022). The persistent drug crisis only piles more pressure on public health and law enforcement, pointing to a need for blended strategies that tackle both substance misuse and its mental health side-effects (Hosen et al., 2023). Understanding how these troubles intertwine remains key for crafting effective forensic interventions (Figure 9.18).

9.3.3. Impact of Substance Abuse on Forensic Evaluations

Substance misuse really complicates the process of forensic evaluations, making everything a lot complicated. When novel psychoactive substances come into play, neurological and psychological signs often show up that can both imitate and hide real mental health issues – something that generally leaves forensic pathologists scratching their heads (Mazurek et al., 2024).

Then there is the mix of rough childhood experiences with drug misuse, which sometimes pushes behavior toward traits like antisocial personality disorder – a factor many experts wind up having to check in their assessments (McPhail et al., 2022). It seems that understanding both the immediate drug effects and the broader, messy backdrop of one's life is key to making sense of forensic interpretations. In most cases, the interplay of neurochemical changes and lasting psychological trauma means that substance abuse can undercut the reliability of forensic evaluations, pointing squarely to why a cross-disciplinary approach in legal assessments is so needed.

9.3.4. Role of Mental Health Professionals in Forensic Settings

Addressing issues of substance abuse in forensic settings is not a solo job—it takes a mix of experts all pitching in with their own kind of know-how (Figure 9.19). Doctors, for instance, usually focus on spotting psychiatric disorders and using meds to stabilize patients—a fundamental first step that lays the groundwork.

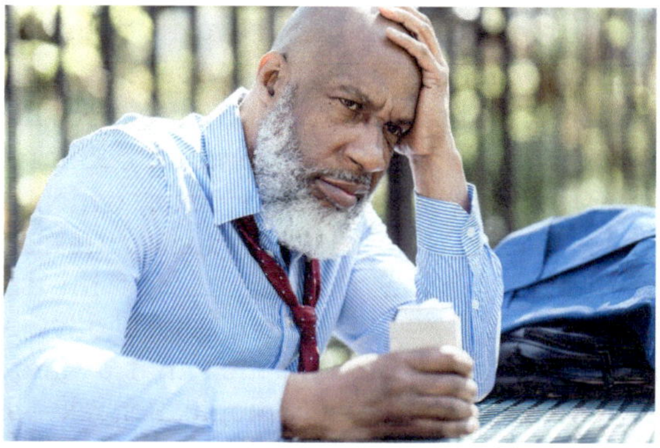

Figure 9.19. Addressing issues of substance abuse in forensic settings is not a solo job—it takes a mix of experts all pitching in with their own kind of know-how.

Source: Roots Recovery. (2023). *Stressed Man Holding Coffee Cup at Outdoor Table.* https://roots-recovery.com/wp-content/uploads/2023/04/pexels-photo-7925823-1024x683.jpeg.

Psychologists, on their part, delve into personal histories so that folks can begin to see recurring behavior linked to their substance use; they often repeat this idea as a means of opening up new ways to understand the problem. Meanwhile, occupational therapists focus on everyday skills that, quite frankly, are essential for recovery, and social workers step in to facilitate community reentry and plan aftercare. Frontline nurses, who sometimes juggle security duties, may lean toward a criminogenic view that focuses on controlling behavior. Even so, communication hiccups and strict hierarchies between these professionals can hinder a smooth, integrated approach—potentially limiting treatment efficacy. Generally speaking, recognizing and bridging these divides is really key to effective risk management and rehabilitation for forensic patients struggling with substance abuse. All in all, this type of multidisciplinary effort highlights the complex yet crucial role that mental health experts play in forensic care (Davies et al., 2006).

9.3.5. Treatment Options for Substance Abuse in Offenders

Taking on substance abuse in offender populations means weighing both the mind and body sides of addiction. Programs often mix medications with talk-therapy methods like cognitive-behavioral approaches to keep relapse numbers down and help with longer-term improvement. Individual treatment plans that factor in gender differences and other mental health hurdles are critical—studies suggest that how symptoms show up and added complications play a significant role in how people engage and recover (Young et al., 2020). Building support networks outside of just clinical settings—for example, teaming up with legal, social, and healthcare agencies—can also facilitate the process of reintegrating people into society. This broad perspective recognizes that substance abuse in forensic groups is complex and calls for ongoing care across different points in life. In most cases, matching therapeutic efforts with current clinical insights and shifting social policies can help the justice system reduce repeat offenses and support lasting recovery among those struggling with addiction (Reed et al., 2016).

9.3.6. Recidivism and Mental Health Treatment Outcomes

Tackling the causes behind repeated offenses remains tricky, especially when drug problems mix with mental health issues. Recent studies have looked into programs like Juvenile Drug Treatment Courts (JDTC) that, in most cases, blend substance use services with mental health care for at-risk youth (Figure 9.20). The results generally show that these courts cut down on cannabis use and repeat offenses a bit while also ramping up access to mental health support for high-risk groups - though uneven implementation still holds back their overall impact (Belenko et al., 2022). Likewise, cognitive-behavioral initiatives such as Moral Reconation Therapy (MRT) have been checked out for their ability to ease criminal thought patterns and reduce reoffending. At the same time, MRT participants did show some progress with issues like criminal associates and legal troubles, its effect on reoffending compared to regular care turned out to be statistically insignificant - a result partly due to low engagement levels, in most cases (Blonigen et al., 2022). Overall, these findings paint a complex picture of treatment effectiveness in forensic settings. They highlight why it is essential to have interventions that are not only tailored to individual needs but also delivered consistently, if we really want to lower both recidivism and mental health challenges.

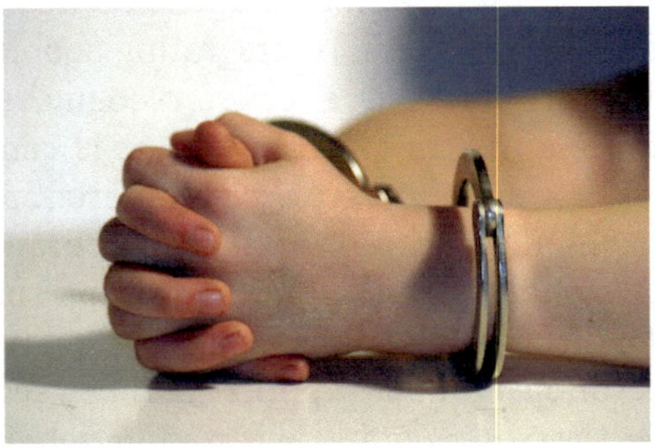

Figure 9.20. Juvenile drug treatment courts (JDTC).

Source: RiverheadLOCAL. (2017). Youth in Handcuffs. https://riverheadlocal.com/wp-content/uploads/2017/02/2017_0213_youth_handcuffs.jpg.

9.3.7. Legal Defenses Based on Mental Health and Substance Abuse

Mental health issues tangled up with substance misuse create a really messy situation in legal cases. People dealing with both a heavy mental condition and a substance problem often face unexpected roadblocks in court—challenges that are not usually part of the regular record. These combined issues can significantly impact how someone thinks or controls their behavior, so legal teams sometimes have to pause and carefully consider what is happening inside. For example, signs that we would expect from PTSD might, in many cases, end up being read as symptoms of a personality issue, which can lead to biased treatment by authorities and, unfortunately, skew the fairness of the trial (Gillette et al., 2011). Courts these days are slowly warming up to the idea that a kind of deep, compassionate psychological check—one that looks at the whole picture in a trauma-aware way—really matters for understanding a defendant's state of mind. In most situations, these assessments can bolster a defense by mitigating the perceived blame or gently shifting the focus toward rehabilitative sentencing rather than just punishment (Erickson et al., 2007). All in all, mixing mental health and substance abuse factors into legal defenses is pretty key to trying to reach a just outcome, even if the process is not always neat.

9.3.8. Importance of Interdisciplinary Approaches in Forensics

Substance abuse issues in forensic settings tend to pull experts from a mix of fields. Rather than simply following a neat textbook method, mental health, behavioral science, toxicology, and legal ideas often collide in ways that matter. Look, even the updated psychiatric guidelines from the ICD-11 (Stein et al., 2020) can sharpen the way we spot substance-related disorders, making it easier for forensic work to stay both clinically solid and globally relevant. At the same time, incorporating everyday psychology skills—such as basic behavioral techniques commonly seen in primary care—helps shape more comprehensive evaluations for individuals involved in forensic cases (McDaniel et al., 2014). These kinds of blended, sometimes unpredictable, connections between science and practice let professionals better untangle how substance abuse twists behavior and decision-making. In the end, integrating these various viewpoints not only enhances the quality of forensic evidence but also supports a justice system that is medically informed, ethically mindful, and attuned to the real context (Figure 9.21).

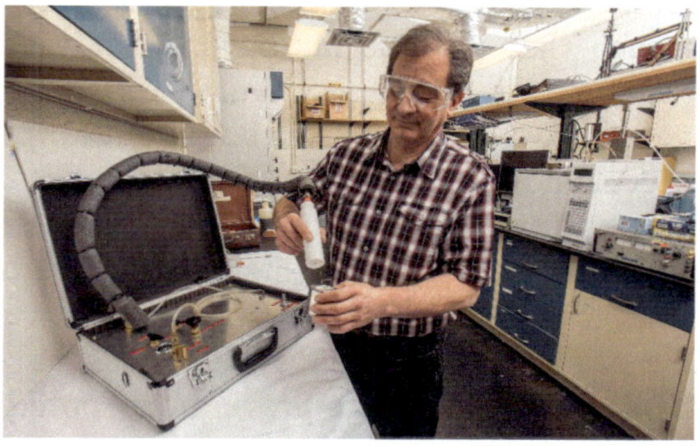

Figure 9.21. Quality of forensic evidence.

Source: National Institute of Standards and Technology. (2018). *Scientist Working in a Laboratory.* https://www.nist.gov/sites/default/files/styles/2800_x_2800_limit/public/images/2018/01/23/15mml017_tom_bruno_2364_hr_resized.jpg?itok=9sji9_LN.

9.3.9. Future Directions for Research on Mental Health and Substance Abuse

Our growing grasp of how mental health and substance use problems play out in forensic groups hints that research should look at both broad system issues and the personal struggles people face. Many folks think long-term studies could really help reveal how these challenges shift over time—especially during reentry phases, when the risk for relapse and repeat offenses tends to spike.

It is essential, in most cases, to mix in methods that see how well forensic counselling works, particularly when there's evidence (Dadashazar et al., 2017) suggesting that solid mental health support can keep ex-offenders from slipping back into crime. At the same time, one must also wonder how state public health agencies are teaming up with correctional systems to create treatment plans that blend jail-based care with community support, reflecting the mix of organizational dynamics and accountability noted in some public health analyses. By honing in on specialized training for forensic mental health pros and sticking with practices that have a firm evidence base, future studies may well cut down substance abuse-related crime and improve rehabilitation outcomes in these challenging settings.

Test Your Knowledge

1. How does substance abuse contribute to the development of mental health disorders?
2. How can depression and anxiety lead to or worsen substance dependence?

9.4. Prevention and Intervention Strategies

Learning Outcome

1. Understand community-based prevention programs
2. Explain the role of law enforcement in substance abuse prevention
3. Focus on education and awareness campaigns
4. Perform screening and early intervention in forensic settings
5. Learn about collaboration between forensic and health professionals
6. Describe policy implications for substance abuse prevention
7. Know the effectiveness of rehabilitation programs
8. Identify challenges in implementing prevention strategies
9. Focus on case studies of successful intervention programs

Early on, identifying potential issues and providing personalized treatment plays a significant role in forensic work—it is not just a checklist, but a blend of early detection, hands-on education, and treatment plans tailored to each case. Forensic fields generally call for a mix of ideas; a lot is left to frontline folks, like emergency nurses, who not only pick up on signs of substance misuse but also work to secure key forensic evidence, even though studies suggest they often do not get the specialized training they really need (Donaldson et al., 2020). Closing that training gap through focused forensic education could, in most cases, boost both confidence and competence, paving the way for better patient care and clearer legal proceedings. Evidence-inspired approaches, combined with community support, appear to promote rehabilitation and even reduce repeat offenses—sometimes, it feels like a small miracle when everything comes together. Technological strides and data-based programs, on the other hand, sharpen risk assessments and help target interventions more precisely (Tennessee. Department of Finance & Administration, 2015). In the end, a cooperative effort that weds insights from healthcare, forensic experts, and law enforcement proves pretty essential for tackling substance abuse challenges in these contexts, balancing recovery with justice even if the process is not ever perfectly smooth.

9.4.1. Community-Based Prevention Programs

Substance abuse today requires a multifaceted approach that extends far beyond traditional institutional interventions (Figure 9.22). It is not just about top-down policies but about tapping into local know-how and resources to tackle the unique cultural, social, and sometimes economic factors that drive substance use. Forensic reports, for instance, often reveal links between abuse patterns and larger systemic issues – a reminder that grassroots prevention, rooted in community engagement, can be key.

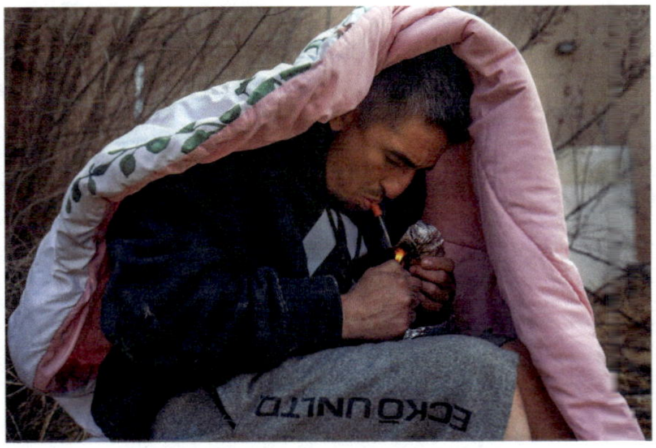

Figure 9.22. Substance abuse today requires a multifaceted approach that extends far beyond traditional institutional solutions.

Source: Sullivan, K. (2025). *Fentanyl in New Mexico Town*. Los Angeles Times.

Local programs, mainly shaped by community input, can offer education that truly fits the culture, identify those at risk early, and provide easy-to-access support services; all of these efforts help reduce both the frequency and severity of substance-related problems. In most cases, analyses of public health roles show that local agencies play a crucial part in putting these measures into action. Research focusing on indigenous populations, in most cases, confirms that flexible, community-driven models not only improve the detection and treatment of issues but also build long-term wellness and resilience against substance abuse (Service et al., 1997).

9.4.2. Role of Law Enforcement in Substance Abuse Prevention

Substance abuse is not solved by a single, neat fix—it actually requires a combination of strong legal rules and active public health efforts. Law enforcement, for example, is busy breaking up drug trafficking rings while keeping a close eye on regulations that restrict access to illegal substances. In places like Jammu & Kashmir, where drug challenges seem to escalate, the police often find themselves juggling shifting usage trends and even newer substances that throw a wrench in both spotting issues and taking action (Ullah et al., 2025).

Generally speaking, when officers, community voices, and health officials pool their efforts, early-warning measures get a boost, and harm reduction tactics slowly cut down narcotics demand. Out in spots such as Cibening village, local law enforcement and officials are right at the front line—using focused, sometimes even improvised, interventions to stop drugs from leaping past urban areas (Restu et al., 2024). Ultimately, combining forensic science with active police work becomes essential; this union not only strengthens legal proceedings by providing solid evidence, but it also paves the way for proactive, forward-thinking steps to effectively curb substance abuse.

9.4.3. Education and Awareness Campaigns

Tackling drug misuse is not solved by just relying on police work or forensic tests. In many cases, mixing different approaches seems to do the trick—education and awareness efforts really shape how people view and act about drugs. Sharing straightforward facts about the dangers and consequences of substance abuse can kickstart early prevention and even trim down the demand for illegal substances. At the same time, targeted outreach, aimed at specific groups or regions, often highlights unique patterns in drug use – you can even see these shifts over various time periods and places (Ambre et al., 2013). Some policymakers argue that it is essential to scrub any political bias from drug classifications so that the educational content stays rooted in solid science rather than political spin. All in all, broad education initiatives paired with evidence-based policies not only help forensic experts get a better grip on drug trends, but they also work toward lowering the overall harm drugs inflict on society (Figure 9.23).

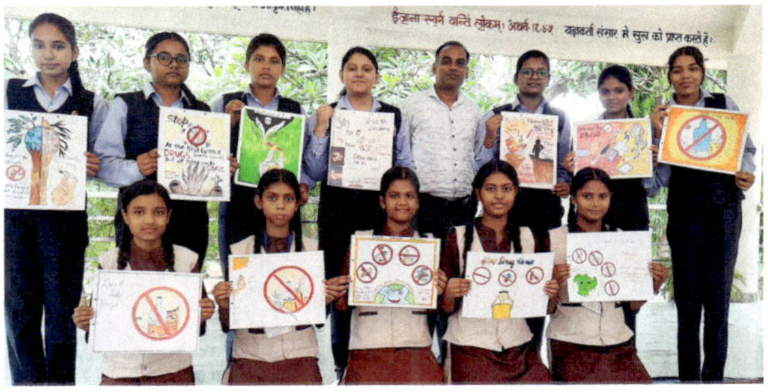

Figure 9.23. Education and awareness campaigns.

Source: DAV Nandraj Public School. (2024). *Poster Making Competition on Occasion of Drug Abuse Awareness Campaign.* https://i0.wp.com/davnrps.com/wp-content/uploads/2024/06/WhatsApp-Image-2024-06-19-at-2.39.53-PM.jpeg?fit=1280%2C631&ssl=1.

9.4.4. Screening and Early Intervention in Forensic Settings

Managing substance misuse in forensic groups calls for quick, on-the-spot detection and responses that take into account both physical needs and the messy social circumstances. New technology—such as wearable electrochemical sensors—is emerging, offering continuous, non-invasive checks on drug levels while helping to tailor treatment plans and monitor adherence in real-time (Teymourian et al., 2020). In most cases, these breakthroughs not only improve patient outcomes but also provide law enforcement with handy tools for on-site drug screening and support immediate clinical decisions. At the same time, community efforts remind us that partnerships across different sectors and integrating mental health services into forensic settings can significantly enhance early detection and prevention (Castillo et al., 2019). All in all, the blend of innovative devices with strong community ties generally shapes a more rounded screening and early intervention approach that, ultimately, cuts down on reoffending and improves rehabilitation success for those battling substance abuse.

9.4.5. Collaboration Between Forensic and Health Professionals

Substance abuse management in forensic settings is not just about following set rules—it really depends on a close collaboration of forensic and health experts, each bringing their own expertise to meet the complex needs. Forensic nurses, who are often on the front lines, require more than just basic training; they need specialized education to handle tasks such as preserving evidence and managing legal issues that arise in conjunction with emergency healthcare (Donaldson et al., 2020). In correctional environments, psychiatric care also shows just how crucial it is for everyone to team up, especially when you are dealing with challenges like juggling multiple medications and the chance for medication misuse in jail. Health professionals, in most cases, need to communicate openly with their forensic colleagues to develop safe, evidence-based medication plans—especially during those critical moments when care transitions from one stage to another (Ellis et al., 2024). All in all, this kind of teamwork not only helps improve outcomes for patients but also keeps legal processes and public safety on track, ensuring that every health decision takes into account the forensic aspect in a balanced and ethical manner (Figure 9.24).

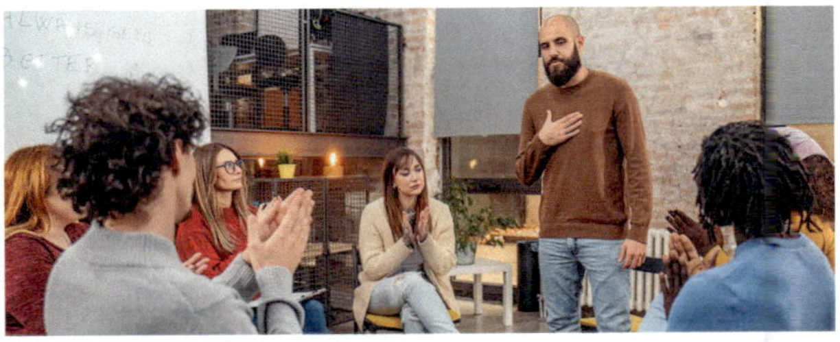

Figure 9.24. Collaboration between forensic and health professionals in substance abuse management.

Source: DAV Nandraj Public School. (2024). *Poster Making Competition on Occasion of Drug Abuse Awareness Campaign.* https://dpjh8al9zd3a4.cloudfront.net/sites/default/files/styles/rti_masthead_with_image_large_image/public/emerging-issues-hero-images/microsoftteams-image_75.png.webp?itok=e0BBrJ4v.

9.4.6. Policy Implications for Substance Abuse Prevention

Preventing substance misuse in forensic settings generally needs policies built on solid risk assessments and a mix of expertise from various fields. Tools like the Short-Term Assessment of Risk and Treatability (START) often demonstrate that identifying high-risk individuals while easing restrictions on those deemed lower risk can inform a more balanced intervention plan (Dickens et al., 2015). At the same time, policies must tackle the tangled challenges of assisting people with intellectual disabilities who also display offending behaviors—a situation that, in many cases, leads to unnecessarily extended institutional stays due to worries over community risk and legal limits (Alexander et al., 2015). Blending hospital care with community treatment options under a legal and ethical umbrella may open up more tailored, humane approaches that favor rehabilitation over strict containment. Therefore, preventive strategies should not only manage risk but also work on strengthening bonds between institutions and communities, nurture individualized care plans, and ensure that resource allocation truly reflects both public safety and the recovery needs of patients in forensic settings.

9.4.7. Effectiveness of Rehabilitation Programs

Rehabilitation programs in forensic settings matter a lot—they help address both substance misuse and criminal behavior (Figure 9.25). Treatments typically rely on evidence-based approaches, targeting risk factors while considering individual needs. Sometimes, studies into Buddhist practices like mindfulness and vipassana show that even small changes in how people view substance use, manage their emotions, and value themselves (especially among those incarcerated) can make a difference. Admittedly, while these studies have some methodological quirks, in most cases, they suggest that tailoring treatment to unique offender challenges may be effective (Griffiths et al., 2013). Juvenile rehabilitation, too, often focuses on assessing risks and meeting specific needs early on, which can help identify and address deep-seated behavioral and social issues before they escalate (Day et al., 2004). All in all, these mixed approaches suggest that successful rehabilitation is not one-size-fits-all—it usually needs a blend of solid planning and genuinely personalized care to curb both substance abuse and criminal conduct.

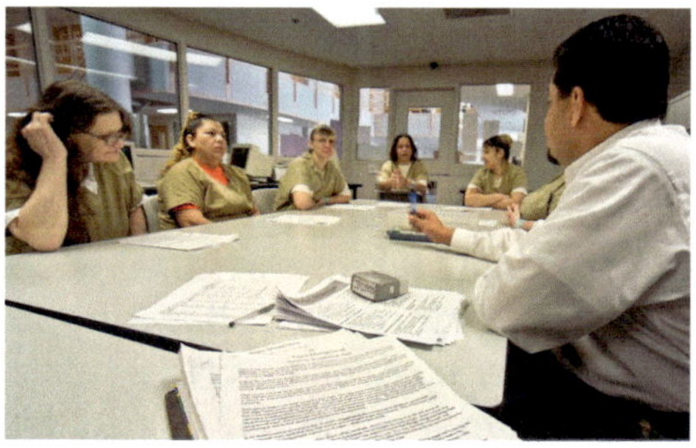

Figure 9.25. Rehabilitation programs in forensic settings matter a lot—they help address both substance misuse and criminal behavior.

Source: National Institute on Drug Abuse. (n.d.). *Women in Treatment Program.* https://nida.nih.gov/sites/default/files/images/women-in-treatment-program.jpg.

9.4.8. Challenges in Implementing Prevention Strategies

Substance abuse prevention hits a bunch of everyday hurdles—both system-wide problems and hands-on issues come into play, especially in forensic settings. Public health services are scattered across various organizations, with roles and accountability often left unclear, which makes it difficult for teams to synchronize and share resources effectively. Frontline care providers, like emergency nurses, usually lack that specific forensic know-how, so catching substance misuse early on before it turns into a legal or health crisis becomes even more challenging (Donaldson et al., 2020). When forensic training is not up to standard, evidence is mishandled and clinical advice falls short, which compromises prevention methods that rely on accurate identification and prompt action. The legal side of things is not any simpler either—a maze of complicated laws and shifting frameworks complicates the effort to create sound prevention policies. All in all, these varied obstacles suggest that better education, clearer roles, and a dose of cross-field teamwork are pretty key to tackling substance abuse issues in forensic contexts.

9.4.9. Case Studies of Successful Intervention Programs

Substance abuse intervention is becoming more crucial, especially when legal issues twist the recovery process in forensic settings. People are now mixing in advanced tools like AI to sort out treatment plans, flag relapse risks, and boost support structures – notably for folks often left out, like the homeless. Generally speaking, this technology shows a lot of promise by focusing on individual needs and enhancing service delivery, all while encouraging us to keep ethics and fair access at the forefront (Yusuff et al., 2025). At the same time, family-centered approaches, which may seem outdated, have also been gaining traction. Strengthening the family's role can really shift the balance, and programs like the Brief Intervention Program for addiction prevention in families have brought about fundamental changes in how households handle tension, build consensus, and develop coping strategies (Cabrera-Perona et al., 2025). In short, blending technology with a strong family focus seems to offer a well-rounded way to tackle substance abuse in these complicated forensic arenas.

Test Your Knowledge

1. How can mental health screening in schools and workplaces aid in early intervention?
2. What is the role of rehabilitation centers in preventing relapse?

SUMMARY

Substance abuse in forensic settings throws up a host of challenges that usually call for a mix of different viewpoints. Obtaining accurate analysis and effective intervention is not as simple as relying on a single method—often, combining insights from multiple fields works best. Think about how drug use leaves physical traces (for instance, subtle changes in oral health) that can serve as forensic hints, really helping to back up investigations and even legal processes. Then there's WBE, which, in most cases, provides a fresh and almost real-time way to track how substances are consumed across communities; this method offers a broader, population-level insight that traditional techniques might overlook. By blending hands-on clinical observations with solid forensic expertise and a few new technological advances, it becomes possible to enhance the overall trustworthiness of detecting and interpreting substance abuse. And when dental professionals, forensic scientists, and toxicologists team up—even if their approaches vary slightly—they not only sharpen diagnostic precision but also catch early signs of substance misuse, ultimately strengthening both our public health efforts and justice systems (Da Nğlıoğlu et al., 2024; Nilendu, 2024).

Tackling substance abuse in forensic cases is not a one-track deal; it twists into a puzzle that refuses simple answers. Substance issues often hang around psychological quirks like ADHD, with symptoms showing up in all sorts of ways among different ages and genders (Kooij et al., 2018; Young et al., 2020). Accurate diagnosis matters a lot—when you get it right, it pretty much sets the course for both intervention steps and the legal side of things, although, honestly, it can be a messy process. Forensic experts, in most cases, face challenges like gender biases and symptoms that hide or morph unexpectedly, which can trip up both treatment and rehabilitation. Looking at the whole picture over a person's lifetime becomes key since clinical signs and social factors tend to change over time. A smart approach usually involves combining medication, counseling, and social support in an overall, evidence-based plan aimed at reducing repeat issues and enhancing long-term recovery in forensic settings—even if the path forward sometimes seems a bit bumpy.

KEY TERMS FROM THIS CHAPTER

- Alcohol
- Cannabis
- Counseling
- Depression
- Mucosal lesions
- Opioids
- Stimulants
- Anxiety
- Cocaine
- Dental cavities
- Methamphetamine
- Nicotine
- Psychosis
- Stress

CRITICAL THINKING QUESTIONS

1. **Which of the following is commonly used to assess recent drug use in forensic toxicology?**
   a. Blood glucose level
   b. Hair follicle analysis
   c. Chest X-ray
   d. Electrocardiogram (ECG)
2. **What is a common symptom seen in forensic psychiatric evaluations of chronic alcohol abusers?**
   a. Hyperalertness
   b. Visual hallucinations
   c. Photophobia
   d. Manic episodes
3. **Substance abuse is most often associated with which type of criminal behavior?**
   a. White-collar crime
   b. Environmental crime
   c. Violent crime and theft
   d. Intellectual property crime
4. **Which of the following substances is classified as a central nervous system depressant?**
   a. Cocaine
   b. Methamphetamine
   c. Heroin
   d. LSD
5. **In forensic cases, which biological sample is considered best for detecting chronic substance abuse?**
   a. Saliva
   b. Blood
   c. Urine
   d. Hair

Short Answer Questions

1. How do specific substances like methamphetamine or cocaine contribute to aggressive or erratic behavior?
2. What role does substance abuse play in drug-facilitated crimes, such as sexual assault?
3. Can substance abuse be considered a mitigating factor in criminal responsibility?
4. How does the legal system differentiate between crimes committed under the influence vs. with intent?
5. What are common patterns of recidivism among offenders with substance use disorders?
6. How do drugs contribute to organized crime and gang-related violence?
7. How effective are rehabilitation programs in reducing drug-related criminal behavior?
8. How do socioeconomic factors influence the link between substance abuse and criminal acts?
9. What is the role of toxicological analysis in establishing drug use during a criminal offense?
10. How are juvenile offenders with substance abuse issues treated legally and medically?

Answers to Critical Thinking Questions

1. (b); 2. (b); 3. (c); 4. (c); 5. (d)

REFERENCES

1. Alexander, R., Chester, V., Devapriam, J., McCarthy, J., et al. (2015). "Why can't they be in the community?" A policy and practice analysis of transforming care for offenders with intellectual disability. *Advances in Mental Health and Intellectual Disabilities*. https://core.ac.uk/download/41990943.pdf (accessed on 9th May 2025).
2. Ali, H. S., & Mohammed, S. H. (2024). Impact of psychological abuse, physical abuse, sexual abuse, and neglect during childhood on criminal behavior among prisoners at forensic mental health department. *South Eastern European Journal of Public Health*. https://www.semanticscholar.org/paper/fd83aa7e295af141a1f8e9c0f7eb114eca0e826f (accessed on 9th May 2025).
3. Ambre, A., Banta-Green, C., Bellis, M., Boyd, R., Chiaia, A., Cohen, M., et al. (2013). Profiles of illicit drug use during annual key holiday and control periods in Australia: Wastewater analysis in an urban, a semi-rural and a vacation area. *Addiction*, *108*(3), 556–565. https://core.ac.uk/download/15154526.pdf (accessed on 9th May 2025).
4. Apodaca, R. F. D., Stevens, L., & Blake, B. T. (2015). When can forensic psychologists comment on the credibility of criminal defendants. *Journal of Arts and Humanities, 4*, 39–46. https://www.semanticscholar.org/paper/d7c848c5ed90cdf9e32fd85762c5791355295b1b (accessed on 9th May 2025).
5. Belenko, S., Dennis, M., Hiller, M., Mackin, J., Cain, C., Weiland, D., Estrada, B. D., et al. (2022). The impact of juvenile drug treatment courts on substance use, mental health, and recidivism: Results from a multisite experimental evaluation. *The Journal of Behavioral Health Services & Research, 49*, 436–455. https://www.semanticscholar.org/paper/6848b05e508864cad82d07c709aeaccf3ad21e2e (accessed on 9th May 2025).
6. Blonigen, D., Cucciare, M. A., Byrne, T., Shaffer, P. M., Giordano, B. L., Smith, J., Timko, C., et al. (2022). A randomized controlled trial of moral reconation therapy to reduce risk for criminal recidivism among justice-involved adults in mental health residential treatment. *Journal of Consulting and Clinical Psychology*. https://www.semanticscholar.org/paper/c2969f835853de11858fbf5c63cd2318a60c6a0f (accessed on 9th May 2025).
7. Brandt, S. D., King, L. A., & Evans-Brown, M., (2014). The new drug phenomenon. *Drug Testing and Analysis, 6*, 587–597. https://doi.org/10.1002/dta.1686.
8. Brennan, T., (2019). *Identification of Psychosocial Factors in the Development of Serial Killers in the United States*. https://core.ac.uk/download/235714179.pdf (accessed on 9th May 2025).
9. Cabrera-Perona, V., Moriano, J., Lloret-Irles, D., González-Galnares, I., & Ordoñez, A., (2025). Assessing the impact of a family-based intervention program on family dynamics: A pilot study in the context of indicated substance abuse prevention. *Family Process, 64*(1), e70024. https://www.semanticscholar.org/paper/1064420f2164053a6cb9a244fc0f28acbd03313b (accessed on 9th May 2025).
10. Castillo, E. G., Ijadi-Maghsoodi, R., Shadravan, S., Moore, E., Mensah, M. O., Docherty, M., Aguilera Nunez, M. G., et al. (2019). Community interventions to promote mental health and social equity. *Current Psychiatry Reports, 21*. https://doi.org/10.1007/s11920-019-1017-0 (accessed on 9th May 2025).
11. Dadashazar, N., (2017). *Offender Recidivism: A Quantitative Study of Motivational Risk Factors*

and Counseling. https://core.ac.uk/download/147838412.pdf (accessed on 9th May 2025).

12. Dağlıoğlu, N., Aydin, A. A., Güzel, E. Y., & Ertas, B. S. (2024). Wastewater analysis of illicit substances as a means of detecting substance abuse. *Emanate – Highlights from the Drug Abuse and Addiction Studies Sessions*. https://www.semanticscholar.org/paper/ca6a8be04ad64dc25810690ff02d9fb06fc8bb27 (accessed on 9th May 2025).
13. Davies, J., Godin, P., Heyman, B., Reynolds, J., et al. (2006). The problems of offenders with mental disorders: A plurality of perspectives within a single mental health care organization. *Social Science and Medicine, 63*(4). 1097–1108. https://core.ac.uk/download/57061.pdf (accessed on 9th May 2025).
14. Day, A., Howells, K., & Rickwood, D., (2004). *Current Trends in the Rehabilitation of Juvenile Offenders.* http://hdl.handle.net/10536/DRO/DU:30020615 (accessed on 9th May 2025).
15. Dickens, G. L., & O'Shea, L. E. (2015). Predictive validity of the START for unauthorized leave and substance abuse in a secure mental health setting: A pseudo-prospective cohort study. International *Journal of Nursing Studies*. https://core.ac.uk/download/228177184.pdf (accessed on 9th May 2025).
16. Dominik, P., Waßmer, M. P., Soyka, M., & Franke, A., (2022). Stimulant abuse as a coping strategy—Forensic and criminal consequences of stimulant abuse for neuroenhancement. *Frontiers in Public Health, 10*. https://www.semanticscholar.org/paper/f0f19228b2a65044decd4132123fd3198ca54358 (accessed on 9th May 2025).
17. Donaldson, A., (2020). *New Zealand Emergency Nurses' Knowledge About Forensic Science and Its Application to Practice*. https://core.ac.uk/download/322841929.pdf (accessed on 9th May 2025).
18. Ellis, K. A., Petreca, V., & Harding, S. L. (2024). *Psychiatric Deprescribing: Case Studies and Clinical Implications in Forensics: Psychiatric Deprescribing*. https://core.ac.uk/download/641909572.pdf (accessed on 9th May 2025).
19. Erickson, S. K. (2007). *Mind Over Morality*. https://core.ac.uk/download/236348372 pdf (accessed on 9th May 2025).
20. Focardi, M., Defraia, B., Bianchi, I., Gori, V., Romanelli, M., Ferretti, G., Nanni, L., et al. (2025). Sexual abuse or traffic accidental trauma? Analysis of a case. *La Clinica Terapeutica, 176*(Suppl 1(2)), 1–3. https://www.semanticscholar.org/paper/dcd6c61c8f35ceaf33411542cc96adc204417bba (accessed on 9th May 2025).
21. Forsythe, L., (2013). *Measuring Mental Health in Criminology Research: Lessons from the Drug Use Monitoring in Australia Program*. https://core.ac.uk/download/pdf/30677468.pdf (accessed on 9th May 2025).
22. Gillette, K. E. (2011). *The Psychological and Emotional Experiences of Pregnant and Postpartum Incarcerated Women*. https://core.ac.uk/download/231078138.pdf (accessed on 9th May 2025).
23. Giorgetti, A., & Boscolo-Berto, R., (2025). Investigating gender dynamics in forensic toxicology: The role of masculinity and femininity in alcohol and drug abuse. *Advances in Clinical and Experimental Medicine: Official Organ Wroclaw Medical University*. https://www.semanticscholar.org/paper/eeff63aa72a760c4a7bc9452f4693b19bfda779d (accessed on 9th May 2025).

24. Griffiths, M. D., Shonin, E., Slade, K., Van Gordon, W., et al. (2013). *Mindfulness and Other Buddhist-Derived Interventions in Correctional Settings: A Systematic Review.* https://core.ac.uk/download/30639514.pdf (accessed on 9th May 2025).

25. Hansen, A., Dahl, L., Olson, G., Thornton, D., Grung, B., & Thayer, J., (2015). A long-term fatty fish intervention improved executive function in inpatients with antisocial traits and a history of alcohol and drug abuse. *Scandinavian Journal of Psychology, 56*(5), 467–474. https://www.semanticscholar.org/paper/1040302e320f2664df91b75759888ab5d4f73676 (accessed on 9th May 2025).

26. Haslam, N., Holland, E., & Kuppens, P., (2011). Categories *versus* dimensions in personality and psychopathology: A quantitative review of taxometric research. *Psychological Medicine, 42*, 903–920. https://doi.org/10.1017/s0033291711001966.

27. Heinsvig, P. J., Holler, K. R., Lindholst, C., & Nielsen, T. S. (2024). Detection of substance use in clinical forensic cases: Urine analysis of victims and perpetrators. *Forensic Science, Medicine, and Pathology*. https://www.semanticscholar.org/paper/8c9609cfd57088b84a620229521f98ac0d33f999 (accessed on 9th May 2025).

28. Helverschou, S. B., Rasmussen, K., Steindal, K., Søndanaa, E., Nilsson, B., & Nøttestad, J. A. (2015). Offending profiles of individuals with autism spectrum disorder: A study of all individuals with autism spectrum disorder examined by the forensic psychiatric service in Norway between 2000 and 2010. *Autism, 19*, 850–858. https://doi.org/10.1177/1362361315584571 (accessed on 9th May 2025).

29. Idemudia, E., (2014). Journal abstracts from current research in the field of child and adolescent mental health. *Journal of Child & Adolescent Mental Health, 26*, 265–268. https://www.semanticscholar.org/paper/6e7f33b44d6e2c940fa05e716212d7982750129b (accessed on 9th May 2025).

30. Imrankhan, M., Cse, D. E. O., Vinayagar, M., Viji, M., Sathishkumar, R., Gnanaprakash, T., Karthik, R., et al. (2024). Blockchain-based digital forensic data for unbreakable trust and security. In *2024 International Conference on System, Computation, Automation and Networking (ICSCAN)*. https://www.semanticscholar.org/paper/778a539ea06fa596ad3da913ac068fd2cab5bab2 (accessed on 9th May 2025).

31. Indian Health Service, Office of Public Health Staff, Office of Planning, Evaluation and Research, & National Indian Justice Center. (1997). *Child Abuse and Neglect in American Indian/Alaska Native Communities and the Role of the Indian Health Service*. https://core.ac.uk/download/151599917.pdf (accessed on 9th May 2025).

32. Kooij, J. J. S., Bejerot, S., Blackwell, A. D., Caci, H., Casas, M., Carpentier, P. J., Edvinsson, D., et al. (2010). European consensus statement on diagnosis and treatment of adult ADHD: The European Network Adult ADHD. *BMC Psychiatry, 10*. https://doi.org/10.1186/1471-244x-10-67.

33. Kooij, J. J. S., Bijlenga, D., Salerno, L., Jaeschke, R., Bitter, I., Balázs, J., Thome, J., et al. (2018). Updated European consensus statement on diagnosis and treatment of adult ADHD. *European Psychiatry, 56*, 14–34. https://doi.org/10.1016/j.eurpsy.2018.11.001.

34. Kulnides, N., & Lorsirigool, A., (2023). The role of veterinarians in forensic science: A review. *World's Veterinary Journal*. https://www.semanticscholar.org/paper/4843c979b93d148eb5a5eb6a3d98f1b343dbba88 (accessed on 9th May 2025).

35. Kycler, M., Rzepczyk, S., Teżyk, A., & Żaba, C., (2024). Forensic aspects of salbutamol overdose – doping, abuse, and suicide. *European Journal of Clinical and Experimental Medicine*. https://www.semanticscholar.org/paper/5716c0e8e6820b0ff70e37e82bd439bc8cdc4cf5 (accessed on 9th May 2025).

36. Majd Al-Soleiti, Munipalli, B., Morris, A., & Rummans, T., (2024). COVID-19: Ramifications of the pandemic on mental health and substance abuse. *Frontiers in Public Health, 12*. https://www.semanticscholar.org/paper/55a26d6347f50345c0ef4050c08895bb9089acdd (accessed on 9th May 2025).

37. Manley, G. T., Gardner, A. J., Schneider, K., Guskiewicz, K. M., Bailes, J. E., Cantu, R. C., Castellani, R. J., et al. (2017). A systematic review of potential long-term effects of sport-related concussion. *British Journal of Sports Medicine, 51*, 969–977. https://doi.org/10.1136/bjsports-2017-097791.

38. Marshall, L., Kletzka, N., Kanitz, J., Opperman, K. J., & Rockwell, J., (2024). Effectiveness of dialectical behavior therapy (DBT) in a forensic psychiatric hospital. *The Journal of the American Academy of Psychiatry and the Law, 52*, 196–206. https://www.semanticscholar.org/paper/febf6eda419380ad023f8ccb6135248b49217f48 (accessed on 9th May 2025).

39. Mazurek, A., & Bolster, M., (2024). Trends in novel psychoactive substance use and the impact of Irish legislative efforts. *UCC Student Medical Journal*. https://www.semanticscholar.org/paper/6d3c70377325f92dfa12fbee976737b638f32515 (accessed on 9th May 2025).

40. McDaniel, S. H., Grus, C. L., Cubic, B., Hunter, C. L., Kearney, L. K., Schuman, C. C., Karel, M. J., et al. (2014). Competencies for psychology practice in primary care. *American Psychologist, 69*, 409–429. https://doi.org/10.1037/a0036072.

41. McPhail, E., Meggison, N., Yanson, I., Majumder, P., & Sales, C. P. (2022). Exploring the effects of early trauma in a forensic high secure population: Evaluating associations between adverse childhood experiences (ACEs) and diagnosis of antisocial personality disorder (ASPD). *BJPsych Open, 8*, S60. https://www.semanticscholar.org/paper/c8835d0c09a5a02b10e2170cc3abefb8313c179f (accessed on 9th May 2025).

42. Negro, F., Di Trana, A., & Marinelli, S., (2022). The effects of the COVID-19 pandemic on the use of performance-enhancing drugs. *PubMed, 92*, e2021401. https://doi.org/10.23750/abm.v92i6.12377.

43. Nilendu, D., (2024). Oral pathophysiology in substance abuse: A systematic analysis of recreational and medicinal drug impact with forensic correlations. *Clinical Pathology & Research Journal*. https://www.semanticscholar.org/paper/0be2b27e24f8c03648b6934d9bd02e20a2f2d2f4 (accessed on 9th May 2025).

44. Ojansuu, I., Latvala, A., Kautiainen, H., Forsman, J., Tiihonen, J., & Lähteenvuo, M., (2023). General and violent recidivism of former forensic psychiatric patients in Finland. *Frontiers in Psychiatry, 14*. https://www.semanticscholar.org/paper/c18e73d6879d999016f552200bb5dba8f4b14f86 (accessed on 9th May 2025).

45. Patel, H. A., Heshmati, K., Ryan, K. A., Yarbrough, K. L., Mixon, L. M., Williams, D. E., Kittner, S., et al. (2024). Abstract WP277: Stroke etiology in young adults with substance abuse. *Stroke*. https://www.semanticscholar.org/paper/8fdbd57cc7950d446c5b8012e7e426fe9d96f28e (accessed on 9th May 2025).

46. Quansah, L., & Sulley, Y. S. (2022). *Assessing the State of Forensic Support to Criminal Investigations in Ghana: A Case Study in the Greater Accra Region*. https://core.ac.uk/download/524766463.pdf (accessed on 9th May 2025).

47. Reed, G. M., Drescher, J., Krueger, R. B., Atalla, E., Cochran, S. D., First, M. B., Cohen-Kettenis, P. T., et al. (2016). Disorders related to sexuality and gender identity in the ICD-11: Revising the ICD-10 classification based on current scientific evidence, best clinical practices, and human rights considerations. *World Psychiatry, 15*, 205–221. https://doi.org/10.1002/wps.20354.

48. Restu, D. D., Daming, S., & Lestari, N., (2024). The participation of the Cibening Village apparatus, Pamijahan District, Bogor District in the prevention and manage of narcotics abuse. *Jurnal Mahasiswa Yustisi*. https://www.semanticscholar.org/paper/024cae340c1add82be5c69fef4d8b9c2168d3c54 (accessed on 9th May 2025).

49. Sacco, M. A., Gualtieri, S., Spiliopoulou, C., Tarallo, A. P., Verrina, M. C., & Aquila, I., (2025). The role of toxicology investigations in overdose deaths. *Cureus, 17*. https://www.semanticscholar.org/paper/df5a8e68f24a90c3e9c3e844b39ae54131c3e5b5 (accessed on 9th May 2025).

50. Saglam, I., Aslan, R., Akgür, S., & Kurtulmuş, Y., (2025). Abuse of gabapentinoids in individuals with substance use disorders. *Journal of Forensic Sciences*. https://www.semanticscholar.org/paper/287fcc72c4976fbe4851a335be4faca75e86c865 (accessed on 9th May 2025).

51. Salari, S., (2007). *Patterns of Intimate Partner Homicide Suicide in Later Life: Strategies for Prevention*. https://core.ac.uk/download/pdf/8289097.pdf (accessed on 9th May 2025).

52. Sami Ullah, & Khan, F., (2025). Emerging substance abuse trends in Jammu & Kashmir: Shifts, forensic challenges and strategic responses. *Forensic Research & Criminology International Journal*. https://www.semanticscholar.org/paper/3d49dcbc33779935bf855f5a4f765a365281b37a (accessed on 9th May 2025).

53. Sherman, E. M. S., Slick, D. J., & Iverson, G. L. (2020). Multidimensional malingering criteria for neuropsychological assessment: A 20-year update of the malingered neuropsychological dysfunction criteria. *Archives of Clinical Neuropsychology, 35*, 735–764. https://doi.org/10.1093/arclin/acaa019.

54 Sistrunk, C., (2022). *The Effect of Trauma on the Mental Health of Forensic Scientists*. https://core.ac.uk/download/539106877.pdf (accessed on 9th May 2025).

55 Stein, D. J., Szatmári, P., Gäebel, W., Berk, M., Vieta, E., Maj, M., De Vries, Y. A., et al. (2020). Mental, behavioral and neurodevelopmental disorders in the ICD-11: An international perspective on key changes and controversies. *BMC Medicine, 18*. https://doi.org/10.1186/s12916-020-1495-2.

56. Tambuzzi, S., Gentile, G., Primavera, R., Muccino, E., & Zoja, R., (2024). Pilot application of SEM/EDX analysis on suspected cigarette burns in a forensic autopsy case of child abuse. *The American Journal of Forensic Medicine and Pathology*. https://www.semanticscholar.org/paper/0077e72458c7926d55b329f5b67449133ed2373f (accessed on 9th May 2025).

57. Teicher, M. H., & Parigger, A., (2015). The 'Maltreatment and Abuse Chronology of Exposure' (MACE) scale for the retrospective assessment of abuse and neglect during development. *PLoS ONE, 10*, e0117423. https://doi.org/10.1371/journal.pone.0117423.

58. Tennessee. Department of Finance & Administration. (2015). *Office of Criminal Justice Programs Annual Report 2013–2014*. https://core.ac.uk/download/588405703.pdf (accessed on 9th May 2025).

59. Teymourian, H., Parrilla, M., Sempionatto, J. R., Montiel, N. F., Barfidokht, A., Van Echelpoel, R., De Wael, K., et al. (2020). Wearable electrochemical sensors for the monitoring and

screening of drugs. *ACS Sensors, 5*, 2679–2700. https://doi.org/10.1021/acssensors.0c01318.

60. The College at Brockport, College Senate. (2008). *Forensic Science Minor*. https://core.ac.uk/download/233580026.pdf (accessed on 9th May 2025).

61. Titova, N., (2024). Peculiarities of modern expert and forensic studies of "criminal drugs," abuse of which leads to addiction. *SSP Modern Pharmacy and Medicine*. https://www.semanticscholar.org/paper/1520c4d1c1b6b7251f9b035f30b64642263c6f2a (accessed on 9th May 2025).

62. Tseng, W., Matthews, D. B., & Elwyn, T., (2004). *Cultural Competence in Forensic Mental Health: A Guide for Psychiatrists, Psychologists, and Attorneys*. https://www.semanticscholar.org/paper/a1cf452a0c39a6a2c5b341c990d4c8eb6af387a9 (accessed on 9th May 2025).

63. Van Hosen, J., (2023). *Real-Time Surveillance of the Drug Epidemic: An Assessment and Comparative Visualization of Substance Abuse in the Commonwealth of Kentucky*. https://core.ac.uk/download/564070940.pdf (accessed on 9th May 2025).

64. Wootton, A., (2016). *AB 109 and Its Impact on Prison Overcrowding and Recidivism: A Policy Analysis*. https://core.ac.uk/download/70427284.pdf (accessed on 9th May 2025).

65. Young, S., Adamo, N., Ásgeirsdóttir, B. B., Branney, P., Beckett, M., Colley, W., Cubbin, S. et al. (2020). Females with ADHD: An expert consensus statement taking a lifespan approach providing guidance for the identification and treatment of attention-deficit/hyperactivity disorder in girls and women. *BMC Psychiatry, 20*. https://doi.org/10.1186/s12888-020-02707-9.

66. Yusuff, M., Akinsola, O., Olabiyi, M., Anioke, S. C., Agbasiere, C., & Kamwesiga, J., (2025). Leveraging AI in drug and substance abuse recovery: A systematic approach to reintegration and rehabilitation for the homeless. *Journal of Medicine and Health Research*. https://www.semanticscholar.org/paper/46d67a71b83b8f68aa0b556617dad4404200d186 (accessed on 9th May 2025).

67. Zhu, X., & Wang, X. P. (2014). Risk assessment of mentally ill patients are urgently needed in China. *Journal of Forensic Research, 5*, 1, 2. https://www.semanticscholar.org/paper/f2f64122d9c910ec6674853d3b4d477e1c6ffd04 (accessed on 9th May 2025).

DNA FINGERPRINTING AND BIOTECHNOLOGY

10

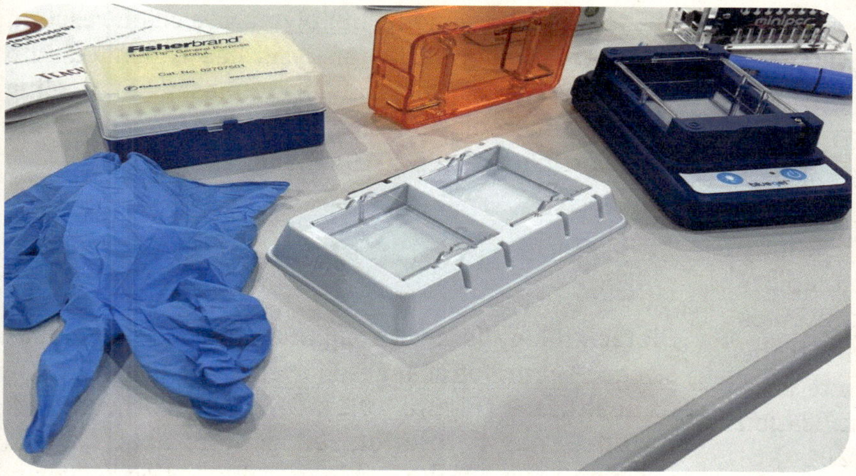

LEARNING OBJECTIVES

After studying this chapter, you will be able to:

1. Explain principles of DNA fingerprinting
2. Focus on applications of DNA fingerprinting
3. Know advances in biotechnology related to DNA fingerprinting
4. Identify the challenges and controversies associated with DNA fingerprinting and biotechnology.

Introduction

Over the last few decades, forensic science has taken a big leap by mixing in biotechnology, especially with DNA fingerprinting. Experts in molecular biology and chemistry join forces in ways that are not always by the book, making tests both faster and more accurate; in most cases, this shift has turned traditional investigations on their head. Forensic biotechnology continues to evolve, opening up unexpected paths in genomics and even microbial forensics, which reminds us that having advanced tools is nearly a necessity. DNA analysis, for example, clearly shows this change—it not only helps crack crimes but also influences farming practices. One study on cotton's genetic diversity revealed that fingerprinting could pinpoint key polymorphisms to fine-tune breeding strategies (Ijaz et al., 2024; Sunny et al., 2025). Ultimately, where DNA fingerprinting meets biotechnology, we find a major frontier that is reshaping both crime-solving and agriculture, leaving a profound mark on society.

Definition of DNA Fingerprinting

The genetic makeup of living things is surprisingly varied, and this complexity has prompted people to devise clever, sometimes unexpected methods for distinguishing one individual from another (Figure 10.1). Take DNA fingerprinting – it uses molecular techniques to identify those unique patterns in our DNA, allowing us to differentiate individuals with remarkable precision. This method shines particularly in forensics, where it helps establish identities in criminal cases or resolve paternity disputes. Additionally, it is crucial for identifying genetic differences among species, which enables the development of more effective conservation plans (Karp, 2000). Its use is not just confined to legal boxes; it extends into areas such as agriculture and medicine, where understanding genetic details can significantly enhance biotechnological advances. As our ability to detect even tiny genetic differences continues to improve, DNA fingerprinting remains at the heart of where biology and technology intersect, driving progress in both individual identification and biodiversity conservation (Khan, 2014).

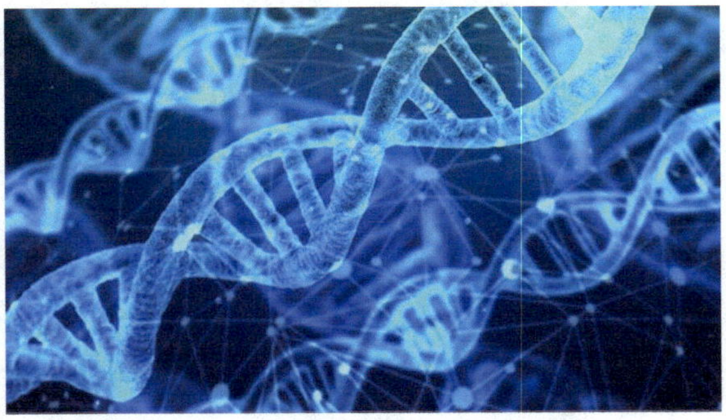

Figure 10.1. Genetic makeup.

Source: University of Connecticut. (2023). Genetic makeup of new strains of West Nile virus identified. *Technology Networks*.

Historical Background of DNA Fingerprinting

DNA fingerprinting marked a huge turning point where biology meets technology. In the past, forensic science employed broad profiling methods that often overlooked the fine details required in criminal cases. Back in the early 1980s, a technique called restriction fragment length polymorphism (RFLP) showed up unexpectedly, helping scientists compare DNA samples with much more accuracy—this really shifted how things were done. Sir Alec Jeffreys, daring in his approach, applied DNA profiling to legal matters in 1986, and his work, in most cases, ultimately transformed criminal justice. Today, with ongoing advancements in molecular techniques—including improvements in polymerase chain reaction (PCR) technology—DNA analysis has expanded into numerous areas, from solving crimes to unraveling complex microbial puzzles in diverse environments (Franco-Duarte et al., 2019; Shang et al., 2018).

Importance of Biotechnology in Modern Science

Biotechnology is now a significant force in modern science—it drives changes in everything from farming to healthcare (Figure 10.2). DNA fingerprinting, for instance, has revolutionized genetic analysis and forensic work, making it generally easier to verify identities and solve complex criminal cases. At the same time, this field advances methods for quickly identifying microbes—a significant benefit for both industrial and medical labs.

Traditional approaches still get the job done, but they tend to be slow and labor-intensive modern molecular techniques, however, significantly reduce that waiting time, which in most cases means that identifying microorganisms becomes easier and helps boost bioremediation efforts. Take microbial-assisted phytoremediation as an example—it tackles environmental contaminants like lead in a way that is both sustainable and good for keeping our food safe and our public health intact (Franco-Duarte et al., 2019; Kumar et al., 2020). All these twists and turns really highlight biotech's crucial role in solving some of today's toughest challenges.

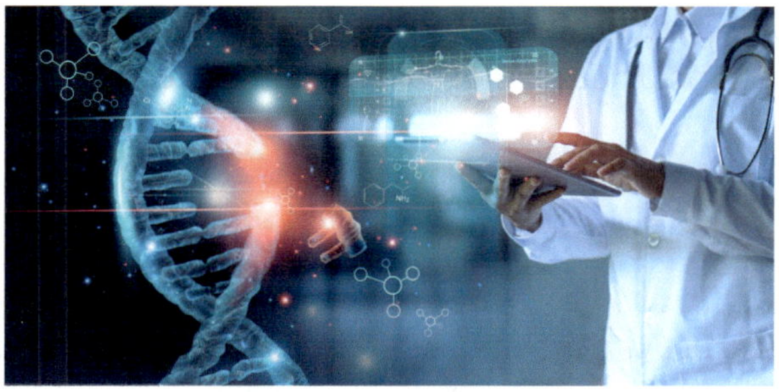

Figure 10.2. Biotechnology is now a major force in modern science—it drives changes in everything from farming to healthcare.

Source: JD Bots. (2023). *1-1.png.* https://i0.wp.com/jd-bots.com/wp-content/uploads/2023/08/1-1.png?fit=1000%2C488&ssl=1.

Overview of the Relationship Between DNA Fingerprinting and Biotechnology

DNA fingerprinting really changed biotechnology. It all started with noticing the tiny quirks in each person's DNA, so that we can pinpoint genetic material with a level of precision that was just not possible before; this has, in most cases, opened up a bunch of new applications across different fields. Take health informatics - a few recent studies (Ravi et al., 2016) show that combining DNA fingerprinting with machine learning yields robust predictive models and personalized medicine strategies that may significantly alter our expectations for healthcare. There has also been a growing buzz around newer methods, such as aqueous two-phase systems, which highlights the flexibility of biotech in extracting and analyzing genetic material. These methods, as noted, offer both economic and environmental benefits (Iqbal et al., 2016). All in all, the way DNA fingerprinting and biotechnology come together not only shines a light on fresh breakthroughs in genetics but also kicks off what looks like a whole new chapter in medicine, forensic science, and agriculture.

Key Terms and Concepts

DNA fingerprinting and biotechnology converge in ways that demonstrate how molecular biology has transformed numerous sectors. Scientists have begun to enhance identification methods by utilizing DNA profiling, which utilizes short tandem repeat (STR) markers to pinpoint genetic uniqueness, rather than relying on outdated techniques. This kind of pinpoint precision is evident in forensic science, agriculture, and medicine, underscoring, in most cases, the profound impact of biotech on society. Then there is the rise of methods like targeting induced local lesions in genomes (TILLING) which hints at clever new ways to tweak plant genomes for better traits (Brannigan, 2015). As technology continues to evolve, gaining a solid understanding of fundamentals like genetic markers and molecular approaches is crucial, enabling researchers to navigate the complex landscape of genetic details. All in all, mixing these ideas not only offers fresh depth to scientific inquiry but also charts a course for what the future holds in biotechnology and applied sciences (Brannigan, 2015).

Relevance to Current Scientific Research

Biotechnology has come a long way these days—DNA fingerprinting, for instance, really grabs your attention across a whole range of areas. It is not just a tool for solving crimes or settling paternity tests; in most cases, it is also used in medical diagnostics and exploring genetic oddities. When you apply this method to pharmaceutical research, it begins to identify genetic markers associated with various ailments, which generally advances the development of more targeted treatments. Recent research (Padhy et al., 2020) suggests that these techniques help unravel the complex network of biological systems, while opening doors to new treatment ideas. The way biotech and forensics overlap shows just how varied its use can be (Brannigan, 2015)—a reminder that the blending of different fields can really shift how we tackle both everyday and theoretical challenges. Ultimately, this combination of approaches underscores that DNA fingerprinting is not merely a niche practice; it is a transformative force deeply ingrained in modern science.

10.1. Principles of DNA Fingerprinting

Learning Outcome

1. Understand basic concepts of DNA structure
2. Identify techniques used in DNA extraction
3. Explain the polymerase chain reaction (PCR)
4. Focusing on gel electrophoresis methodology
5. Describe short tandem repeats (STR) analysis
6. Know the comparison of DNA samples
7. Learn the interpretation of DNA profiles
8. Discuss limitations of DNA fingerprinting
9. Focus on ethical considerations in DNA analysis

DNA fingerprinting has really changed things—not just forensics but also biotech, among other areas. Researchers now look at the unique twists in someone's DNA to sort out identity, check paternity, and even trace ancestry with striking precision. This breakthrough rests on markers like short tandem repeats (STRs) and single-nucleotide polymorphisms (SNPs); these elements, which differ widely between individuals, serve as the core of the method. At the same time, storing such a large amount of genetic data in biobanks raises significant ethical questions. Issues like privacy, consent, and the risks of misusing genetic info keep cropping up. Generally speaking, discussions often lean on values tied to the common good and respect for human rights (Stewart et al., 2006). And when you start thinking about how the loss of genetic diversity might affect key crops such as Coffea arabica, it becomes clear that pushing innovation must go hand-in-hand with solid ethical care (Aga et al., 2005).

10.1.1. Basic Concepts of DNA Structure

DNA's design is impressively complex—it is not just a neat instruction manual, but it also lays the groundwork for modern biotech and genetic studies. Picture two strands that run in opposite directions, twisting together in what we call a double helix; each is built from nucleotide sequences that hold our genetic code. Each nucleotide comes together with a phosphate blob, a deoxyribose sugar, and one of four nitrogenous bases—adenine, thymine, cytosine, or guanine. In most cases, adenine tends to pair with thymine, while cytosine pairs with guanine, a setup that helps cells copy their DNA accurately when they divide. This pattern is not confined to theory; it also plays a role in real-world tasks, such as DNA fingerprinting. By poking at the , slight differences in DNA sequences (using methods like inter-simple sequence repeat (ISSR) analysis), researchers can spot genetic diversity among species, which gives us deeper insights into gene preservation and sparks further biotechnological advances (D'Elia et al., 2024). All of this, in one way or another, underscores the groundbreaking promise of recombinant DNA technologies (Chokheli et al., 2022) (Figure 10.3).

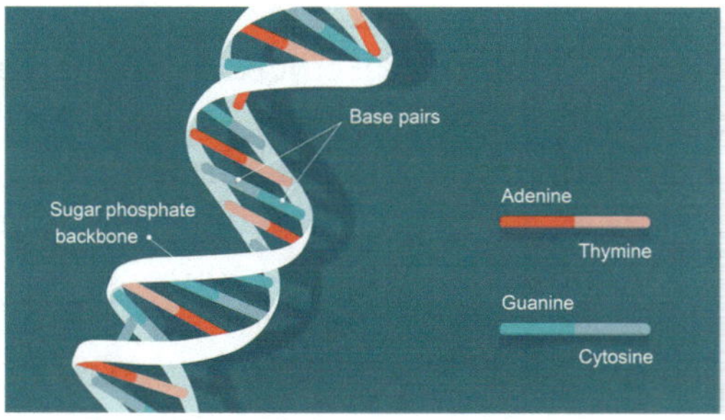

Figure 10.3. DNA structure.

Source: Healthline. (2019). *DNA Structure Illustration.* https://post.healthline.com/wp-content/uploads/2019/08/DNA-01.jpg.

10.1.2. Techniques Used in DNA Extraction

DNA extraction stands as one of the core routines in molecular biology—it is the step that initiates everything from DNA fingerprinting to biotech experiments. How you extract the DNA can significantly impact the outcome, often determining the purity and quantity of the sample you end up with. Take the old-school phenol-chloroform method, for instance; it is effective but comes with its fair share of risks and is pretty slow, which is not always ideal. Nowadays, many labs rely on ready-made kits that are celebrated for their speed and safety; however, recent studies suggest that in most cases, they may not always provide the genomic DNA quality required for certain projects (Ražná et al., 2015). Then there is the CTAB method—a technique that is been getting noticed for its knack at isolating DNA from tricky plant tissues with a decent yield and quality (Ribeiro et al., 2019). Generally speaking, as these techniques continue to evolve, the ongoing challenge appears to be establishing protocols that are more accessible and flexible, ensuring that areas such as forensic science and genetic research can consistently rely on robust outcomes—even if the details may shift slightly in practice.

10.1.3. Polymerase Chain Reaction (PCR)

PCR truly revolutionized molecular biology by providing a method to amplify specific bits of DNA with a speed and accuracy that still astounds many researchers. Many labs utilize it in applications such as DNA fingerprinting—essentially matching genetic profiles for forensic work and paternity tests—although its benefits also extend to other areas. In most cases, this versatility even paved the way for real-time PCR, a method that monitors the amplification process as it unfolds, making it a trusted tool for diagnostics when spotting pathogens like the emerging SARS-CoV-2 (Artika et al., 2022). Furthermore, advancements in PCR have led to innovative applications, such as DNA-based encryption, where the intricate patterns of DNA sequencing are cleverly utilized to enhance information security (Zhang et al., 2017). All in all, PCR continues to prove its worth across biotechnology and forensic science, continuously reaffirming its central role in modern research and diagnostic laboratories (Figure 10.4).

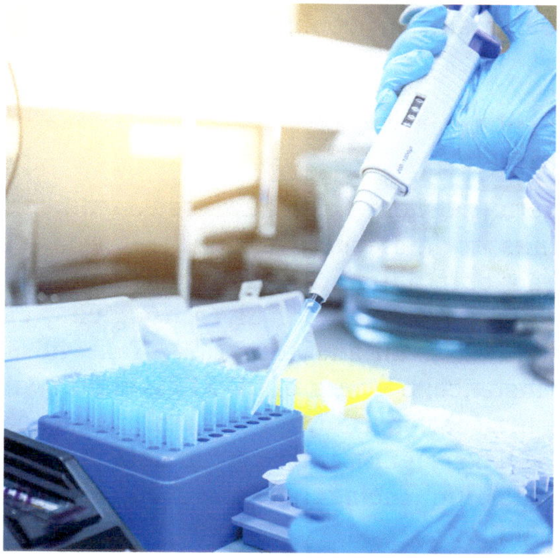

Figure 10.4. Polymerase chain reaction (PCR).

Source: AirClean Systems. (n.d.). *Polymerase Chain Reaction (PCR) - Hormones Application.* https://marvel-b1-cdn.bc0a.com/f00000000275470/aircleansystems.com/img/applicationnotes/Polymerase%20-Chain-Reaction-Hormones-Application.jpg.

10.1.4. Gel Electrophoresis Methodology

Microbial biotechnology has come a long way, and now gel electrophoresis is at the heart of DNA fingerprinting. This process helps separate nucleic acids simply by their size and charge. In many labs, this fundamental step enables researchers to visualize DNA fragments produced by PCR, a crucial step in pinpointing microbes. You may notice that the pattern on the gel provides clues about which organisms are present, and these patterns sometimes even hint at the specific microbial groups responsible for cleaning up pollutants (Sharma et al., 2022). Often, this technique's speed and ease outdo older methods, which is why so many modern studies lean on it (Franco-Duarte et al., 2019). At its core, gel electrophoresis provides a quick and clear glimpse into genetic diversity, demonstrating its value in both biotechnology research and environmental stewardship.

10.1.5. Short Tandem Repeats (STR) Analysis

Genetic markers have advanced significantly thanks to molecular techniques that now impact both animal and human genetics. STRs exhibit a great deal of diversity, giving each individual a unique signature. Take horses, for instance; a group of 17 STRs, endorsed by the International Society for Animal Genetics (ISAG), has significantly helped decipher horse lineages, influencing trade and even the creation of studbooks.

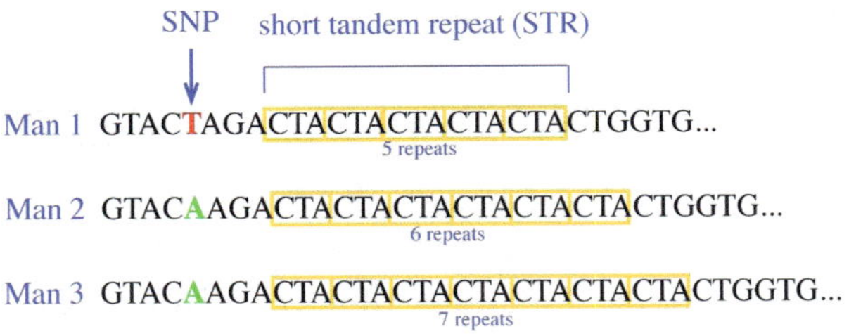

Figure 10.5. Short tandem repeats (STR) analysis.

Source: MoCoGenSo Webmaster. (2021). *Monterey County Genealogy Society*. https://mocogenso.wordpress.com/wp-content/uploads/2021/06/snp_str.jpg.

Researchers, tweaking these markers with multiplex PCR, have often found a cheaper route for genotyping, which in turn makes tracing pedigrees in horses more doable (Mustafa et al., 2024). In forensics, STR analysis is generally the go-to method for identifying people, as it can reliably build profiles from even low-concentration touch DNA samples—demonstrating its versatility and solid performance across different biotech applications (Saamia et al., 2024) (Figure 10.5).

10.1.6. Comparison of DNA Samples

Genetic research can reveal surprising life stories. Studying DNA allows scientists to catch glimpses of nature's diversity and see how species are interconnected in unexpected ways. Researchers often compare DNA samples using tools like ISSR and SRAP—methods that, in most cases, have pushed our grasp of genetic variation further. In fact, some studies suggest that ISSR markers exhibit more polymorphic regions than SRAP; the work on Chrysopogon aciculatus (Zhang et al., 2016) supports this finding quite well. Plus, RAPD has proven itself, capturing subtle phenotypic differences across various environments and hinting at its potential in biotech ventures. Overall, these approaches do more than map out genetic details; they also help advance conservation efforts and fuel new strategies in plant breeding.

10.1.7. Interpretation of DNA Profiles

Decoding genetic information opens up numerous opportunities, whether in forensic science or simply exploring biodiversity in nature (Figure 10.6). Interpreting DNA profiles—basically analyzing certain genetic markers to figure out everything from someone's identity to their evolutionary ties—is one of those key moves. For example, in most cases, DNA barcoding has proven useful for identifying and verifying plant species, which significantly enhances quality control in areas such as herbal medicine (Patel et al., 2024). Then there are tools such as Tn5 transposase, which by shuttling DNA around more efficiently, help us delve into genome-wide studies and unravel what makes genetic architectures tick (Penkov et al., 2023). These methods not only speed up identification but also steadily add to the broader effort of understanding genetic diversity and the messy interrelations among species. All in all, reading DNA profiles is pretty much the cornerstone for things ranging from crime-solving to ecological research, highlighting, generally speaking, its many roles in contemporary biotech.

Figure 10.6. Decoding genetic information opens up a lot of doors, whether you are talking about forensic science or just checking out biodiversity in nature.

Source: INTEGRA Biosciences. (n.d.). *DNA Fingerprinting.* https://www.integra-biosciences.com/sites/default/files/images/dna-fingerprinting-web.jpg.

10.1.8. Limitations of DNA Fingerprinting

DNA fingerprinting is now a widely used method in forensics and biomedical research, but it comes with challenges that often go unnoticed. A significant concern is that samples may become contaminated during collection or analysis – a mistake that can easily lead to errors and, in some cases, result in wrongful convictions. DNA does a great job at confirming identity, yet it is not foolproof; natural differences in our genetic makeup can sometimes result in confusing or even misleading conclusions about family ties. The complex interplay of genes with environmental factors—something we can clearly see when discussing the exposome—shows that our inherited traits are not entirely divorced from our surroundings (Wild, 2012). Meanwhile, new approaches, such as deep learning, are emerging to tackle data analysis in health informatics, although their true impact on making DNA fingerprinting more reliable is still under debate (Ravì et al., 2016). In most cases, acknowledging these issues is absolutely key to using DNA fingerprinting responsibly.

10.1.9. Ethical Considerations in DNA Analysis

Biotechnology is advancing rapidly, particularly with our new methods for decoding DNA. This rapid progress brings along a range of ethical puzzles—issues such as consent, privacy, and even potential discrimination—that demand a closer examination. In many cases, when companies introduce workplace genetic testing, it raises a range of privacy issues; for instance, your genetic traits might be used in ways you never intended (see policy chatter, Muthuchidambaram, 1993). At the same time, while our ability to read the genetic code is only getting stronger, it is not clear that we are taking the time to think about the bigger picture. Generally speaking, the idea that "if we can, we should" can sometimes backfire, hinting that unchecked scientific progress might have unexpected downsides. This calls for ongoing, open-ended discussions between scientists, lawmakers, and ethicists—something that echoes the warnings from past biotechnological breakthroughs (Buchholz et al., 2011).

Test Your Knowledge

1. What is DNA fingerprinting?
2. What are short tandem repeats (STRs) and how are they used in DNA profiling?

10.2. Applications of DNA Fingerprinting

Learning Outcome

1. Understand forensic science and criminal investigations
2. Explain paternity testing and family relationships
3. Learn the identification of missing persons
4. Focus on wildlife conservation and poaching preventio
5. Describe medical diagnostics and genetic disorders
6. Focus on agricultural biotechnology and crop improvement
7. Know ancestry and genealogical research
8. Learn biobanking and preservation of genetic material
9. Describe the role in personalized medicine

DNA fingerprinting is not just a tool for solving crimes—it is become something that touches a lot of fields, from farming to medicine. In agriculture, for example, this method helps reveal the genetic variety among crops, which is pretty essential when breeders try to boost yields or ward off diseases. It even accelerates the process of introducing improved plant types into use and facilitates the incorporation of key genes into them, thereby advancing sustainable farming (Tchatchoua et al., 2016).

In the medical world, DNA fingerprinting has significantly transformed how criminal cases are investigated, while also enhancing our ability to detect genetic disorders and infections (Diwakar et al., 2012). Taken all together, it demonstrates that DNA fingerprinting not only meets immediate needs but also lays the groundwork for longer-term breakthroughs in biotechnology, paving the way for innovative solutions in diverse areas.

10.2.1. Forensic Science and Criminal Investigations

Forensic science and law often intersect in ways that raise significant ethical questions—DNA profiling in criminal cases is a prime example. DNA techniques are continually evolving, transforming raw biological evidence into usable information for courts, and this change inevitably raises complex civil rights issues. It is curious how personal biological materials, once strictly private, enter the public arena; this really shows the push and pull between individual privacy and the power of the state. Different practices in forensic genetics (*see* Toom et al., 2012) sometimes lead to varied interpretations of what civil rights mean, which raises questions about whether our traditional legal standards require a second look. Take Singapore's method, for example; safety is prioritized over personal liberty, a sign that the approach may lean toward authoritarian ideas (Toom et al., 2014). All in all, forensic science is not just about lab results—it weds itself with legal principles and can reshape societal norms, clearly signaling that careful oversight is necessary (Figure 10.7).

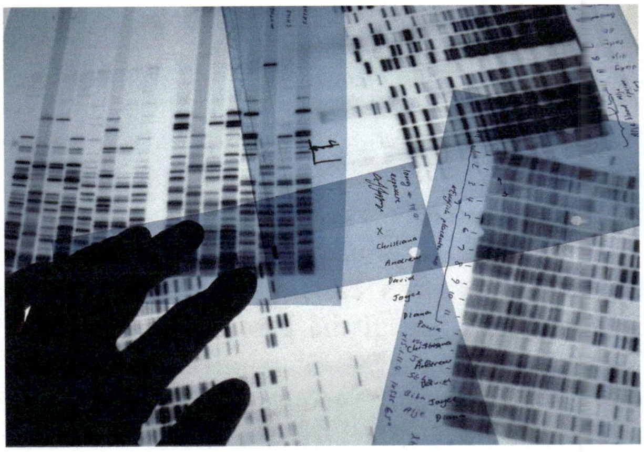

Figure 10.7. DNA profiling in criminal cases.

Source: National Library of Medicine. (n.d.). *Illustration of Forensic Science Techniques.* https://www.nlm.nih.gov/exhibition/visibleproofs/media/detailed/iii_d_220.jpg

10.2.2. Paternity Testing and Family Relationships

DNA fingerprinting really flipped the script on paternity testing, shaking up the way we see family ties—sometimes in ways that catch you off guard. Instead of a formal, step-by-step procedure, it delves straight into our genetic code to reveal who is actually related, with a precision that is quite uncommon. It is not merely about determining parentage; by revealing genetic links, this method often uncovers profound truths that can challenge long-held family roles. Take Alec Jeffreys, for example. His early work—spotting those curious hypervariable repeats in our DNA—did not just open doors for paternity checks; it paved the way to peek into broader family connections, confirming bonds or, at times, revealing discrepancies (Chambers et al., 2014). Additionally, there are observational studies, such as one conducted with the Madurese, which found that using sibling indices based on shared alleles can reliably indicate familial ties, supported by solid statistical evidence (Nzilibili et al., 2021). All in all, DNA fingerprinting is not just a lab tool; it is a game-changer in how we confirm and even question what we think of as family, nudging us to reconsider personal identities and social connections in unexpected ways.

10.2.3. Identification of Missing Persons

Identifying missing persons is not always a straightforward process, especially when traditional methods are insufficient (Figure 10.8). Catastrophic events, such as plane crashes or severe natural disasters, tend to wipe out standard biometric clues—think fingerprints and the like—making it difficult to use conventional techniques. Forensic dentistry, with its focus on sturdy dental records and bones, now steps in as a promising alternative for piecing together victim identities (Yazdanian et al., 2022). At the same time, breakthroughs in biotechnology—such as nanoparticle-based methods—tweak biological recognition so that it works faster and with greater precision, even in the most challenging scenarios (Akhter et al., 2021). All in all, combining DNA fingerprinting with these innovative biotech approaches generally points to a significantly improved method for tracking down missing individuals.

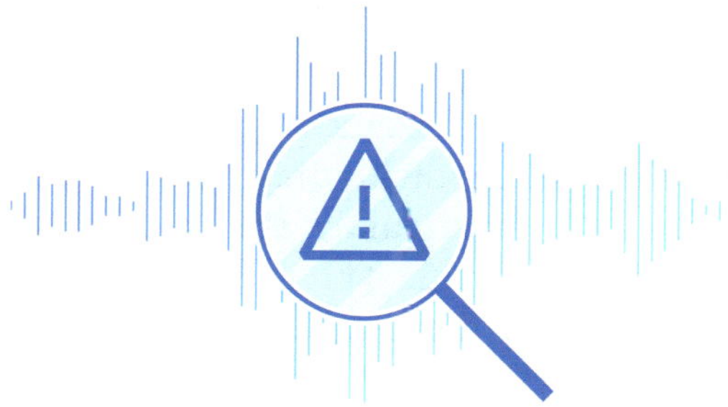

Figure 10.8. Identifying missing persons.

Source: Cloudflare. (2023). *Disruption.* https://blog.cloudflare.com/content/images/2023/01/Disruption.png.

10.2.4. Wildlife Conservation and Poaching Prevention

Technology and nature join forces in surprising ways to address urgent issues such as poaching and the protection of wild creatures. DNA fingerprinting—a cutting-edge breakthrough in biotechnology—has become a key tool for tracking animals taken by poachers, providing a significant boost to on-the-ground conservation efforts. When conservation teams examine genetic material, they can often trace confiscated items—such as ivory or parts from endangered species—back to their origins, which in most cases makes the legal case against poachers that much stronger. The sharp precision of these DNA methods lets experts keep a closer watch on biodiversity; this means decisions about habitat protection and reviving struggling species can be more informed, generally speaking. You might say the benefits extend beyond immediate fixes;

advances in understanding how DNA carries traits add an extra layer to the broader story of life and our responsibility to protect it from human-made harm (Sulley et al., 2022). All in all, using biotechnology is not just a handy move for saving wildlife—it is a fundamental piece in the broader puzzle of achieving sustainable development.

10.2.5. Medical Diagnostics and Genetic Disorders

Biotechnology breakthroughs have revolutionized medical diagnostics—genetic disorders, in particular, are undergoing a significant overhaul (Figure 10.9). Rather than sticking to the old step-by-step routine, tools like next-generation sequencing (NGS) now enable researchers to dive straight into identifying genetic variations associated with a host of diseases. NGS, by scanning millions of DNA strands simultaneously, reveals the intricate details of genetic issues in a way that was previously inaccessible (Satam et al., 2023).

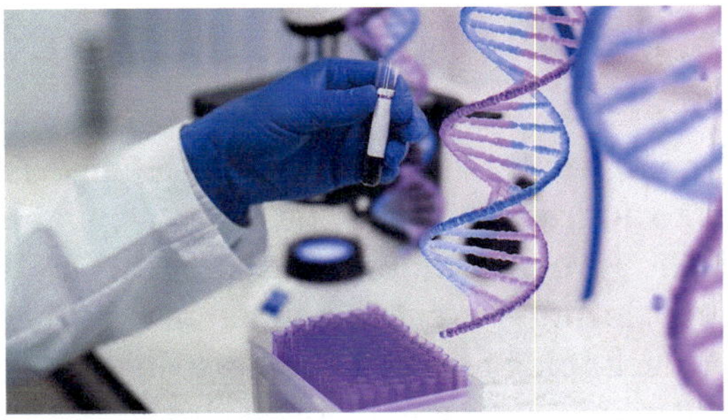

Figure 10.9. Biotechnology breakthroughs have flipped the script on medical diagnostics—genetic disorders, in particular, are seeing a major overhaul.

Source: BioSpectrum India. (n.d.). *Gene Sequencing Technology.* https://www.biospectrumindia.com/uploads/articles/gene-25304.jpg.

On a similar note, metabolomics has emerged as a key player, showing that these tiny metabolites act as informal messengers, nudging various bodily functions and even shifting disease pathways. This expanding cache of knowledge not only hones the precision of condition diagnosis but also sparks the creation of personalized therapies crafted to match individual genetic profiles (Wishart, 2019). When you combine these innovative methods, the result is a promising preview of how diagnostics and treatment strategies for genetic disorders might be revolutionized.

10.2.6. Agricultural Biotechnology and Crop Improvement

Climate challenges and food shortages are hitting us hard these days, making inventive agricultural biotech a real must-have. DNA fingerprinting is not just a fancy term—it is a hands-on approach to identifying and modifying crop traits to enhance their ability to withstand pests, unpredictable weather, and other environmental stresses. With erratic rainfall and hotter days becoming the norm, biotechnological methods are earning their keep as we aim for crops that can withstand these shocks. Researchers are even getting curious about plant and microbe teamwork; for instance, using plant growth-promoting rhizobacteria (PGPR) has shown some promise in boosting growth when drought strikes (Niu et al., 2018). This mix of innovative, down-to-earth approaches not only helps keep our farms productive but also works in step with practices that preserve our natural ecosystems amid persistent climate crisis issues (Raza et al., 2019).

10.2.7. Ancestry and Genealogical Research

DNA fingerprinting has come a long way and now plays a massive role for anyone curious about their family history (Figure 10.10). What was once used mainly in forensic labs has, over time, made its way into home genealogy, allowing people to trace their lineage with a level of precision that is unprecedented. Generally speaking, when someone takes a genetic test, they often uncover a mix of migration stories and identity shifts that mirror larger social trends. This process can sometimes feel as winding as it is fascinating. Commercializing these tests has opened the door to genetic insights for many, yet it also stirs debates about the ethical handling of our personal data, especially regarding who collects it and how it is used. Looking back at historical migration, it is interesting to see DNA profiling acting both as a connector between people and, in some cases, as a sort of regulatory mechanism, linking our personal identity to broader political narratives (Bivins, 2022). All in all, ancestry research now tends to blend a personal look into family history with the steady march of scientific progress (Xu et al., 2022).

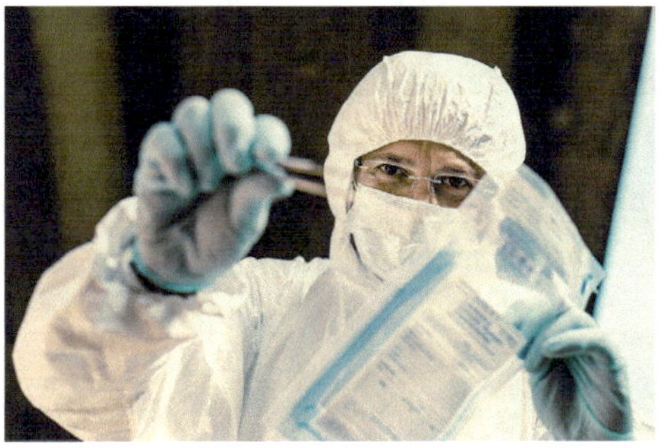

Figure 10.10. DNA fingerprinting has come a long way and now plays a huge role for anyone curious about their family history.

Source: INTEGRA Biosciences. (n.d.). *Sample Collection Process.* https://www.integra-biosciences.com/sites/default/files/styles/large/public/images/sample-collection-web.jpg?itok=l02Q8YF_.

10.2.8. Biobanking and Preservation of Genetic Material

Preserving genetic material is becoming a vital cornerstone in modern biotech—biobanking, really, is at its core. Methods for collecting and freezing samples, such as bird semen, have come a long way; these techniques now aim to protect our biodiversity and sometimes even counteract species decline. Bezerra et al. (2023) even highlight several approaches under research that try to boost post-thaw performance, though issues such as contamination and low sample volumes still rear their head. DNA fingerprinting, on the other hand, has significantly reshaped forensic science by refining identification methods; it is now crucial for roles in forensics and paternity testing alike. It is also intriguing how teeth can retain DNA despite degradation—as mentioned in Qadri et al. (2023)—which hints at their special role in forensic odontology. All in all, biobanking is not just a conservation tool; it also lays the groundwork for genetic and forensic research, which in many cases brings broad benefits to society.

10.2.9. Role in Personalized Medicine

Biotechnology has really reshaped both medical research and the way we approach personal healthcare (Figure 10.11). Using methods like DNA fingerprinting, doctors can now match treatments to a person's unique genetic blueprint, which generally boosts therapy success while reducing unwanted side effects. This targeted approach helps them identify key biomarkers—sometimes even uncovering new ways to manage diseases more effectively. For example, recent attention has been given to tiny particles in human breast milk called exosomes; these little carriers, packed with vital bioactive molecules, seem to offer clues that can help shape personalized nutrition plans for infants (Rudloff et al., 2024). Several studies, in most cases, indicate that combining genomics with proteomics offers new insights into disease mechanisms, ultimately leading to healthcare solutions tailored to each patient's genetic profile (Safeena et al., 2013). All in all, the combination of DNA fingerprinting and modern biotechnology serves as a key driver in advancing personalized medicine.

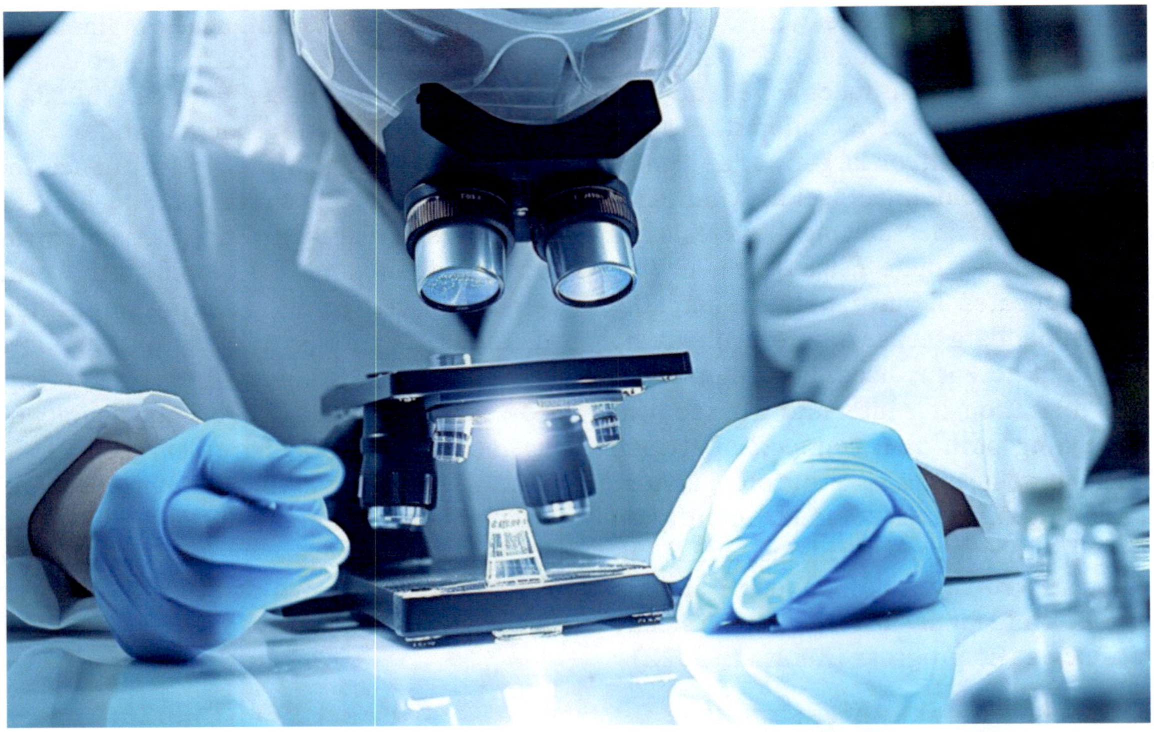

Figure 10.11. Biotechnology has really reshaped both medical research and the way we approach personal healthcare.

Source: INTEGRA Biosciences. (n.d.). *Sample Collection Process.* https://tcgibp.com/wp-content/uploads/2024/01/01-1200x800px-image-resizing.jpg.

Test Your Knowledge

1. How is DNA fingerprinting used to identify suspects in criminal cases?
2. In what ways does DNA help in linking a suspect to a crime scene?

10.3. Advances in Biotechnology Related to DNA Fingerprinting

Learning Outcome

1. Explain next-generation sequencing technologies
2. Understand CRISPR and gene editing applications
3 Discuss bioinformatics and data analysis
4 Focus on synthetic biology and its implication
5 Learn the development of new biomarkers
6 Describe the integration of AI in genetic research
7. Understand advances in cloning techniques
8. Know the ethical implications of biotechnological advancements
8. Escribe future trends in biotechnology

Genomic research has taken a wild turn over the years—driven mainly through leaps in NGS and some fresh biopharma methods. NGS now enables scientists to rapidly analyze massive amounts of DNA, allowing them to identify genetic variations that are crucial in fields such as forensic work and family tree research, which is at the core of DNA fingerprinting. At the same time, biotechnology is mixing with innovative drug techniques. Before you know it, the biosimilar scene pops up, offering treatments that keep costs down without skimping on strict quality checks based on key characteristics. This mashup of faster sequencing and evolving pharmaceutical strategies marks a significant shift in how DNA fingerprinting is utilized in both medical testing and crime labs. In most cases, these ongoing upgrades not only deepen our understanding of genetic material but also expand the practical applications of DNA fingerprinting across various fields, underscoring its significant impact on modern science and society (Nupur et al., 2022; Satam et al., 2023).

10.3.1. Next-Generation Sequencing (NGS) Technologies

Genomic data is becoming increasingly complex these days, so scientists are being pushed to find more efficient ways to work with it—especially when it comes to DNA fingerprinting and other biotech projects (Figure 10.12). NGS has revolutionized genetic research by enabling researchers to read entire genomes at lightning speed, which in most cases results in a vast amount of data that is becoming indispensable for personalized medicine. It is not just about moving fast; these improvements also help identify subtle structural changes and copy number differences that play a crucial role in understanding genetic diseases, ultimately enhancing our ability to conduct thorough genomic profiling (Pellegrini et al., 2016). There are also new systems emerging that utilize resistive pulse sensing technology to examine single molecules without the need for added labels, providing unexpected insights into the fine details of molecular interactions (Harrer et al., 2015). All in all, NGS has become a cornerstone in modern biotech, opening up fresh paths for breakthroughs in both diagnostics and therapies.

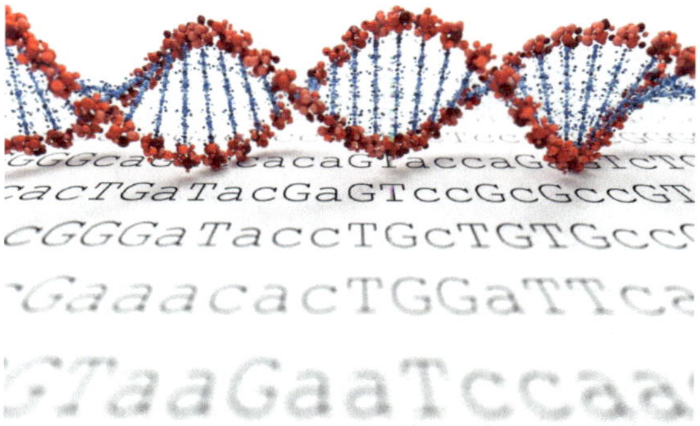

Figure 10.12. Next-generation sequencing (NGS).

Source: Novogene. (2021). *Next Generation Sequencing (NGS): A Beginner's Guide.*

10.3.2. CRISPR and Gene Editing Applications

Biotechnology has been advancing at a rapid pace, resulting in a range of powerful tools that significantly alter our understanding of gene editing. One striking example is CRISPR (that is short for Clustered Regularly Interspaced Short Palindromic Repeats); it is famous for being sharp and flexible when it comes to editing genes, so researchers can make concrete changes at the genome level. This tech shows a lot of promise—in biomedical research, it might help tackle genetic disorders, and in farming, it is already playing a role in creating crops that fight off disease and even boost yields. Then there is the cool work with smart nanoparticles (*as noted in* Sun et al., 2023), which seem to mix with CRISPR to deliver drugs in a very targeted way for cancer treatment. At the same time, strategies mentioned in Singh et al. (2020) suggest that gene editing could accelerate the improvement of crop species, helping to meet global food needs while nudging us toward sustainability. All in all, these developments, in many cases, highlight the transformative potential of CRISPR across various fields.

10.3.3. Bioinformatics and Data Analysis

Computational tools have significantly transformed the way we approach biology—DNA fingerprinting and biotechnology, for instance, are no longer the same as they used to be. New bioinformatics methods let us dive into massive datasets from NGS, making it possible to spot genetic quirks like copy number variations (CNVs) and tandem repeats. Usually, these markers tend to align with key bodily functions or diseases, which makes precise data analysis crucial in clinical labs. At the same time, advanced algorithms that search for patterns in genomic sequences are playing a significant role, as researchers attempt (in many cases) to unravel those complex genetic relationships that could shed light on how diseases work or hint at new treatment strategies. There is also some buzz about these breakthroughs opening doors for fresh forensic DNA analysis applications, as seen in recent studies (Anastassopoulos, 2006; Pellegrini et al., 2016). All in all, bioinformatics stands out as the cornerstone in transforming raw genomic data into insights that can have a real-world impact (Figure 10.13).

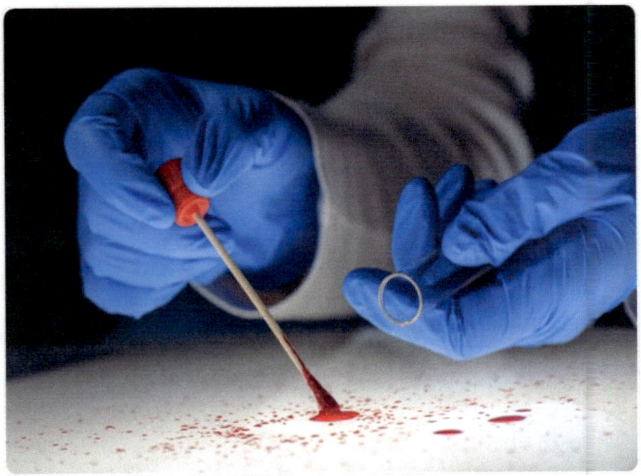

Figure 10.13. Bioinformatics and data analysis in forensics.

Source: Bits and Splits. (2016). *Forensic Technician Taking DNA Sample from Blood Stain at Crime Scene.* https://d1g9yur4m4naub.cloudfront.net/image-handler/picture/2020/7/shutterstock_521221120.jpg.

10.3.4. Synthetic Biology and Its Implications

Synthetic biology is shaking up biotech in ways we had not expected—it is changing how we view genetic manipulation and applying it everywhere. We can now mix and match biological parts and systems like assembling a custom kit, opening new doors in disease diagnosis and treatment. Recent studies have even shown that relying on specific biomarkers can, in most cases, significantly enhance disease management (Ahmad et al., 2023). Different disciplines, working side by side, have come up with innovative solutions that may well change everyday life and healthcare routines (Betz et al., 2023). As this field grows, we are not only seeing technical upgrades; there are also pressing ethical issues to consider, like genetic privacy, concerns about biosafety, and even the risk of bioterrorism. As synthetic biology becomes increasingly intertwined with techniques like DNA fingerprinting, it highlights a pressing need for robust, carefully considered rules that safeguard both individual rights and the broader public interest.

10.3.5. Development of New Biomarkers

Innovative technology in molecular genetics has significantly impacted biotech, particularly in the development of new biomarkers (Figure 10.14). These biomarkers, you see, end up being central in many areas—take plant protection for example, where both DNA and RNA have now become unexpected heroes in insecticides.

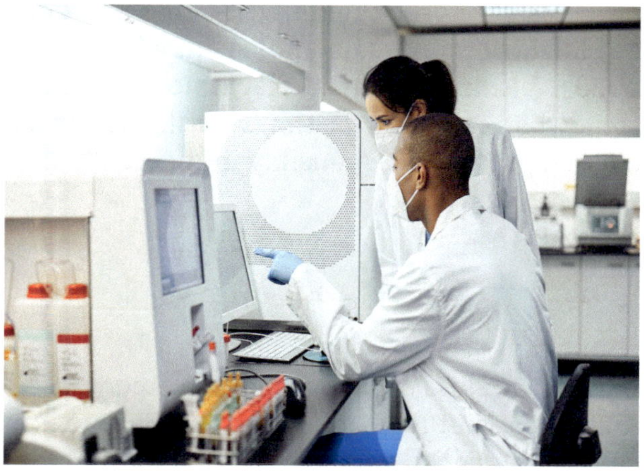

Figure 10.14. Innovative technology in molecular genetics has significantly impacted biotech, particularly in the development of new biomarkers.

Source: Smile. (2021). *Nurse with Patient.*

They boost pest control through techniques like RNA interference and even the antisense DNA approach. In most cases, these biomolecular methods appear to be paving the way for a rapidly evolving landscape in agricultural biotechnology, potentially offering solutions that are not only highly specific but also more environmentally friendly (Oberemok et al., 2024). Recent advances in DNA fingerprinting have also helped us gain a better understanding of genetic diversity in plant species. Studies on Elaeagnus angustifolia germplasm, for instance, have provided clearer insights into its genetic background and even laid the groundwork for breeding standout varieties. At the same time, they remind us—quite subtly—that DNA-based techniques serve multiple roles in our ecological and economic landscapes (Wang et al., 2024).

10.3.6. Integration of AI in Genetic Research

Artificial intelligence and genetic research are merging in ways that have led to significant breakthroughs in DNA fingerprinting and biotechnology. Generally speaking, deep learning systems now delve into vast genomic datasets—data produced by NGS—that help us unravel how genetic variations are linked to various diseases. It is not just about identifying disease markers; this mix of technology also makes crafting personalized medicine a smoother process. Interestingly, AI-powered smart nanoparticles have emerged as promising platforms for targeted drug delivery, capable of responding to specific biological cues, as indicated by recent studies (Sun et al., 2023). When you blend traditional biotech strategies with new AI innovations, researchers are often better-equipped to tackle challenges in oncology and genetic disorders, leading to more nuanced analyses and genuinely inventive solutions tailored to individual needs (Satam et al., 2023). All in all, this fusion is poised to reshape both research methods and therapeutic approaches in genetics completely.

10.3.7. Advances in Cloning Techniques

Genetic research is in full flux these days—tech breakthroughs are shaking up cloning in ways we never expected. NGS now lets scientists look into DNA with an almost revolutionary intensity. Instead of the old, clunky methods, researchers can spot tiny differences in the genetic blueprint, helping them pick traits for clones, which generally makes agricultural biotech and biodiversity efforts work a bit smoother. NGS is not just about zooming in on genomes; it is a tool that enables experts to combine classic cloning with fresh insights into genetic variation. Meanwhile, new tricks for tweaking the microbiome are broadening cloning's reach in the animal sector—poultry included. Take sustainable poultry production as an example: knowing more about the gut microbiota, that critical sidekick for nutrient absorption and immune health, really makes a difference. As progress continues to unfold in unexpected ways, blending cloning techniques with refined genetic knowledge appears poised to open up a range of new research avenues and practical biotech applications (Shang et al., 2018; Satam et al., 2023) (Figure 10.15).

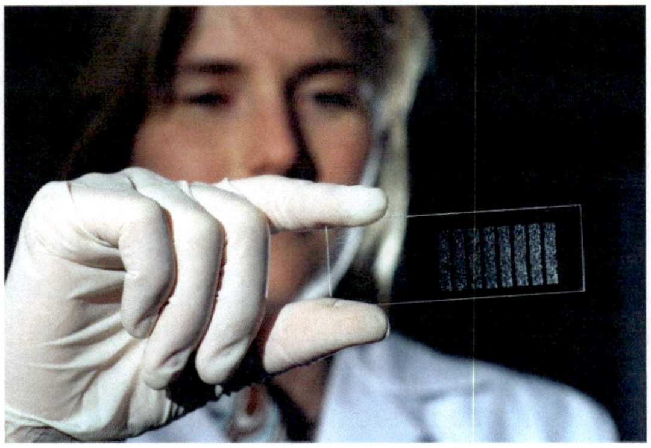

Figure 10.15. Genetic research.

Source: Encyclopaedia Britannica. (n.d.). *Microarray DNA Slide.* https://cdn.britannica.com/40/262340-050-9FBD8959/Microarray-DNA-slide-genetics.jpg.

10.3.8. Ethical Implications of Biotechnological Advancements

Biotechnological breakthroughs are advancing rapidly these days – DNA fingerprinting stands as just one vivid example, sparking ethical debates that we cannot ignore. Every new advance offer sweeping potential to transform various industries, but it also comes bundled with risks if things are not adequately managed. Sometimes, when personal genetic data is gathered on a massive scale and run through complex algorithms, it can lead to privacy breaches, unequal treatment, and messy disputes over who really controls our biological material. The picture becomes even murkier when technologies like brain tech join forces with tiny nano biotech systems. Although the benefits can be enormous, unchecked progress may expose users to harm, as noted in discussions about the Metaverse (Bibri, 2023). In most cases, a steady and honest conversation among scientists, policymakers, and the public is key to ensuring that such progress supports human well-being and does not infringe on fundamental rights (Betz et al., 2023). Ultimately, these discussions—even if somewhat scattered at times—will help steer biotech practices responsibly in this constantly evolving landscape.

10.3.9. Future Trends in Biotechnology

Biotechnology is evolving in unexpected ways as innovative methods and eco-friendly practices converge, transforming the way many sectors operate. Take biorefineries—they have been tweaked to process tough plant materials like lignocellulosic biomass, and in many cases, this tweak is creating greener alternatives to the usual products. This idea, using leftovers from agriculture, not only cuts down our reliance on petrochemicals but also reveals how farm waste can be turned into biofuels, biocomposites, and even bioplastics (Mujtaba et al., 2023). Optical meta-surfaces, for example, have made some headway recently; generally speaking, they might change how we handle light for biomedical tasks, computer simulations, and quantum tech, potentially boosting the accuracy of our biotech tools (Cheng-Qiu et al., 2021). Overall, these developments seem to point to a future where biotech both champions environmental sustainability and steps up diagnostic and treatment efforts—DNA fingerprinting included—broadening its reach in medicine and farming alike.

Test Your Knowledge

1. How has Next-Generation Sequencing (NGS) improved forensic DNA analysis?
2. How can bioinformatics tools support DNA fingerprinting in large databases?

10.4. Challenges and Controversies in DNA Fingerprinting and Biotechnology

Learning Outcome

1. Understand privacy concerns and data security
2. Focus on misuse of genetic information
3. Learn the legal implications of DNA evidence
4. Know public perception and acceptance of biotechnology
5. Explain ethical dilemmas in genetic manipulation
6. Discuss regulatory frameworks and policies
7. Describe socioeconomic disparities in access to technology
8. Focus on the environmental impacts of biotechnological practices
9. Identify future challenges in the field

Biotechnology is shaking things up across numerous areas, and DNA fingerprinting—take that for example—is caught in a complex web of challenges and debates. More and more, we rely on DNA methods for forensic work, which raises ethical issues such as privacy concerns and the risk that our genetic information might be misused. Nailing down exactly what a DNA sample really tells us is not always straightforward; at times, this complexity leads to significant discrepancies and even wrongful convictions, a point many still argue about. In the world of plants and microbes, the need for solid good manufacturing practices (GMPs) underscores that failing to employ reliable scientific methods can lead to the production of unsafe products (Upton et al., 2019). And then there is the buzz around probiotics, such as Bacillus—the promise is there. Still, different strains with varying safety profiles only add to public unease and regulatory hurdles (Jżewska-Frąckowiak et al., 2018). All in all, even though DNA fingerprinting and biotech hold game-changing potential, they also force us to weigh ethical, interpretative, and safety concerns carefully.

10.4.1. Privacy Concerns and Data Security

Biotechnology is advancing at a rapid pace these days, making privacy issues increasingly difficult to ignore. DNA fingerprinting is no longer a distant dream—it is now widely available, and with that, concerns about the careless or unauthorized use of our genetic data are growing. Adding artificial intelligence into the picture only ups the risk, as these algorithms sift through details that often are not well protected. People might not fully understand what they are agreeing to when their DNA ends up being analyzed, which leads to real ethical debates about true informed consent. Our security measures seem to be lagging behind too, leaving us exposed to threats like data breaches and making stricter regulation a must. In most cases, as pointed out in recent studies (Dara et al., 2025; Patel et al., 2024), if we do not tackle these privacy concerns head-on, we risk trading the benefits of DNA technology for losses in individual rights and our overall trust (Figure 10.16).

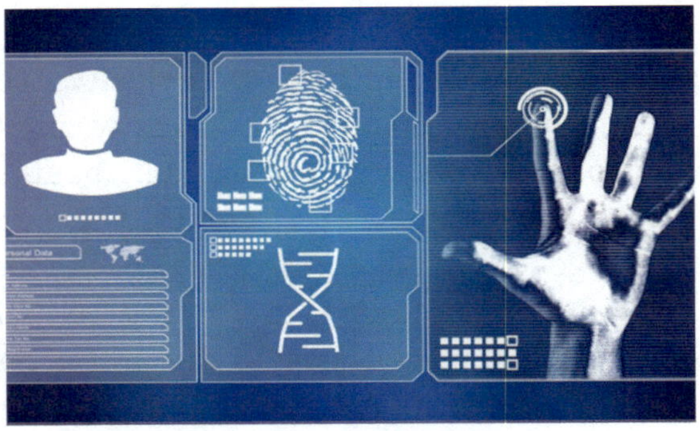

Figure 10.16. Forensic evidence and right to privacy.

Source: Pachauri, S. (2022). *Forensic Evidence and Right to Privacy.*

10.4.2. Misuse of Genetic Information

DNA fingerprinting has advanced at an almost dizzying pace, opening up promising routes in forensic labs and hospitals alike—but it also raises serious ethical concerns about the potential misuse of our genetic blueprints. One major concern is that our genetic data might slip into uses far removed from proper criminal investigations—raising flags for privacy breaches and even discrimination. In most cases, this issue comes into sharper focus when we look at efforts like the DNA Technology (Use and Application) Regulation Bill 2019; this bill, aiming to set some ground rules, insists on keeping the tech strictly for legal, legitimate purposes (Juyal et al., 2021). Then there is the matter of DNA databanks, which store genetic information for future research. In some instances, this may open a can of worms by encouraging studies into genetic hints of criminal behavior, which could unintentionally entrench damaging stereotypes and label people unfairly (Kaye et al., 2006). All in all, it is pretty clear that robust, well-thought-out regulations are needed to balance the real benefits of biotechnology with its potential pitfalls.

10.4.3. Legal Implications of DNA Evidence

Biotechnology and the law are getting tangled up these days, largely because DNA evidence has taken center stage in both criminal and civil cases. DNA fingerprinting keeps improving, and with it come a host of questions about privacy, consent, and whether the genetic data even speaks the truth.

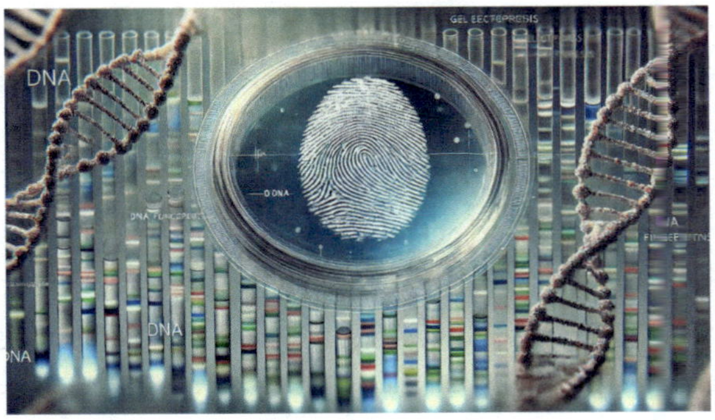

Figure 10.17. DNA fingerprinting keeps improving, and with it come a host of questions about privacy, consent, and whether the genetic data even speaks the truth.

Source: WP Engine. (n.d.). *DNA Fingerprinting.* https://wpengine-lmg-cl-blog.s3.amazonaws.com/wp-content/uploads/DNA-Fingerprinting.jpg.

Courts often have to scratch their heads over whether to admit this kind of evidence, usually weighing how solid the testing methods really are. Some studies—one looking at DNA fingerprinting in farming contexts, for example—that point to a growing trend of leaning on genetic info to shape policies, hinting that tougher legal rules are needed (Hodson et al., 2020). Additionally, as NGS becomes more prevalent in debates, regulators now face the challenge of determining whether food products are sufficiently authentic and traceable to ensure consumer safety (Haynes et al., 2019) (Figure 10.17).

10.4.4. Public Perception and Acceptance of Biotechnology

Biotechnology gets its kick from what people think, especially when it comes down to stuff like DNA fingerprinting. High-profile criminal cases on TV, for example, pull the public into the criminal justice drama; but these stories often pump-up forensic science way more than reality would suggest (Santos et al., 2012). This hype makes it hard for many to believe that results are as fast and flawless as portrayed—leading to a fair bit of doubt about these techniques. There is also the mix of worries about ethics, privacy concerns, and even the risk of genetic discrimination that muddle the picture further. In most cases, figuring out these complex feelings is crucial for having honest conversations about biotech. Ultimately, that kind of conversation can sway how groundbreaking innovations like DNA fingerprinting are accepted, even if folks still eye them with a bit of hesitation (Hadi et al., 2017).

10.4.5. Ethical Dilemmas in Genetic Manipulation

Biotechnology is speeding ahead, especially when it comes to tweaking genes, and it stirs up some deep moral puzzles that really deserve a closer, careful look. Scientists are exploring various gene-editing methods; while these innovative ideas hold considerable promise, they also raise concerns about their implications for our identity and the structure of our communities. Think about altering our genetic blueprint—it might accidentally widen social gaps or even lead to tricky cases like so-called designer babies. Gene doping in sports, for example, shows how pushing genetic limits can mess with fair play and overall health, which is why we still need those strict detection methods (de Boer et al., 2019). And as mix-and-match technologies emerge, issues like vast data collection and algorithm-led oversight bring more ethical challenges, clearly pointing to the need for rules that keep human well-being at the forefront (Bibri, 2023) (Figure 10.18).

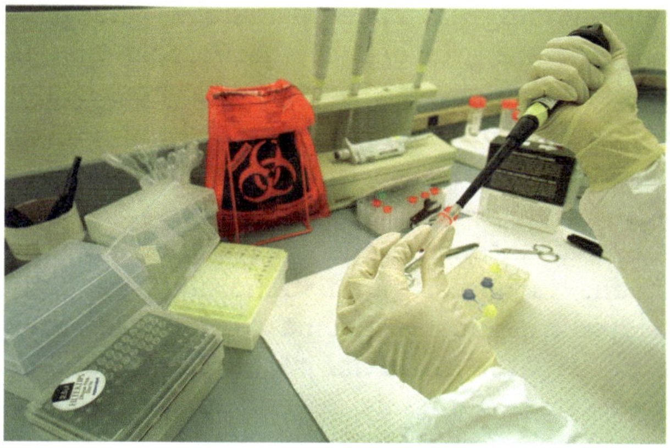

Figure 10.18. Ethical dilemmas in genetic manipulation in forensics.

Source: King, R. (2000). *Civilian Scientist Working in the Broward County Crime Lab Handles Processed DNA Extractions.*

10.4.6. Regulatory Frameworks and Policies

Biotechnology is moving at a breakneck pace these days – take DNA fingerprinting, for instance, which really stands out. New methods like these spark a host of issues, from privacy concerns and debates about proper consent to worries over how genetic info might be misused. Oversight bodies are now stuck balancing the push for fresh innovation with the need to keep public safety in check. Every genetic sample tends to have its own quirks, so in most cases, risks get evaluated on a case-by-case basis—be it in law enforcement or in medical diagnostics. Increasingly, policies are blending old rules with modern tactics, like using machine learning and harmonized datasets, to tackle the many-layered challenges these advances bring. All in all, combining cutting-edge technology with careful oversight signals a broader, more interconnected perspective on how biotechnology impacts society and the environment (Joseph et al., 2023).

10.4.7. Socioeconomic Disparities in Access to Technology

Biotechnology is speeding ahead, and DNA fingerprinting is one of those tools that is shaking things up in areas like healthcare, criminal work, and even tracking family roots. But with such exciting progress comes a downside—usually, the folks who need these advancements the most do not have the means to access them. Generally speaking, people from lower-income backgrounds may not have the financial resources to access these state-of-the-art genetic tools, resulting in unequal opportunities both at home and in the workplace. This uneven distribution does not just hold back individual potential; it plugs directly into larger, systemic issues of injustice. Machado and Granja have even noted that when genetic tech collides with the criminal justice system, marginalized groups end up facing even tougher challenges (Granja et al., 2020). In most cases, if we ignore these access gaps, we risk cementing longstanding inequalities that ripple throughout society (National Center for HIV, STD, and TB Prevention, 2025). Rethinking how we share and use these technologies might be exactly what is needed to help level the playing field for everyone.

10.4.8. Environmental Impacts of Biotechnological Practices

Biotechnological practices are turning agriculture upside down in ways that touch both our natural world and the economy (Figure 10.19). A striking case is transgenic *Bacillus thuringiensis* (Bt) cotton, which many folks praise for cutting back on insecticides and slashing production costs, thereby unlocking both environmental and financial perks (Ijaz et al., 2024). Still, it is essential to monitor the genetic diversity among these Bt cotton strains; if we slack on this, issues such as seed adulteration and reduced benefits can arise, a concern that particularly affects developing countries like Pakistan (Ijaz et al., 2024). Meanwhile, beneficial microorganisms are making their mark in everything from bioremediation to sustainable farming—they boost nutrient cycling and improve soil health, yet there is an undercurrent of concern about possible ecological disruptions and even the rise of antibiotic resistance. All in all, this messy mix of promise and pitfalls generally calls for a careful, ongoing review of these technologies so that bold innovation stays in step with protecting our environment.

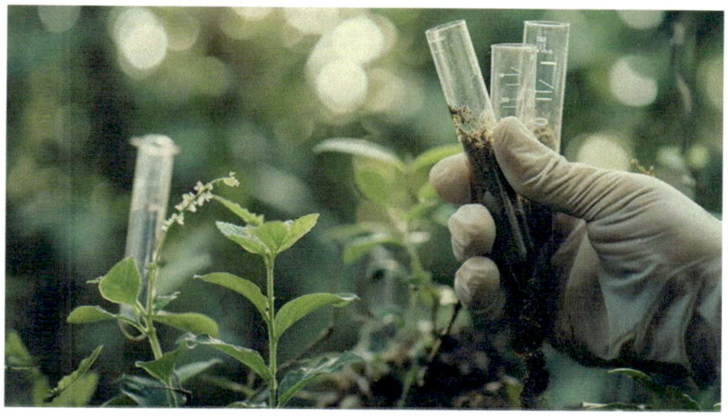

Figure 10.19. Biotechnological practices are turning agriculture upside down in ways that touch both our natural world and the economy.

Source: Team EMB. (2024). *Trends in Biotechnology in 2024: What's Next?*

10.4.9. Future Challenges in the Field

DNA fingerprinting and biotechnology are pushing ahead at a wild pace. With all this progress comes challenges that call for creative fixes and careful ethical thought—old methods just do not cut it anymore. Genetic data is only getting more tangled, and our usual techniques are starting to fall short; we now need sharper computational tools to sift through mountains of info and catch those subtle gene interactions and epigenetic hints (Álvarez-Venegas et al., 2016). Then there is the whole mix-up of different biological layers—genomic, transcriptomic, proteomic, and even metabolomic data—which throws up its own set of tech and interpretation puzzles (Woyke et al., 2015). At the same time, questions about gene editing and who truly owns the genetic information are emerging, especially as these techniques become more widespread. In most cases, handling these powerful tools responsibly is key to unlocking their potential while still keeping public trust and biodiversity intact. How we end up facing these issues will, in many ways, steer the future of the field and shape society in ways we are only beginning to see.

Test Your Knowledge

1. What are the major limitations of DNA fingerprinting in forensic investigations?
2. How can contamination of DNA samples affect the outcome of a criminal case?

SUMMARY

DNA fingerprinting breakthroughs are shaking things up across a range of fields – criminal justice, biotechnology, and more. In most cases, researchers lean on methods like polymerase chain reaction (PCR), a quick and cost-friendly trick to spot microbes, to dodge the old, slow, and labor-intensive ways (Franco-Duarte et al., 2019). Sometimes, examining complex systems—such as the gastrointestinal microbiota in poultry—reveals that these new methods not only enhance food production but also advance public health through improved animal care practices (Shang et al., 2018). The deeper we dive into our genetic codes via fingerprinting, the more likely it seems to unlock unexpected paths that strengthen forensic work and boost farm productivity. Ultimately, the mix of DNA fingerprinting and biotechnology appears set to play a key role in shaping tomorrow's scientific landscape, pushing progress in ways we are only beginning to see.

Biotechnology breakthroughs have flipped forensic science on its head—DNA fingerprinting sits right at the center of it all. It boosts our ability to identify individuals and plays a big part in cracking cases and, in a roundabout way, delivering justice. Studies, in most cases, point out that tweaks in DNA methylation and shifts in gene expression are pretty crucial for understanding a whole range of health issues; for example, some recent work links these changes to acute myocardial infarction (AMI) (Luo et al., 2022). Researchers investigating genetic variations often encounter potential biomarkers that could lead to earlier diagnoses and more effective treatment plans. A neat twist is seen in methods like 2D-DNA fingerprinting, which some industries now use to catch counterfeit operations (Mims et al., 2022). All in all, these pieces, when put together, really highlight the transformative power of combining modern biotech with DNA fingerprinting in both healthcare and security realms.

KEY TERMS FROM THIS CHAPTER

- Adenine
- Cytosine
- Gel electrophoresis
- Genetic markers
- Inter-simple sequence repeat (ISSR) analysis
- Paternity tests
- Short tandem repeats
- Cells
- Deoxyribose sugar
- Genetic code
- Guanine
- Nucleotide
- Polymerase Chain Reaction (PCR)
- Thymine

CRITICAL THINKING QUESTIONS

1. Which of the following is the primary method used for DNA amplification in forensic DNA fingerprinting?

a. Gel electrophoresis

b. Polymerase chain reaction (PCR)

c. Southern blotting

d. Fluorescent *in situ* hybridization (FISH)

2. The process of separating DNA fragments by size and charge is called:

a. Gene editing

b. Electrophoresis

c. DNA denaturation

d. Transcription

3. Which of the following is true about STR (Short Tandem Repeat) markers used in DNA profiling?

a. They are regions with non-repetitive sequences of DNA

b. They are unique to each individual, making them highly reliable for identification

c. They do not vary significantly between individuals

d. They are not found in human DNA

4. Which of the following technologies allows for high-throughput DNA analysis in forensic science?

a. Next-Generation Sequencing (NGS)

b. Fluorescence *in situ* hybridization (FISH)

c. Restriction Fragment Length Polymorphism (RFLP)

d. Southern blotting

5. Which of the following is an ethical concern related to the use of DNA fingerprinting in forensics?

a. Accuracy of DNA evidence

b. Misidentification of suspects

c. Invasion of privacy in DNA database storage

d. Contamination of DNA samples

Short Answer Questions

1. What role does polymerase chain reaction (PCR) play in DNA fingerprinting?
2. How is restriction fragment length polymorphism (RFLP) used in DNA analysis?
3. What are the main steps involved in the process of DNA fingerprinting?
4. How does gel electrophoresis help in separating DNA fragments?
5. What type of samples can be used for DNA fingerprinting?
6. How is contamination prevented in forensic DNA analysis?
7. What is the importance of control samples in DNA profiling?
8. How can DNA fingerprinting establish paternity or biological relationships?
9. In what ways is DNA evidence used in criminal investigations?
10. What are the ethical concerns surrounding DNA fingerprinting?

Answers to Critical Thinking Questions

1. (b); 2. (b); 3. (b); 4. (a); 5. (c)

REFERENCES

1. Aga, E., (2005). *Molecular Genetic Diversity Study of Forest Coffee Tree (Coffea arabica L.) Populations in Ethiopia: Implications for Conservation and Breeding.* https://core.ac.uk/download/11694916.pdf (accessed on 9th May 2025).
2. Ahmad, A., Imran, M., & Ahsan, H., (2023). Biomarkers as biomedical bioindicators: Approaches and techniques for the detection, analysis, and validation of novel biomarkers of diseases. *Pharmaceutics, 15*, 1630. https://doi.org/10.3390/pharmaceutics15061630.
3. Akhter, M. H., Khalilullah, H., Gupta, M., Alfaleh, M. A., Alhakamy, N. A., Riadi, Y., & Md, S., (2021). Impact of protein corona on the biological identity of nanomedicine: Understanding the fate of nanomaterials in the biological milieu. *Biomedicines, 9*, 1496. https://doi.org/10.3390/biomedicines9101496.
4. Álvarez-Venegas, R., & De-la-Peña, C., (2016). Editorial: Recent advances of epigenetics in crop biotechnology. *Frontiers in Plant Science, 7.* https://www.semanticscholar.org/paper/6639bd7919afea75d1bb6cbe744aa27e350b4412 (accessed on 9th May 2025).
5. Anastassopoulos, E., (2006). *DNA Fingerprinting in Plants: Principles, Methods, and Applications* (2nd ed., Vol. *60*, p. 97. https://www.semanticscholar.org/paper/bedbc594232eed040bfa574531378a8f1e111c37 (accessed on 9th May 2025).
6. Antil, S., & Vandana, J., (2025). Biotechnology in forensic science: Advancements and applications. *Journal of Forensic Science and Research.* https://www.semanticscholar.org/paper/8bfaf77700dfb382cbd6d326001b8d9e2c434b4f (accessed on 9th May 2025).
7. Artika, I., Dewi, Y., Nainggolan, I., Siregar, J. E., & Antonjaya, U., (2022). Real-time polymerase chain reaction: Current techniques, applications, and role in COVID-19 diagnosis. *Genes, 13.* https://www.semanticscholar.org/paper/f28da843608b9a14454426b2a92500bd7e4d4929 (accessed on 9th May 2025).
8. Betz, U. A. K., Arora, L., Assal, R. A., Azevedo, H., Baldwin, J., Becker, M., Bostock, S., et al. (2023). Game changers in science and technology – now and beyond. *Technological Forecasting and Social Change, 193*, 122588. https://doi.org/10.1016/j.techfore.2023.122588 (accessed on 9th May 2025).
9. Bezerra, L. G., Oliveira, R. E., Comizzoli, P., & Silva, A. R. (2023). Collection, handling, and preservation of wild bird semen: Current status, challenges, and perspectives. *Biopreservation and Biobanking.* https://www.semanticscholar.org/paper/92a539fe21c3d79ab87e208a[illegible]f2b11ac6c35d92 (accessed on 9th May 2025).
10. Bibri, S. E. (2023). The metaverse as a virtual model of platform urbanism: Its converging AIoT, XReality, neurotech, and nanobiotech and their applications, challenges, and risks. *Smart Cities, 6*, 1345–1384. https://doi.org/10.3390/smartcities6030065.
11. Bivins, R., (2022). Forgone, not forgotten: "DNA fingerprinting," migration control and Britain's DNA profiling pilot project. *Science Technology & Human Values, 49*, 3–27. https://doi.org/10.1177/01622439221139877.
12. Brannigan, V., (2015). Mobile geolocation – a technico-legal revolution. *ISIS.* https://www.semanticscholar.org/paper/845c580ca39b2e2323fc6d719d6d793ede2f9a19 (accessed on 9th May 2025).

13. Buchholz, K., & Collins, J., (2011). *Concepts in Biotechnology: History, Science and Business.* https://www.semanticscholar.org/paper/1e6b52bb4db4a4a253206645f27d5bf9ba4aeaba (accessed on 9th May 2025).

14. Chambers, G. K., Curtis, C., Huynen, L., Lambert, D. M., et al. (2014). *DNA Fingerprinting in Zoology: Past, Present, Future.* https://core.ac.uk/download/43369146.pdf (accessed on 9th May 2025).

15. Chokheli, V. A., Shmaraeva, A., Kornienko, I., Stepanenko, V. V., Rajput, V., Singh, A., Kumari, A., et al. (2022). Assessment of genetic diversity and DNA fingerprinting of rare species of the genus *Crambe* (Brassicaceae). *Crop and Pasture Science, 74*, 1014–1022. https://www.semanticscholar.org/paper/80eaeec5db227627a75f59a19326ccf42f1df26b (accessed on 9th May 2025).

16. D'Elia, T., & Carroll, M., (2024). Plant biotechnology. *The American Biology Teacher.* https://www.semanticscholar.org/paper/5ff88d360ed324ed4853f6d6a3df95e996ad42a0 (accessed on 9th May 2025).

17. Dara, M., & Azarpira, N., (2025). Ethical considerations emerge from artificial intelligence (AI) in biotechnology. *Avicenna Journal of Medical Biotechnology, 17*, 80, 81. https://www.semanticscholar.org/paper/f0fbd6f92d182581ff435858155c24bf2f55157c (accessed on 9th May 2025).

18. de Boer, E. N., van der Wouden, P. E., Johansson, L., van Diemen, C. C., & Haisma, H. J. (2019). A next-generation sequencing method for gene doping detection that distinguishes low levels of plasmid DNA against a background of genomic DNA. *Gene Therapy, 26*, 338–346. https://doi.org/10.1038/s41434-019-0091-6.

19. Diwakar, S., Achuthan, K., Nedungadi, P., & Nair, B., (2012). *Biotechnology Virtual Labs: Facilitating Laboratory Access Anytime-Anywhere for Classroom Education.* https://www.semanticscholar.org/paper/1fbfe8e4fc22f15b5c9d6a8c6a9ccc5bffb66f65 (accessed on 9th May 2025).

20 Franco-Duarte, R., Černáková, L., Kadam, S., Kaushik, K. S., Salehi, B., Bevilacqua, A., Corbo, M. R., et al. (2019). Advances in chemical and biological methods to identify microorganisms—From past to present. *Microorganisms, 7*, 130. https://doi.org/10.3390/microorganisms7050130.

21. Granja, R., & Machado, H., (2020). *Forensic Genetics in the Governance of Crime.* https://core.ac.uk/download/289102108.pdf (accessed on 9th May 2025).

22. Hadi, A., Azwanis, A., Hafidzi, A., Farhana, N., Mustapha, M., Syuhada, N., Pasi, H., et al. (2017). *Prevalence of Depression and Anxiety and Stress Among HIV Patients in Kuantan.* https://core.ac.uk/download/300448903.pdf (accessed on 9th May 2025).

23. Harrer, S., Harrer, S., Kim, S. C., Schieber, C., Kannam, S., Gunn, N., Moore, S., et al. (2015). Label-free screening of single biomolecules through resistive pulse sensing technology for precision medicine applications. *Nanotechnology, 26.* https://www.semanticscholar.org/paper/b9ca11a2c9ec5eaf9db7f4725f0946fe7baa5b92 (accessed on 9th May 2025).

24. Haynes, E., Jiménez, E., Pardo, M. Á., & Helyar, S., (2019). The future of NGS (next generation sequencing) analysis in testing food authenticity. *Food Control, 101*, 134–143. https://doi.org/10.1016/j.foodcont.2019.02.010.

25. Hodson, D., Jaleta, M., Tesfaye, K., Yirga, C., Beyene, H., Kilian, A., Carling, J., et al. (2020). Ethiopia's transforming wheat landscape: Tracking variety use through DNA fingerprinting. *Scientific Reports, 10*. https://doi.org/10.1038/s41598-020-75181-8.

26. Ijaz, S., & Abubakkar, M., (2024). Tracing the diversity of cultivated transgenic cotton in Pakistan by SSR based DNA fingerprinting. *Agricultural Sciences Journal*. https://www.semanticscholar.org/paper/5addf227896eff6f3e7f79177b597dbc78a30c0f (accessed on 9th May 2025).

27. Iqbal, M., Tao, Y., Xie, S., Zhu, Y., Chen, D., Wang, X., Huang, L., et al. (2016). Aqueous two-phase system (ATPS): An overview and advances in its applications. *Biological Procedures Online, 18*. https://doi.org/10.1186/s12575-016-0048-8.

28. Jeżewska-Frąckowiak, J., Seroczyńska, K., Banaszczyk, J., Wozniak, D. J., Żylicz-Stachula, A., & Skowron, P. M. (2018). The promises and risks of probiotic *Bacillus* species. *Acta Biochimica Polonica*. https://doi.org/10.18388/abp.2018_2652.

29. Joseph, T. M., Mahapatra, D. K., Esmaeili, A., Piszczyk, Ł., Hasanin, M. S., Kattali, M., Haponiuk, J. T., et al. (2023). Nanoparticles: Taking a unique position in medicine. *Nanomaterials, 13*, 574. https://doi.org/10.3390/nano13030574.

30. Juyal, R., (2021). *Regulation & Use of DNA Profiling in India*. https://core.ac.uk/download/477975916.pdf (accessed on 9th May 2025).

31. Karp, A., (2000). *Molecular Tools for Detecting Genetic Diversity*. https://www.semanticscholar.org/paper/bfc7886887f9cc84e470470f5dd287a769549a1a (accessed on 9th May 2025).

32. Kaye, D. H. (2006). *Behavioral Genetics Research and Criminal DNA Databases*. https://core.ac.uk/download/62553467.pdf (accessed on 9th May 2025).

33. Khan, F., (2014). *Biotechnology in Medical Sciences*. https://www.semanticscholar.org/paper/849804049d3bf6f6059428b745e5f329025a19af (accessed on 9th May 2025).

34. Kumar, A., Kumar, A., Cabral-Pinto, M. M. S., Chaturvedi, A. K., Shabnam, A. A., Subrahmanyam, G., Mondal, R., et al. (2020). Lead toxicity: Health hazards, influence on food chain, and sustainable remediation approaches. *International Journal of Environmental Research and Public Health, 17*, 2179. https://doi.org/10.3390/ijerph17072179.

35. Luo, X., Hu, Y., Shen, J., Liu, X., Wang, T., Li, L., & Li, J., (2022). Integrative analysis of DNA methylation and gene expression reveals key molecular signatures in acute myocardial infarction. *Clinical Epigenetics, 14*. https://www.semanticscholar.org/paper/da0349e6a3b2e17bc1e8453132e3050a40ebd96e (accessed on 9th May 2025).

36. Mims, W. H., Temple, M., & Mills, R., (2022). Active 2D-DNA fingerprinting of WirelessHART adapters to ensure operational integrity in industrial systems. *Sensors (Basel, Switzerland), 22*. https://www.semanticscholar.org/paper/8b018819cb0592ff1c84ffa6144ad3d22881e5e1 (accessed on 9th May 2025).

37. Muhammad, S. M., & Jega, B., (2024). A review on environmental impacts and risks of beneficial microorganisms. *Innovative Research in Applied, Biological and Chemical Sciences*. https://www.semanticscholar.org/paper/8a22ef49dd50bdff7ee61e976fb9ea6c24cc99ea (accessed on 9th May 2025).

38. Mujtaba, M., Fraceto, L. F., Fazeli, M., Mukherjee, S., Savassa, S. M., de Medeiros, G. A., Pereira, A. E. S., et al. (2023). Lignocellulosic biomass from agricultural waste to the circular economy:

A review with focus on biofuels, biocomposites and bioplastics. *Journal of Cleaner Production, 402*, 136815. https://doi.org/10.1016/j.jclepro.2023.136815.

39. Mustafa, U., Zaroon, S., Shoukat, S., Juveria, J., & Hussain, M., (2024). Optimization of autosomal STR markers for equine genotyping using multiplex PCR. *Futuristic Biotechnology*. https://www.semanticscholar.org/paper/914963fe2b1a0a105d0b0380f6525598a8ef120b (accessed on 9th May 2025).
40. Muthuchidambaram, S., (1993). *Genetic Testing at the Workplace: Scientific, Legal and Ethical Considerations*. https://www.semanticscholar.org/paper/0578401075ba0d78032f86e972f7d8190acc80a0 (accessed on 9th May 2025).
41. National Center for HIV, STD, and TB Prevention (U.S.), Division of Tuberculosis Elimination. (2025). *Ending Neglect: The Elimination of Tuberculosis in the United States*. https://core.ac.uk/download/144201085.pdf (accessed on 9th May 2025).
42. Neh, N., Joshi, S., Gulliarme, D., & Rathore, A. S. (2022). Analytical similarity assessment of biosimilars: Global regulatory landscape, recent studies and major advancements in orthogonal platforms. *Frontiers in Bioengineering and Biotechnology, 10*. https://doi.org/10.3389/fbioe.2022.832059.
43. Niu, X., Song, L., Xiao, Y., & Ge, W., (2018). Drought-tolerant plant growth-promoting rhizobacteria associated with foxtail millet in a semi-arid agroecosystem and their potential in alleviating drought stress. *Frontiers in Microbiology, 8*. https://doi.org/10.3389/fmicb.2017.02580.
44. Nzilibili, S. M. M., Setiawan, F., & Yudianto, A., (2021). Sibling indices as comparisons in personal identification process through short tandem repeats [STR] loci CSF1PO, TH01, TPOX, vWA of Maduranese ethnic in Surabaya. *Journal of Tropical Biodiversity and Biotechnology, 6*(2):60318. https://core.ac.uk/download/478167590.pdf (accessed on 9th May 2025).
45. Oberemok, V., & Gal'chinsky, N. V. (2024). Oligonucleotide insecticides (contact unmodified antisense DNA biotechnology) and RNA biocontrols (double-stranded RNA technology): Newly born fraternal twins in plant protection. *bioRxiv*. https://www.semanticscholar.org/paper/1dd0d1de98f36cf4417b1903457f4c1da4b043aa (accessed on 9th May 2025).
46. Padhy, I., Mahapatra, A. P., Saraswat, D., & Song, J., (2020). *Role of Biotechnology in Pharmaceutical Research: A Comprehensive Review*. https://www.semanticscholar.org/paper/ea01210dda74a86283f9b2158dcddc1edb939f77 (accessed on 9th May 2025).
47. Patel, N., Otieno, W. O., Gawande, N. D., Parmar, S., Karthik, H. N., & Sankaranarayanan, S., (2024). DNA barcoding-based molecular profiling of *Bougainvillea*, *Dianthus*, and *Plumeria* using matK locus. *Journal of Applied Biology & Biotechnology*. https://www.semanticscholar.org/paper/dadc823a7e543470538f8ee44ff8abe9d7f324dd (accessed on 9th May 2025).
48. Patel, U. H., & Gera, K., (2024). Biometric security systems enhanced by AI: Exploring concerns with AI advancements in facial recognition and other biometric systems have security implications and vulnerabilities. *International Journal of Innovative Science and Research Technology (IJISRT)*. https://www.semanticscholar.org/paper/81054c8bc82197611ea1e7b72d65170a382d0c70 (accessed on 9th May 2025).
49. Pellegrini, M., Magi, A., & Iliopoulos, C., (2016). Editorial: Repetitive structures in biological sequences: Algorithms and applications. *Frontiers in Bioengineering and Biotechnology, 4*. https://www.semanticscholar.org/paper/0cfc16a1dc7638fec83ba1b9726c056f2f78bb05 (accessed on 9th May 2025).

50. Penkov, D., Zubkova, E., & Parfyonova, Y., (2023). Tn5 DNA transposase in multi-omics research. *Methods and Protocols, 6*. https://www.semanticscholar.org/paper/2809e74a5d8ede703a86c330cac93223382a9142 (accessed on 9th May 2025).

51. Qadri, A. W., Yadav, S., Jain, A., Shetty, D., & Gulati, N., (2023). Tooth as a vital source of DNA in forensic odontology: Recent perspective. *Journal of Academy of Dental Education*. https://www.semanticscholar.org/paper/483669bc1d3b131151e89c7f8d4208016b3c87f3 (accessed on 9th May 2025).

52. Qiu, C. W., Zhang, T., Hu, G., & Kivshar, Y. S. (2021). Quo Vadis, metasurfaces? *Nano Letters, 21*, 5461–5474. https://doi.org/10.1021/acs.nanolett.1c00828.

53. Ravì, D., Wong, C., Deligianni, F., Berthelot, M., Andreu-Pérez, J., Lo, B., & Yang, G. Z. (2016). Deep learning for health informatics. *IEEE Journal of Biomedical and Health Informatics, 21*, 4–21. https://doi.org/10.1109/jbhi.2016.2636665.

54. Raza, A., Razzaq, A., Mehmood, S. S., Zou, X., Zhang, X., Lv, Y., & Xu, J., (2019). Impact of climate change on crops adaptation and strategies to tackle its outcome: A review. *Plants, 8*, 34. https://doi.org/10.3390/plants8020034.

55. Ražná, K., Hlavačková, L., Bežo, M., Žiarovská, J., Habán, M., Sluková, Z., & Pernišová, M., (2015). Application of the RAPD and miRNA markers in the genotyping of *Silybum marianum* (L.) Gaertn. *Acta Fytotechnica et Zootechnica, 18*, 83–89. https://www.semanticscholar.org/paper/f4a34921c7a3e5a5f3d1ba7fe6d8acc4c03acc97 (accessed on 9th May 2025).

56. Ribeiro, G. A., Pereira, L. E., & Costa, G. C. (2019). DNA fingerprint: A lab protocol for high school students. *Revista de Ensino de Bioquímica*. https://www.semanticscholar.org/paper/d2e7445eac17bd62ac550686d00cad084cd47a92 (accessed on 9th May 2025).

57. Rudloff, B. E. (2024). *Fingerprinting Breast Milk; Insights Into Milk Exosomics*. https://core.ac.uk/download/621166844.pdf (accessed on 9th May 2025).

58. Saamia, V., Yudianto, A., Nurjayadi, M., Novitasari, N., & Furqoni, A., (2024). Limit detection of short tandem repeats (STR) analysis on touch DNA samples. *Indonesian Journal of Chemistry*. https://www.semanticscholar.org/paper/0c784902379c168d090714be1c26647a26323fb4 (accessed on 9th May 2025).

59. Safeena, M. I. S. (2013). *A Review with Special Reference to Sri Lanka*. https://core.ac.uk/download/143654052.pdf (accessed on 9th May 2025).

60. Santos, F., (2012). *The Dissemination and Popularization of Surveillance Technologies: Five Case Studies of Criminal Cases*. https://core.ac.uk/download/55625930.pdf (accessed on 9th May 2025).

61. Satam, H., Joshi, K., Mangrolia, U., Waghoo, S., Zaidi, G., Rawool, S., Thakare, R. P., et al. (2023). Next-generation sequencing technology: Current trends and advancements. *Biology, 12*, 997. https://doi.org/10.3390/biology12070997.

62. Shang, Y., Kumar, S., Oakley, B. B., & Kim, W. K. (2018). Chicken gut microbiota: Importance and detection technology. *Frontiers in Veterinary Science, 5*. https://doi.org/10.3389/fvets.2018.00254 (accessed on 9th May 2025).

63. Sharma, P., Bano, A., Singh, S. P., Dubey, N. K., Chandra, R., & Iqbal, H. M. N. (2022). Microbial fingerprinting techniques and their role in the remediation of environmental pollution. *Cleaner Chemical Engineering, 2*, 100026. https://doi.org/10.1016/j.clce.2022.100026 (accessed on 9th May 2025).

64. Singh, R. K., Prasad, A., Muthamilarasan, M., Parida, S. K., & Prasad, M., (2020). Breeding and biotechnological interventions for trait improvement: Status and prospects. *Planta, 252*. https://doi.org/10.1007/s00425-020-03465-4.

65. Stewart, J. A. (2006). *DNA, Data and Ethics*. https://core.ac.uk/download/55367.pdf (accessed on 9th May 2025).

66. Sulley, Y. S., Seidu, O. A., Lawal, M., Oboakoh, I., Murtala, S., Dauda, M., & Quansah, L., (2022). The national significance of a DNA revolution: A call for policy action towards sustainable development goals (SDGs). *Journal of Human Earth and Future, 3*, 247–262. https://doi.org/10.28991/hef-2022-03-02-010.

67. Sun, L., Liu, H., Ye, Y., Yang, L., Islam, R., Tan, S., Tong, R., et al. (2023). Smart nanoparticles for cancer therapy. *Signal Transduction and Targeted Therapy, 8*. https://doi.org/10.1038/s41392-023-01642-x.

68. Tchatchoua, D., Tchoundjeu, Z., & Caspa, R., (2016). Application of biotechnology for the domestication of *Dacryodes edulis* (G. Don) H. J. Lam in Cameroon: A review. *African Journal of Biotechnology, 15*, 1177–1183. https://www.semanticscholar.org/paper/2a394f2209b98aaea7e07acc4d5705368d5958bd (accessed on 9th May 2025).

69. Toom, V., (2012). *Bodies of Science and Law: Forensic DNA Profiling, Biological Bodies, and Biopower*. https://core.ac.uk/download/9987119.pdf (accessed on 9th May 2025).

70. Upton, R., David, B., Gafner, S., & Glasl, S., (2019). Botanical ingredient identification and quality assessment: Strengths and limitations of analytical techniques. *Phytochemistry Reviews, 19*, 1157–1177. https://doi.org/10.1007/s11101-019-09625-z.

71. Wang, Z., Zeng, Z., Qin, X., Li, Z., Tong, Y., Liu, K., & Li, Q., (2024). Genetic diversity and fingerprinting of *Elaeagnus angustifolia* based on SSR molecular markers. *Sheng Wu Gong Cheng Xue Bao = Chinese Journal of Biotechnology, 40*(10), 3530–3547. https://www.semanticscholar.org/paper/1c9bce1da5cd6a7fe7e89fc62ffb5643a9af4997 (accessed on 9th May 2025).

72. Wild, C. P. (2012). The exposome: From concept to utility. *International Journal of Epidemiology, 41*, 24–32. https://doi.org/10.1093/ije/dyr236.

73. Wishart, D. S. (2019). Metabolomics for investigating physiological and pathophysiological processes. *Physiological Reviews, 99*, 1819–1875. https://doi.org/10.1152/physrev.00035.2018 (accessed on 9th May 2025).

74. Woyke, T., & Jarett, J., (2015). Function-driven single-cell genomics. *Microbial Biotechnology, 8*, 38, 39. https://www.semanticscholar.org/paper/c479bf6ce7762555b079a7cace4e887e5533c415 (accessed on 9th May 2025).

75. Xu, Y., Allen, E. B., Wang, L., & Wen, S., (2022). Identifying human remains from 20th century warfare: A state of the field essay. *Frontiers in Bioscience-Landmark, 27*. https://doi.org/10.31083/j.fbl2709271.

76. Yazdanian, M., Karami, S., Tahmasebi, E., Alam, M., Abbasi, K., Rahbar, M., Tebyaniyan, H., et al. (2022). Dental radiographic/digital radiography technology along with biological agents in human identification. *Scanning, 2022*, 1–30. https://doi.org/10.1155/2022/5265912.

77. Zhang, X., Liao, L., Wang, Z., Bai, C., & Liu, J., (2016). Analysis of genetic diversity in *Chrysopogon aciculatus* using intersimple sequence repeat and sequence-related amplified polymorphism markers. *HortScience, 51*, 972–979. https://www.semanticscholar.org/paper/c31315d8538a03621682e26816dfd6d0563d2987 (accessed on 9th May 2025).

78. Zhang, Y., Wang, Z., Wang, Z., Liu, X., & Yuan, X., (2017). A DNA-based encryption method based on two biological axioms of DNA chip and polymerase chain reaction (PCR) amplification techniques. *Chemistry, 23*(54), 13387–13403. https://www.semanticscholar.org/paper/2baed4b0caf636a6bc1e794057d2003c1a957359 (accessed on 9th May 2025).

MEDICAL ETHICS AND PROFESSIONAL CONDUCT

11

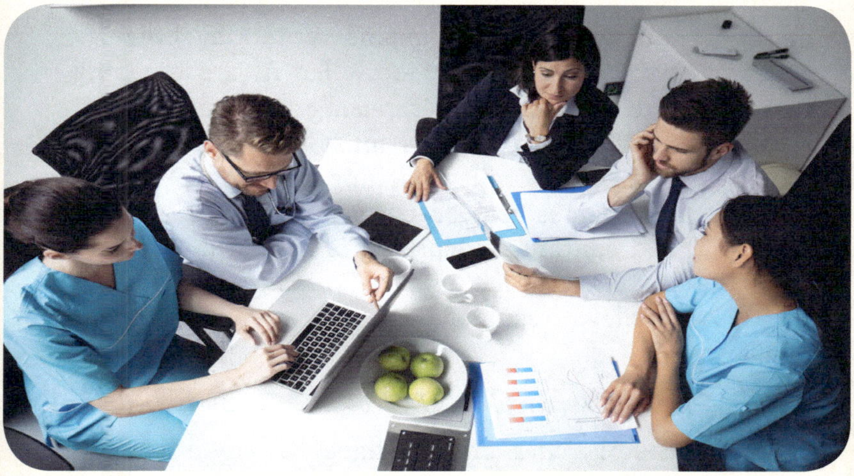

LEARNING OBJECTIVES

After studying this chapter, you will be able to:

1. Understand ethical principles in forensic medicine.
2. Explain professional conduct standards.
3. Identify challenges in forensic ethics.
4. Learn case studies in forensic ethics..

Introduction

In forensic work, the mix of medical ethics and professional behavior is a tricky affair that can sway legal decisions and shape public opinion. Practitioners often stumble into moral dilemmas that push them to stick to their routines and test their personal integrity in unexpected ways. It is crucial to understand what ethical decision-making really means – after all, these tough moments force a closer look at one's commitment to doing what's right. As forensic science continues to evolve rapidly, thanks to new technologies and updated methods, having a solid ethical framework is becoming increasingly essential. Research generally suggests that blending ethical ideas into forensic education and training readies professionals to face challenges in a fair, principled manner (Ranade et al., 2024), while exploring how a professional identity is built in medical education can shed light on how experts pick up the skills needed to steer through these murky ethical territories effectively (Sarraf-Yazdi et al., 2024).

Importance of Ethics in Forensics

Forensics relies on ethical behavior—its outcomes really affect both court decisions and how much the public trusts the whole process (Figure 11.1). Sometimes, a small slip-up, such as mishandling evidence or allowing personal bias to influence analysis, can lead to grave errors—wrongful convictions or even letting the guilty go free—and this undermines the very foundations of justice. Generally speaking, sticking to long-accepted ethical rules helps build transparency and accountability and, in turn, keeps a professional's credibility intact. When dealing with cases that often involve people who are vulnerable, respecting their rights and dignity is not just a nice add-on, it is absolutely crucial.

Now, as advanced tech like artificial intelligence starts playing a bigger role in forensic work, updating these ethical guidelines becomes even more important to manage new risks and hidden biases (Sallam, 2023). All in all, a strong ethical base not only makes forensic evidence more reliable but also upholds our society's commitment to real justice (Tğitcanlar et al., 2020).

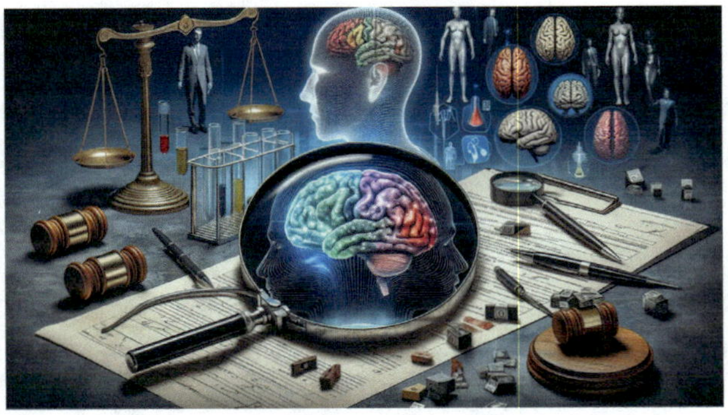

Figure 11.1. Forensics relies on ethical behavior—its outcomes really affect both court decisions and how much the public trusts the whole process.

Source: Cognizavest. (2024). Trends in Biotechnology in 2024: What's Next?

Overview of Professional Conduct

Forensic science runs on the simple rule that doing what's right is not optional—it is everything. Professionals sticking to a solid, if sometimes winding, ethical guide not only shape the outcomes of investigations but also shape the community's trust in this field. In many areas, especially those new and buzzing like investigative genetic genealogy (IGG) (Kling et al., 2021), the tricks we use to piece together relationships need to be both tough and squarely ethical, even if it means rethinking how we work. Additionally, tools like AI are creeping into healthcare, often raising biases and ethical puzzles that experts must untangle (Sallam, 2023). Generally speaking, keeping a culture that values real, on-the-ground ethical choices and continuous learning is key—a messy mix, but one that makes sure forensic work leads to fair legal results.

Historical Context of Medical Ethics

History and culture have heavily reshaped medical ethics – past events and shifting norms have redefined what people expect from healthcare providers. In forensic cases, legal rules, and everyday doctoring mix in unexpected ways, raising old questions rooted in ethical ideas from centuries back. As medicine branches into areas like forensic work, practitioners often end up juggling responsibilities to patients, communities, and the law all at once. Digital tools and new treatment methods now spark debates about consent and personal control, shaking up what we once assumed in medical practice. Overall, this evolving scene clearly demonstrates why solid ethical guidelines are so vital; generally speaking, they serve as a flexible guide for professionals facing new dilemmas. For example, there has been chatter about video therapy during crises – this trend shifts how we see therapeutic bonds and the ethical standards of care (Simpson et al., 2020). Similarly, discussions about old medical records point to the need for a closer read of history; these documents echo the usual stories while also hinting at more offbeat, sometimes subversive interpretations (Zeitlyn, 2012).

Role of Forensic Professionals

Forensic science is not just about mastering technical details—it is also about dealing with a whole mess of ethical issues that pop up along the way. Professionals in this field must balance solid scientific methods with moral considerations, especially when things get complicated during investigations. Today's digital era means that raw data often gets mixed up with opinions, making it harder to tell where ethical lines lie. Take social media, for instance; when professionals post their findings, they have to follow ethical and deontological guidelines—a point a diverse panel hammered home by stressing the need for strong, evidence-based communication (Cortegiani et al., 2024).

Then there's the added twist of new tech like AI systems (ChatGPT, for example), which brings its own set of ethical puzzles into play (Sallam, 2023). Ultimately, maintaining the integrity of forensic work hinges on a consistent, albeit imperfect, commitment to conducting things ethically (Figure 11.2).

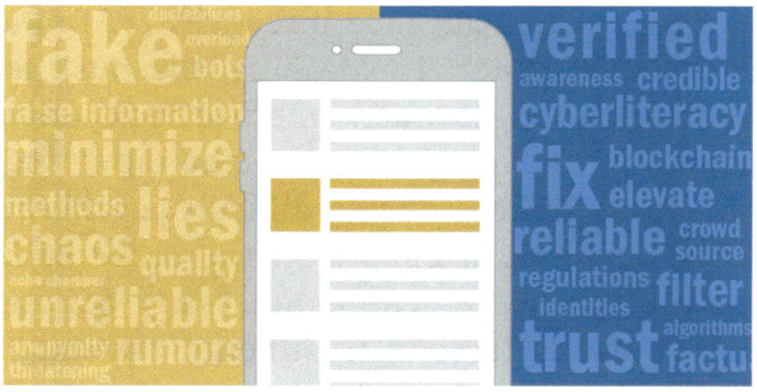

Figure 11.2. Today's digital era means that raw data often gets mixed up with opinions, making it harder to tell where ethical lines lie.

Source: Pew Research Center. (2017). *The Future of Truth and Misinformation Online.*

Ethical Dilemmas in Forensic Practice

Forensic work brings up ethical puzzles every day—it is a messy world. Consent, privacy, and the chance that collected info might be misused all crop up, sometimes unexpectedly. Experts in this field often find themselves working in both law and medicine, and that mix can lead to clashing responsibilities; they are compelled to keep their honesty intact while meeting legal needs. New technologies like AI are now part of forensic methods, sparking debates over who should be held accountable and whether the results can be trusted. Under pressure to produce evidence that stands up, professionals can sometimes see their ethical guard's slip. This jumble of challenges is a lot like other big societal issues, where the pursuit of knowledge and justice bumps heads with ethical values—just as we see in discussions about just war principles and military conduct (Sagan, 2016). In most cases, sorting out these ethical dilemmas calls for a solid approach that balances individual rights with the wider common good (Ali et al., 2023).

11.1. Ethical Principles in Forensic Medicine

Learning Outcome

1. Understand autonomy and informed consent;
2. Explain beneficence and non-maleficence;
3. Describe justice in forensic evaluations;
4. Focus on confidentiality and privacy concerns;
5. Learn professional integrity and honesty;
6. Discuss accountability in forensic practices;
7. 1Know ethical decision-making frameworks;
8. Focus on cultural competence in forensic ethics;
9. Know impact of ethical principles on outcomes.

Forensic medicine is tricky—it needs a firm grip on ethical rules from the get-go. The nature of the work means that even a small error in ethics can really change legal outcomes and affect lives in major ways. Studies show that when medical insights end up on social media, the usual clear-cut ethical lines can get fuzzy; for example, getting proper informed consent may lose ground against the pull of self-promotion (Cortegiani et al., 2024). Generally speaking, legal medicine presents its own set of challenges, prompting us to consider both the broader ethical implications and the specific details of where examinations take place (Sharifi et al., 2022). In the end, these ethical setups work to keep forensic practitioners hitting a high standard of professionalism and accountability, which only adds to the trust that the public and legal folks place in the field.

11.1.1. Autonomy and Informed Consent

Autonomy and informed consent come together as the backbone of ethical practice, especially in forensic settings (Figure 11.3).

Instead of just following a checklist, patients—and even subjects in forensic situations—are expected to decide for themselves how their care should proceed, which really honors their independence. Informed consent is not simply a formality; it stands as a sign of straightforwardness and true respect for an individual's rights. Recent research (Lanka et al., 2025) seems to show that when doctors get these ideas, they naturally show up in their everyday work. As modern medicine keeps throwing unexpected challenges our way, there is generally a noticeable need for ongoing ethics training—particularly in those messy forensic cases (Waseem et al., 2024). All in all, nurturing a culture where informed consent genuinely matters is key to keeping ethical standards solid in forensic medicine.

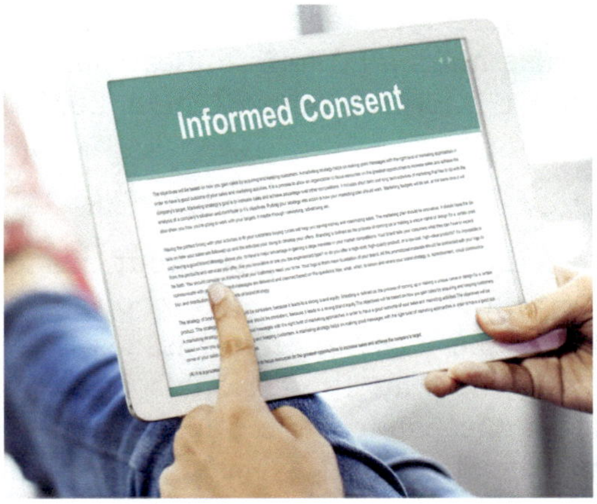

Figure 11.3. Autonomy and informed consent form the backbone of ethical practice, especially in forensic settings.

Source: American Institute of Health Care Professionals. (2024). *Ethics in Healthcare.* https://aihcp.net/main/wp-content/uploads/2024/10/Ethics10-14a.jpg.

11.1.2. Beneficence and Non-Maleficence

Beneficence and non-maleficence sit at the heart of ethical practice in forensics (Figure 11.4). Forensic professionals often rely on these ideas—supporting individual well-being while also minimizing potential harm. Take psychiatric advance directives (PADs) as an example: generally speaking, the push for beneficence nudges practitioners to back patient autonomy, letting people decide how they want to be treated during difficult psychiatric episodes (Karasik, 2023). On the other hand, non-maleficence warns against any actions, such as overly forceful treatments, that might actually worsen a patient's condition (Saputra et al., 2023). By keeping these twin ideas in play, professionals can sort through legal obligations and moral responsibilities with a mix of caution and compassion, ultimately aiming for a more balanced blend of mental health care and legal practice.

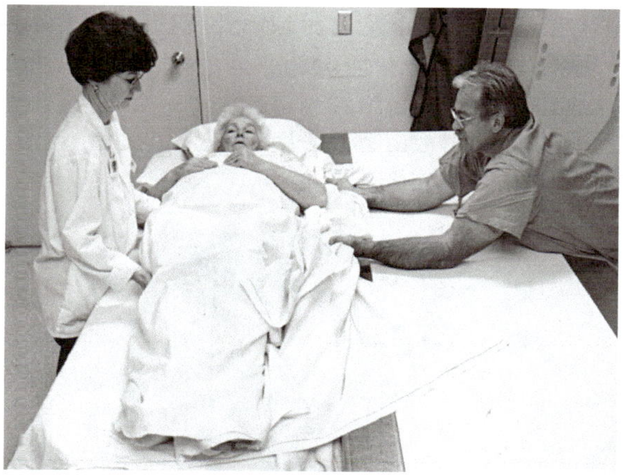

Figure 11.4. Beneficence and non-maleficence sit at the heart of ethical practice in forensics.

Source: Ballinger, P. W., & Frank, E. D. (2007). *Merrill's Atlas of Radiographic Positions and Radiologic Procedures.*

11.1.3. Justice in Forensic Evaluations

Medical assessments and ethical concerns often get really messy, making fairness in forensic settings something we cannot just ignore. If you really dig into processes like figuring out someone's age by looking at their teeth, it becomes clear that mixing different areas of expertise is key—especially for folks who lack proper documents, as Micco et al. (2020) casually points out with its talk on third molar growth. These approaches, you see, stir up a lot of ethical questions—mostly around respecting personal choice and avoiding harm—that need a closer, sometimes even clumsy, look in any forensic review. And then there is the idea of weaving in peer support during mental health checks, which, as (Shalaby et al., 2020) suggests, might help ensure that individuals facing mental health challenges get a fair shake. In most cases, keeping the whole process just is not about ticking boxes; it is about protecting rights and, by and large, keeping the forensic field honest, even if things do not always line up perfectly.

11.1.4. Confidentiality and Privacy Concerns

Sensitive genetic data is now easier to access in our tech-saturated world, which throws fresh privacy and confidentiality challenges at forensic settings (Figure 11.5). Take next-generation sequencing (NGS) as an example – it is completely reshaping how we look at genome data, yet it also sparks up some serious cyber-biosecurity worries. Because this type of data is inherently sensitive, it often invites unauthorized access and unexpected data breaches that can compromise both patient privacy and the ethical standards expected in forensic work (Anjum et al., 2025).

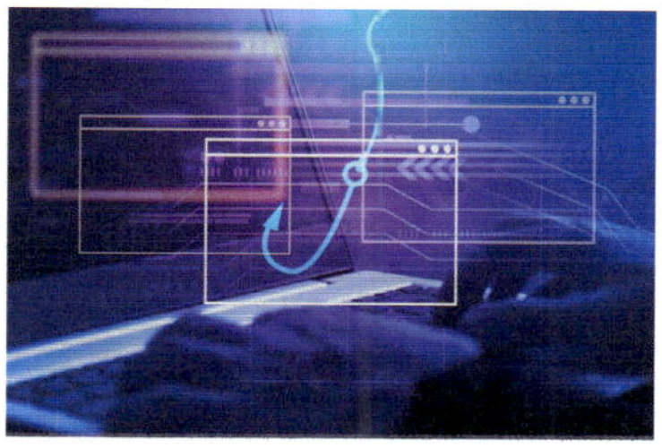

Figure 11.5. Sensitive genetic data is now easier to access in our tech-saturated world, which throws fresh privacy and confidentiality challenges at forensic settings.

Source: janews. (2024). *Cyber Crime Phishing Mail, Security Awareness to Protect Important Data Hacking.*

At the same time, when artificial intelligence is wedded to healthcare, it forces us to take a careful, sometimes painstaking, look at how privacy is maintained at every stage of an AI system's life cycle. Sure, existing legislation offers a bit of a shield, but noticeable gaps finger—pointing to a lack of a complete strategy for handling risks related to data privacy and transparency (Ugleva et al., 2024). The mix of modern technology with long-standing ethical issues seems to call for ongoing dialogue and proactive moves to safeguard individual rights in forensic contexts.

11.1.5. Professional Integrity and Honesty

Trust in forensic medicine really comes down to a steadfast mix of honesty and integrity. Those working in the field must serve up clear, unbiased evidence—a responsibility that can tip legal scales one way or the other. Slip-ups in sticking to solid ethics can have deep consequences; even a single misjudgment might let an innocent face punishment or allow a guilty person to walk free. Recent systematic reviews, in most cases, show that while tools like ChatGPT offer novel twists for healthcare education and practice, they also raise concerns about hidden biases and ethical risks that could erode the trust associated with forensic evaluations (Sallam, 2023). For this reason, it is crucial to nurture a culture of transparency and accountability, ensuring that professionals remain vigilant against ethical missteps while consistently striving for precision in their work (Sallam, 2023).

11.1.6. Accountability in Forensic Practices

Forensic work demands an unwavering commitment to high standards—small mistakes can easily spiral into huge problems like wrongful convictions or leaving people unprotected (Figure 11.6). Experts in this field face a significant ethical burden to maintain the highest standards of data quality and ensure that every method they use adheres to time-tested practices. Their duty does not stop at crunching numbers; sharing clear and honest results builds trust both among scientists and with everyday folks. In most cases, the risk that forensic skills might be misused makes it crucial to emphasize ethical learning, a strategy that helps new professionals navigate complex moral dilemmas more effectively. Creating a culture of accountability in forensic circles further cuts down on misconduct risks, reminding everyone that the know-how these practitioners hold is as much about power as it is about responsibility—an idea echoed in debates over ethical issues in analytical chemistry (Bulska, 2024) and discussions on the need for strong community values (Olivier, 2016).

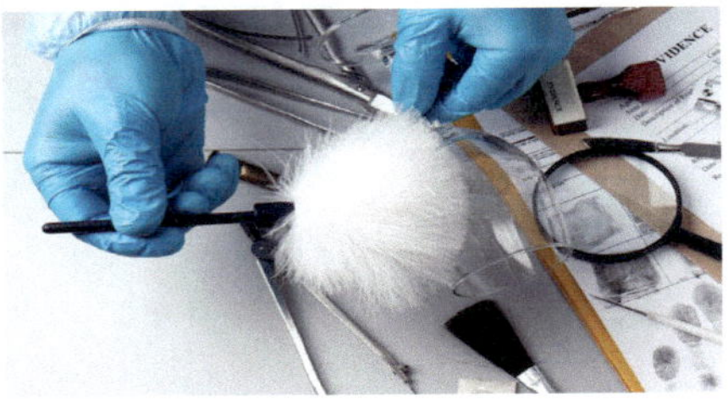

Figure 11.6. Forensic work demands an unwavering commitment to high standards—small mistakes can easily spiral into huge problems like wrongful convictions or leaving people unprotected.

Source: The AP Law Group. (2022). *Forensics.* https://theaplawgroup.com/wp-content/uploads/2022/08/forensics.jpg.

11.1.7. Ethical Decision-Making Frameworks

Forensic medicine is not a neat, tidy field—it is full of twists where ethical choices help sort out messy intersections of care, law, and what society expects. Instead of following a cookie-cutter checklist, these ethical guidelines pop up to assist practitioners in balancing a mix of patient needs, legal duties, and community standards. Generally speaking, the recent buzz about AI and algorithms in hospitals has nudged us to rethink old ethics; nowadays, you might hear folks mention "collaborative tinkering" (Voorst, 2025), an idea where decisions become a joint effort between human judgment and machine input—messing a bit with who is really calling the shots. And then, when studies involve particularly at-risk groups, like kids with Systemic Inflammatory Response Syndrome, issues around informed consent and data privacy come to light once again, making it clear that we need rules that both respect patient rights and allow for flexible, shared decision-making (Stolte et al., 2024). Ultimately, stitching these frameworks together appears crucial for navigating the complex ethical dilemmas encountered throughout forensic work.

11.1.8. Cultural Competence in Forensic Ethics

Forensic work today finds itself wedded to a mix of cultural insight and ethical practice, a blend that is getting more attention in both everyday legal work and medical ethics. When professionals interact with individuals from diverse backgrounds, they often discover that recognizing those subtle cultural cues is crucial if justice and genuine ethical conduct are to prevail.

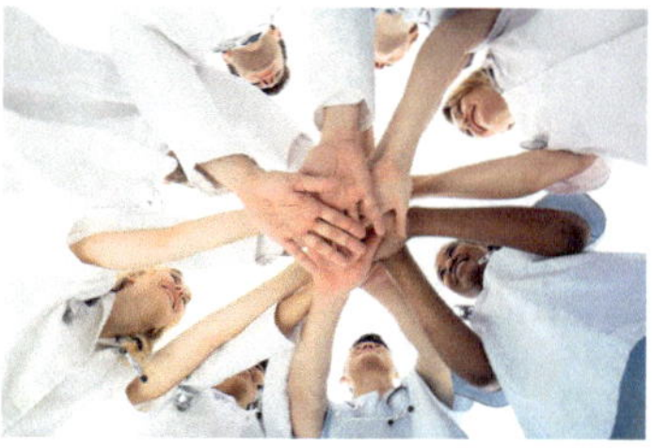

Figure 11.7. Cultural competence in forensic ethics.

Source: Diversity Nursing. (n.d.). *Cultural Competence.* https://blog.diversitynursing.com/hs-fs/hubfs/culturalcompetence.jpg?width=1000&name=culturalcompetence.jpg.

This kind of cultural savvy tends to sharpen assessments and even guide interventions that can boost patient care as well as legal outcomes. It is also true that having a culturally aware perspective helps trim down the risk of bias—which, let us face it, can really mess up the integrity of a forensic evaluation. Various guidelines, in most cases, nudge practitioners toward a commitment to lifelong learning and cultural sensitivity, a sentiment that resonates with the Indian Psychiatric Society's call for upholding high moral standards and patient welfare (Gundugurti et al., 2022). And when you toss in broader problems like corruption and inequality—issues often spotlighted in the Latin American context—it becomes clear that ethical reforms aiming for more inclusive practices just are necessary (Figure 11.7).

11.1.9. Impact of Ethical Principles on Outcomes

Forensic work is not just about following strict procedures—it is really a journey where ethics come first. In practice, professionals who care deeply about being honest and accountable can often nail down more accurate investigations, which generally makes legal findings more solid. This kind of ethical thinking is not simply a set of rules; it guides how experts act and slowly builds the public's trust, a trust that is key when the court system is under scrutiny. Sometimes, sticking to these ethical standards even sparks unexpected teamwork among folks from different fields, leading to more thorough studies that touch on public health issues—a trend you can see in projects like the Global Burden of Diseases, Injuries, and Risk Factors Study (GBD) (Ferrari et al., 2024). At the same time, using modern tools like AI, though exciting, throws new challenges our way, which means setting up clear ethical guidelines becomes even more important to help curb issues like bias and misinformation (Sallam, 2023).

Test Your Knowledge

1. How does the principle of autonomy influence consent in medicolegal examinations?
2. In what situations is beneficence challenged in forensic practice?

11.2. Professional Conduct Standards

Learning Outcome

1. Learn codes of conduct for forensic professionals;
2. Identify the role of professional organizations;
3. Discuss training and education requirements;
4. Know the importance of continuing education;
5. Explain peer review and accountability mechanisms;
6. Reporting unethical behavior;
7. Know the consequences of professional misconduct;
8. Discuss case studies of misconduct in forensics;
9. Explain best practices for maintaining professionalism.

Forensic practice hinges on sticking to a set of professional conduct rules that form the backbone of ethical behavior and fairness in every step of the process. These guidelines not only help build credibility for forensic findings—they also protect the rights of the people involved, a point that, in most cases, gets repeated time and again. In our rapidly changing tech world, where innovations like the Internet of Things and artificial intelligence are becoming increasingly prevalent, professionals are navigating complex ethical landscapes. Take, for instance, the benefits we might see with tools similar to ChatGPT in healthcare; while such innovations offer real advantages, they also push us toward a cautious, sometimes even tentative, implementation that leans on well-established ethical codes to guide decisions (Sallam, 2023). On top of that, the messy challenges linked to digital evidence—especially when privacy and security issues come up—demand that everyone sticks strictly to protocols to keep the investigative process sound (Stoyanova et al., 2020). All in all, when you consider these different aspects together, it is clear that maintaining high professional standards is not just a good idea—it is absolutely essential for ensuring that forensic work remains both trustworthy and reliable.

11.2.1. Codes of Conduct for Forensic Professionals

Forensic investigations are full of twists and require experts to stick to strong ethical guidelines. Clear rules are not just bureaucratic fluff—they keep work accurate, honest, and responsible, especially when even a small slip can sway legal outcomes or public safety.

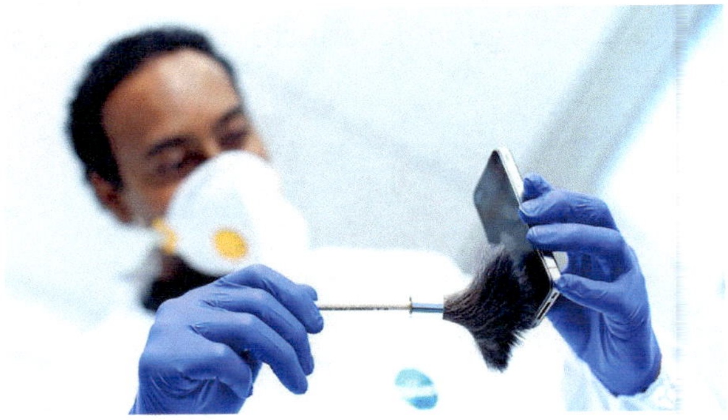

Figure 11.8. Codes of conduct for forensic professionals.

Source: iPleaders. (2016). *Forensics.* https://blog.ipleaders.in/wp-content/uploads/2016/06/forensics.jpg.

These standards do not simply enforce objectivity; they also help professionals determine how to handle new tools like AI and innovative data techniques that continually change the game in ways we had not even imagined. In most cases, the rise of technologies like AI sparks extra worry about fairness and even misinformation (Sallam, 2023), which keeps many in the field debating the best way forward. A solid code of conduct, then, is not just a set of rules—it sparks everyday conversations and builds trust among colleagues across various specialties, which in turn boosts the overall impact of forensic science. Ultimately, these ethical frameworks are vital for making sure that forensic work remains reliable and for keeping the public's trust in our justice system—even if the journey is not always perfectly smooth (Figure 11.8).

11.2.2. Role of Professional Organizations

Professional groups have a big say in how medical ethics unfold within forensics. Take the Indian Academy of Forensic Medicine (IAFM) for example—they are not just bureaucratic bodies, but rather vibrant hubs where ongoing learning and ethical discussions occur in a real, down-to-earth way. They set out guidelines and simple frameworks that do more than establish standards; in most cases, they actively back up the interests of their members. Sometimes, you see this in action: the IAFM recently weighed in on regulatory shifts—its response to the draft regulations from the National Medical Commissions (Mukesh, 2022) clearly shows a shared, almost communal, push to keep ethics tight in the field. These organizations also help different medical disciplines exchange ideas, which ultimately fosters a more comprehensive understanding of the complex forensic issues (Ford, 2000). All in all, through everyday dialogue and steady advocacy, these groups keep the ethical core of forensic medicine alive, even if the process is a bit messy at times.

11.2.3. Training and Education Requirements

Working in forensics is not exactly a walk in the park—it is a realm where split-second decisions mix with weighty ethical questions (Figure 11.9). Lately, innovations such as AI in diagnostics and telemedicine have significantly disrupted traditional routines, prompting us to reassess what constitutes proper practice (Senbekov et al., 2020). In many cases, the COVID-19 outbreak sped up the move toward remote therapeutic services, making it clear that training programs need to keep pace with digital health tools and the ethical baggage they bring along (Simpson et al., 2020). Sometimes, when professionals run smack into unexpected moral challenges, having a solid educational foundation is not just a bonus—it turns out to be absolutely essential. It is not all about mastering the technical side of forensic science; understanding how these new technologies raise complex ethical issues is just as crucial. Generally speaking, blending hands-on technical skills with a genuine awareness of ethics seems to be the best recipe for keeping forensics both responsible and adaptive. All in all, a well-rounded training approach that weaves together both hard science and moral insight is crucial for nurturing real-world professionalism in this challenging field.

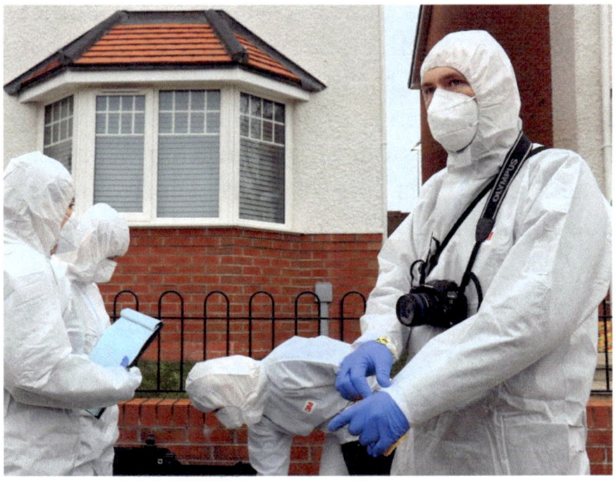

Figure 11.9. Working in forensics is not exactly a walk in the park—it is a realm where split-second decisions mix with weighty ethical questions.

Source: Wrexham University. (n.d.). *Science Laboratory at Wrexham University.* https://wrexham.ac.uk/media/marketing/science/IMG_4088.jpg.

11.2.4. Importance of Continuing Education

Forensics is constantly changing, and ongoing learning plays a huge role here. New technology and innovative methods continue to emerge, so professionals in the field must stay current to maintain the integrity of medical ethics and professional standards. Taking classes and training sessions on a regular basis not only boosts the skills needed for those tricky cases but also builds a steady habit of relying on evidence-based practices that matter a lot for public health. Continuous education encourages professionals to explore innovative approaches, which can help solve crimes more effectively and advance justice. Sometimes, ethical challenges come up unexpectedly in the lab or in the field; having the latest insights means experts are usually better at handling these issues and acting responsibly. Embracing modern tools—like AI systems such as ChatGPT—signals a readiness to adapt, even as one remains cautious about any challenges thrown their way; generally speaking, this mix of new ideas and careful oversight makes ongoing education absolutely essential in this line of work (Ferrari et al., 2024; Sallam, 2023).

11.2.5. Peer Review and Accountability Mechanisms

Forensic science depends on solid peer reviews and clear-cut accountability—it is the backbone of building trust (Figure 11.10). These checks are not just formalities; they work as everyday safety nets that boost confidence in both the results and the methods used. Peer review is not merely about confirming that methods are sound; it also digs into ethical matters so that scientific advances do not endanger people's rights or well-being, generally keeping progress in check. A few recent studies even suggest that a significant amount of research often overlooks legal and ethical considerations, particularly in emerging fields such as algorithmic technology for mental health, which can result in gaps in accountability and transparency (Gooding et al., 2021). Also, discussions about dataset documentation in computer vision suggest that when efficiency is pushed to the front, key ethical values can get overlooked – a reminder that we need frameworks which balance rigorous science with ethical oversight (Scheuerman et al., 2021).

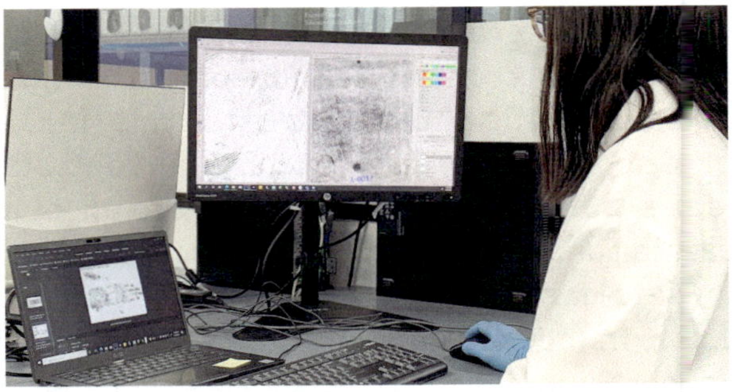

Figure 11.10. Forensic science depends on solid peer reviews and clear-cut accountability—it is the backbone of building trust.

Source: Center for Statistics and Applications in Forensic Evidence. (2022). *Analyzing Prints.* https://forensicstats.org/wp-content/uploads/2022/06/analyzing-prints.jpg.

11.2.6. Reporting Unethical Behavior

Forensics relies on keeping its ethical bar sky-high, especially when odd or shady behavior shows up. Calling out these questionable moves is not just about keeping the public's confidence—it also sets up a kind of accountability system within the field. There is a unique mix here: the way professionals learn about ethics and how they actually report problems seems to shape their overall moral compass. Solid ethical training can spark an openness that makes folks more likely to flag issues; some recent studies (Sivasamy et al., 2024) even point out a need for better training in this regard. A quick look reveals that students and faculty sometimes see unethical behavior in very different lights (Bodinaku et al., 2024), which hints that a bit more awareness and flexible accountability measures might be in order. In the end, having a strong, if not a bit messy, framework to report these issues is key to keeping forensic work both trustworthy and true to its mission.

11.2.7. Consequences of Professional Misconduct

Good forensic practice is key to keeping our public trust and upholding the ethical standards in medicine (Figure 11.11). In most instances, when misconduct among professionals happens, it does not just affect one person—it ripples out, impacting the legal system and even the wider healthcare community. Sometimes, such problematic behavior can call into question whether forensic evidence is really as reliable as it should be; there have been cases when breaches in ethics have compromised the accuracy of investigations, leading to situations where wrongful convictions become a real risk.

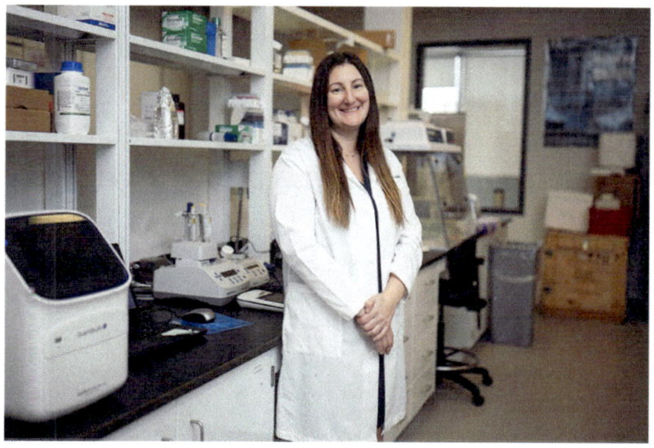

Figure 11.11. Good forensic practice is key to keeping our public trust and upholding the ethical standards in medicine.

Source: University of Toronto Magazine. (2024). *Nicole Novroski in Her Laboratory.* https://magazine.utoronto.ca/wp-content/uploads/2024/04/nicole-novroski-lab.jpg.

This, in turn, weakens the fundamental ideas of justice and fairness that most of us count on in the legal system. Research also suggests that the cultural and ethical environment within organizations generally shapes how professionals behave, which brings along its own set of social and internal challenges (Kashefi et al., 2024). All in all, fostering an environment that truly places ethical conduct first appears essential to lessening the adverse effects of misconduct, aligning well with public health ethics that typically stress fair resource allocation during crises (Novotný et al., 2024).

11.2.8. Case Studies of Misconduct in Forensics

Misconduct in forensic medicine can sometimes hit harder than expected. Even a small slip—intentional or merely careless—might trigger wrongful convictions and, over time, erode public confidence in our justice system. There are cases out there where forensic professionals ended up facing discipline for bending facts or relying on methods that just did not hold up; these examples really drive home the point. You could say that such missteps are best seen in the broader picture of legal rules and labor law expectations that generally point out how medical professionals should act. And now, with new technologies like artificial intelligence in telemedicine, fresh concerns—such as breaches of patient rights and data security—only add another complex layer to this ethical puzzle (Akbar et al., 2024; Razieva, 2025).

11.2.9. Best Practices for Maintaining Professionalism

Professionalism sits at the heart of forensic work, playing a key role in upholding ethics and building trust among people (Figure 11.12). Regular education is a big factor—it nudges us to notice those important bits of medical ethics and proper conduct that might otherwise be missed. Research generally shows that when students dive into clinical settings, their understanding of these values gets a real boost; aspects like communication and confidentiality often come through more clearly in practice (Shaikh et al., 2025). Also, training programs that are thoughtfully designed can, over time, weave these virtues into everyday practice by not only sharing knowledge but also by checking on how one acts in a clinical setup (Shrivastava et al., 2024). Ultimately, adhering to these approaches is essential for maintaining the integrity of forensic medicine and fostering a genuine culture of accountability, respect, and—yes—a human touch that is not entirely predictable.

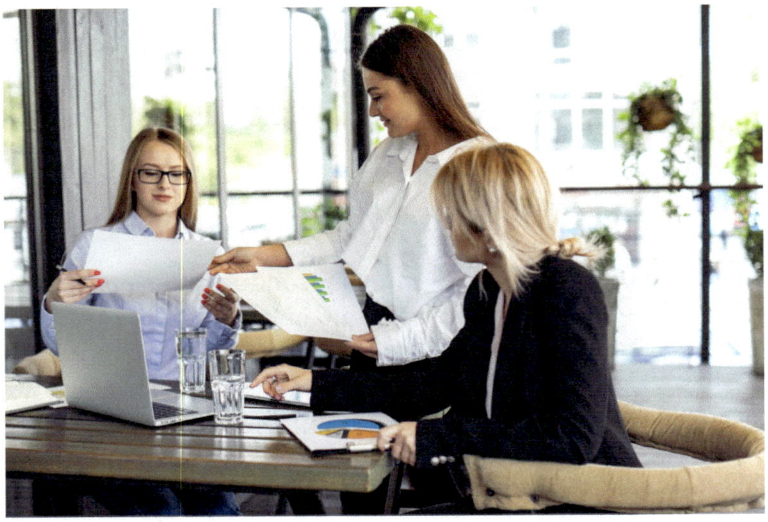

Figure 11.12. Professionalism sits at the heart of forensic work, playing a key role in upholding ethics and building trust among people.

Source: LinkedIn. (n.d.). *Cybersecurity Concept with Digital Padlock.* https://media.licdn.com/dms/image/v2/D4D12AQH9qz7CI7gPEA/article-cover_image-shrink_720_1280/article-cover_image-shrink_720_1280/0/1688128742119?e=2147483647&v=beta&t=w0iEyJAeWEKJvNm9TXTx0J_T4j9Bwoha7bEyDO05J5g.

Test Your Knowledge

1. What is meant by professional conduct in forensic medicine?
2. Why is impartiality crucial in a forensic expert's work?

11.3. Challenges in Forensic Ethics

Learning Outcome

1. Explain conflicts of interest in forensic evaluations;
2. Discuss pressure from law enforcement and legal entities;
3. Focus on media influence on forensic practices;
4. Know ethical dilemmas in expert testimony;
5. Balance scientific evidence and legal standards;
6. Handle sensitive information and vulnerable populations;
7. Discuss the ethical implications of technology in forensics;
8. Address bias and discrimination in forensic work;
9. Identify future challenges in forensic ethics.

Forensic ethics can be a real maze—it throws unexpected challenges at those trying to juggle scientific exactness with moral duties. Practitioners, for instance, constantly face questions about maintaining objectivity, ensuring confidentiality, and the risk that their findings might be misused; these issues are particularly pressing in high-pressure cases where every detail could sway legal outcomes. The increasing use of tools like artificial intelligence and machine learning only deepens the mix, stirring up fresh worries about who's really accountable when evidence interpretation goes off track (Mariani et al., 2021). Recent rules—take the AI Act proposed by the European Commission, for example—add another level of regulatory concern, generally calling for a careful rethinking of risk assessments and enforcement practices (Veale et al., 2021). In most cases, dealing with these varied and sometimes overlapping challenges is not just a matter of keeping standards; it is essential for preserving the trust that forensic science brings to our justice system.

11.3.1. Conflicts of Interest in Forensic Evaluations

Forensic evaluations can be a complex and intricate process. Experts often end up caught between the ironclad rules of the law and their own sense of what's right—so conflicts of interest are not all that surprising. Instead of the usual clinical setting, where patient care takes center stage, forensic work forces professionals to navigate a complex mix of legal demands and ethical expectations; they must maintain honest evaluations while catering to the needs of the court (Bulska, 2024). In most cases, even a small ethical misstep can shake not only the credibility of the findings but the whole idea of justice itself (Kitulwatte et al., 2019). Overall, striking that delicate balance means staying transparent and true to both individual welfare and larger societal trust, even if the path is not always perfectly straight (Figure 11.13).

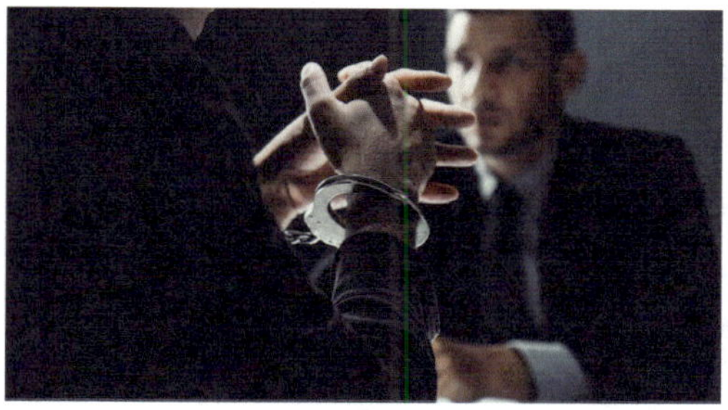

Figure 11.13. Conflicts of interest in forensic evaluations.

Source: The Chicago School of Professional Psychology. (2019). *5 Traits that Can Help Your Success in Forensic Psychology.* https://www.thechicagoschool.edu/insightadmin/2019/06/InstightDigital_1404x766_5-traits-that-can-help-your-success-in-forensic-psychology_24.jpg.

11.3.2. Pressure from Law Enforcement and Legal Entities

Forensic science and the legal system often collide in ways that stir up ethical puzzles—

pressure from law enforcement and legal offices can muddy the waters. In many cases, experts end up being nudged into producing findings tailored to an investigation's needs, and that sometimes means pure scientific objectivity gets a bit compromised. This rush for quick results tends to push accuracy aside, which can chip away at the public's trust in forensic evidence. Additionally, our growing reliance on technology—especially the secretive, black-box side of AI—raises concerns about the transparency and accountability of these methods (Ali et al., 2023); verifying what is produced is not always straightforward. There is also the risk that biased data usage might disproportionately impact marginalized groups, ultimately eroding trust in AI systems (Schwartz et al., 2022). Generally speaking, sticking closely to ethical standards remains essential if we are to keep these pressures in check and preserve the true integrity of forensic evidence.

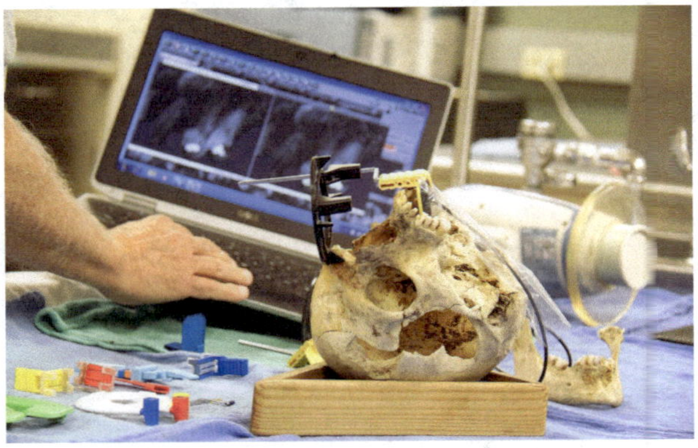

Figure 11.14. Forensics and the media mix in ways that really sway how the public sees things, often stirring up calls for more openness and responsibility in the field.

Source: Medium. (n.d.). *Digital Illustration of a Human Brain with Interconnected Nodes* https://miro.medium.com/v2/resize:fit:4000/1*dLtQrV-yvZ_AFvMR6zP[illegible]Tg.jpeg.

11.3.3. Media Influence on Forensic Practices

Forensics and the media mix in ways that really sway how the public sees things, often stirring up calls for more openness and responsibility in the field (Figure 11.14). In most cases, when news coverage becomes overly dramatic, it can distort what people expect from the careful work of forensic experts—making the entire evidentiary process seem simpler than it actually is. For example, ethical guidelines like those set out by the Indian Psychiatric Society in 1989 generally stress that practitioners must be both skilled and mindful of patient care (Gundugurti et al., 2022). Similarly, legal ideas such as the proposed AI Act remind us to monitor how new technology is applied in forensics - rules need to evolve in tandem with the changing methods of evidence analysis (Veale et al., 2021). Even though the media can, at times, educate the public, its influence also brings extra challenges that demand a careful, sometimes uneven, approach to upholding ethical forensic practices.

11.3.4. Ethical Dilemmas in Expert Testimony

Expert testimony in forensic psychiatry presents some truly challenging ethical dilemmas. Being neutral while shouldering the messy mix of legal and social pressures is no easy feat. Sometimes, these tensions among professionals even spark personal attacks or downright unprofessional behavior that can wreck the whole evaluation process (Rosenbaum et al., 2021). Generally speaking, practitioners often find themselves urged to treat everyone with a basic dose of dignity—a kind of moral nudge that pushes them to respect both clients and colleagues (Mšová et al., 2018). The fallout from biased testimony is not confined to a single case, it often shifts the overall ethical tone of forensic practice in unexpected ways. All in all, sticking to integrity is not merely about checking off boxes—it is really about a firm commitment to professionalism, even when the pressure ramps up.

11.3.5. Balancing Scientific Evidence and Legal Standards

Science and law often bump into each other in forensic work—issues like medical ethics and how professionals behave end up making things real messy. Forensic experts, generally speaking, find themselves juggling solid scientific evidence with the sometimes-rigid legal rules that govern their actions.

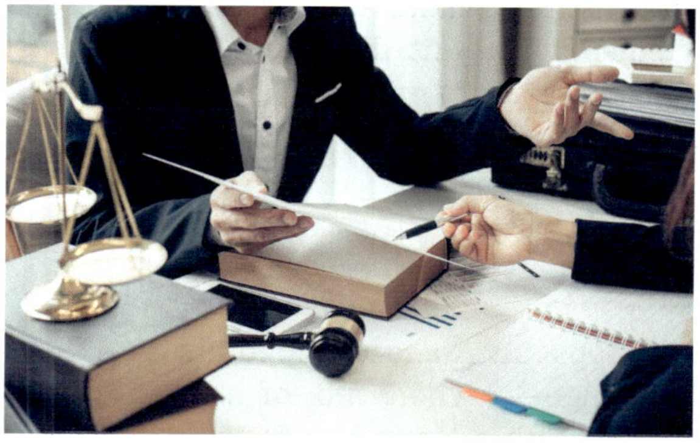

Figure 11.15. Forensic experts, generally speaking, find themselves juggling solid scientific evidence with the sometimes-rigid legal rules that govern their actions.

Source: Amnaj Khetsamtip. (2020). *Businessman and Lawyer Discuss the Contract Document.*

New tech, like artificial intelligence, only adds to this mix; its inner workings tend to be pretty murky, which can make reading evidence a real challenge. Lately, people have been pointing out that Explainable AI (XAI) is needed because, in most cases, understanding how decisions are made helps build trust in forensic results (Ali et al., 2023). There is also the problem of biases creeping into these systems; such slants can hurt individuals' lives and even undermine public confidence in the justice system (Schwartz et al., 2022). All in all, navigating these overlapping demands—balancing science, law, and emerging tech—is key to keeping forensic practice both fair and trustworthy (Figure 11.15).

11.3.6. Handling Sensitive Information and Vulnerable Populations

Ethical guidelines matter a lot when managing sensitive data and helping vulnerable people—it is a challenge that forensic experts face every day. Professionals often find themselves wading through tangled emotions, especially when dealing with individuals who have experienced trauma or exploitation; this constant reminder reinforces that respecting personal privacy and autonomy is not optional but essential. It really comes down to making sure that people feel safe and supported throughout the investigation, a point that cannot be ignored. Furthermore, emerging tools like artificial intelligence introduce new concerns about data privacy and potential bias that could inadvertently harm those already at risk. The current buzz around XAI generally shows that keeping decision-making clear and open is key to earning trust among everyone involved (Ali et al., 2023). In many cases, recent studies suggest that organizations should tread carefully regarding the treatment of personal data—turning it into a commodity might lead to unexpected, sometimes even harmful, outcomes that slowly erode public trust (Schwartz et al., 2022).

11.3.7. Ethical Implications of Technology in Forensics

Tech's entry into forensic work raises numerous ethical questions that cannot be easily brushed aside. With the surge of AI and data crunching methods, one often finds that the shiny benefits must be balanced against risks like inherent bias, murky transparency, and accountability issues. For example, even though these tools can speed up data analysis and smooth out processes, they might just as easily carry forward old biases hidden in their training data. Recent studies generally point out that issues—ranging from spreading misleading information to a lack of genuine originality—can seriously shake the credibility of forensic evidence (Sallam, 2023). Meanwhile, there is an urgent call for clear ethical guidelines so that these innovations serve justice instead of muddling it up (Mariani et al., 2021); in the end, handling these complexities is pretty crucial for keeping the ethical backbone of forensic medicine intact (Figure 11.16).

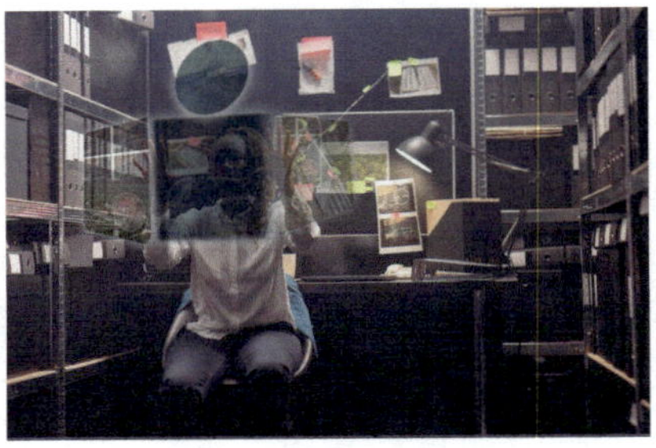

Figure 11.16. Ethical implications of technology in forensics.

Source: ECS Infotech. (2024). *Digital Forensics Investigation in Progress.* https://www.ecsinfotech.com/wp-content/uploads/2024/04/77819.jpg.

11.3.8. Addressing Bias and Discrimination in Forensic Work

Bias and discrimination keep rearing their heads in forensic work, bringing with them some heavy ethical debates that demand real attention. Personal biases can skew evidence interpretation and, in many cases, shift justice outcomes—a problem that hits marginalized folks especially hard. These issues tend to worsen when long-standing inequalities persist in the legal system, leading to different treatment based on factors like race, gender, or socioeconomic standing. Simple training tweaks, such as incorporating elements on implicit bias and cultural awareness, may help forensic professionals recognize and mitigate their own biases. Setting up standard procedures that stress openness and accountability is also a must; after all, clear guidelines can make investigations feel a lot more trustworthy. When forensic practitioners adhere to practices that are fair and balanced, the integrity of their work is upheld, and justice ultimately reaches everyone without undue prejudice. In most cases, taking a hands-on, proactive approach to reducing bias and discrimination in forensic work seems key to nurturing a more just society (Sallam, 2023).

11.3.9. Future Challenges in Forensic Ethics

Tech keeps racing ahead, and forensics is feeling the change—a whole mix of new approaches and fresh ethical puzzles. AI tools and digital evidence gathering compel us, in most cases, to rethink the traditional ethical playbook to maintain the integrity and reliability of forensic work. Remote autopsies and hybrid simulation techniques, while they open up cool educational doors, also bring up tough questions about consent and whether the deceased are treated with the dignity they deserve (Jaramillo-Rincón et al., 2024). Sometimes, the rush to deliver fast answers can lure forensic analysts into bending standards, and that can lead to misinformation that might even tip legal decisions (Bulska, 2024). Balancing these advancements with solid ethical care is, generally speaking, crucial for justice and public confidence as the field twists and turns. Experts, educators, and policymakers must continue to discuss and update these ethical ideas as circumstances evolve.

Test Your Knowledge

1. How should a forensic expert respond to pressure from law enforcement to alter findings?
2. What are the ethical challenges in maintaining confidentiality while fulfilling legal obligations?

11.4. Case Studies in Forensic Ethics

Learning Outcome

1. Understand landmark cases influencing forensic ethics;
2. Know analysis of ethical breaches in high-profile cases;
3. Lessons learned from historical cases;
4. Describe the role of ethics committees in forensic cases;
5. Discuss the impact of case outcomes on public perception;
6. Focus on ethical considerations in wrongful convictions;
7. Learn forensic ethics in international contexts;
8. Compare the analysis of ethical standards globally;
9. Give recommendations based on case study findings.

Case studies bring out how ethics and forensic work really mix in unexpected ways—real situations where professionals often face heartfelt dilemmas. It is not just about following a strict code; sometimes a lapse, however small, or a hint of bias causes real harm, leaving a mark on the credibility and the overall trust in our justice system. In many cases, a single ethical misstep can skew legal outcomes, making people wonder if the process is really fair. As forensic methods change and new technologies—like artificial intelligence and peer support systems—emerge, there is a growing discussion about transparency and who's accountable when things go wrong. Tools like ChatGPT, for example, might boost efficiency and tighten scientific work, but they also force us to look closer at potential risks such as bias and misinformation (Sallam, 2023). Similarly, depending on peer support in labs opens up both promising opportunities and tricky challenges that, in most cases, deserve a second look (Shalaby et al., 2020).

11.4.1. Landmark Cases Influencing Forensic Ethics

Landmark legal cases keep stirring up debates about ethics mixed in with cultural cues in forensic work. In everyday investigations, professionals encounter a wide range of people from diverse cultural backgrounds, and these interactions often carry significant ethical implications (Figure 11.17).

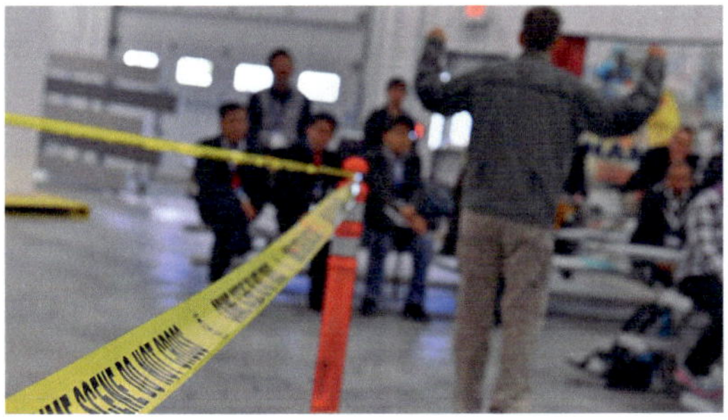

Figure 11.17. In everyday investigations, professionals meet all kinds of people from varied cultural backgrounds, and these encounters bring along some pretty serious ethical baggage.

Source: SciDev.Net. (n.d.). *Forensic Science Main.* https://www.scidev.net/global/wp-content/uploads/Forensic-science-main.jpg.

History shows that not being aware enough of cultural contexts has often led to miscommunications—and even outright ethical slip-ups—during interviews. Researchers, generally speaking, keep reminding us that forensic methods need a healthy dose of cultural insight, especially when dealing with vulnerable groups like survivors of gender-based violence and asylum seekers (Hope et al., 2021). At the same time, the growing influence of data practices in tech-heavy fields such as computer vision raises extra questions about how humans are represented in forensic datasets, pushing experts to juggle efficiency with genuine care for their subjects (Scheuerman et al., 2021). All in all, these varied situations highlight an urgent need for ethical guidelines that are not only formally strict but also truly in tune with the cultural nuances of real-world settings.

11.4.2. Analysis of Ethical Breaches in High-Profile Cases

Ethical breaches in big forensic cases can create serious fallout—not just hurting those directly involved but also chipping away at the public's trust in our health and legal systems. These issues usually crop up from a messy mix of human missteps, institutional pressures, and rapid-fire tech advances, all of which point to why we really need better checks and balance. Sometimes, when evidence is tampered with or conflicts of interest are not properly flagged, the whole legal process can go awry, sometimes even leading to wrongful convictions. One also has to consider how artificial intelligence is becoming involved in forensics; its increasing use sparks new debates about transparency and accountability (Wang et al., 2023). And then there is the case of those opaque machine-learning models—which often function like mysterious black boxes—demanding a careful look to make sure ethical standards are generally met and, ultimately, to keep trust afloat, especially when real lives are on the line (Zhang et al., 2022) (Figure 11.18).

11.4.3. Lessons Learned from Historical Cases

Looking back at many old forensic cases, you see how ethics and professional behavior mix in ways that are not always clear-cut. There were moments—like wrongful convictions built on shaky forensic evidence—that really drive home the need for strict guidelines and real accountability in the field. Nowadays, some new technology even tracks how we perceive things, offering clues into how forensic investigations learn and evolve (Smirnova, 2023). At the same time, as more forensic experts lean on artificial intelligence for assessments, concerns about data integrity and privacy start emerging as major issues (Wang et al., 2023). When you sift through these historical instances, you gain not only a better sense of current practices but also a push to update ethical frameworks, ensuring professionals remain vigilant against the quirks and potential pitfalls of new innovations.

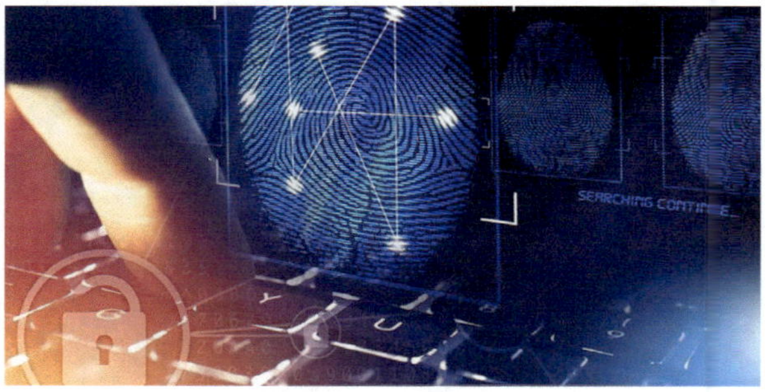

Figure 11.18. Some new technology even tracks how we perceive things, offering clues into how forensic investigations learn and evolve.

Source: BCC Research. (2024). *Forensics Industry Overview.* https://blog.bccresearch.com/hubfs/forensics-industry.webp.

11.4.4. Role of Ethics Committees in Forensic Cases

In forensic psychiatry, keeping ethical standards intact really shapes court decisions and public safety. Ethics committees, almost like behind-the-scenes watchdogs, check on forensic experts to make sure they stick not only to basic rules but also promote a respectful, team-oriented vibe among professionals. It is not just about following a strict list; it is about actually living those values and building trust within the community. Mangiardi and Pelligrino point out that, generally speaking, a commitment to solid ethical research and proper citation of sources is a core duty for individuals in the field (Rosenbaum et al., 2021). Surprisingly, only about 10.9% of medical students seem to know these committees even exist (Chatterjee et al., 2012)—a sign that ethics does not get enough spotlight in forensic training. This gap clearly signals a need for better, more hands-on ethics education in these programs. In short, upholding these principles is not abstract theory; it is a concrete part of ensuring fair justice and safe communities.

11.4.5. Impact of Case Outcomes on Public Perception

Forensic case verdicts really shape how people view both their doctors and our entire justice system (Figure 11.19). When high-profile cases conclude with either complete exoneration or a clear stamp of malpractice, they can significantly alter public sentiment - investigations into malpractice claims support this (Pérez-Puentes et al., 2024).

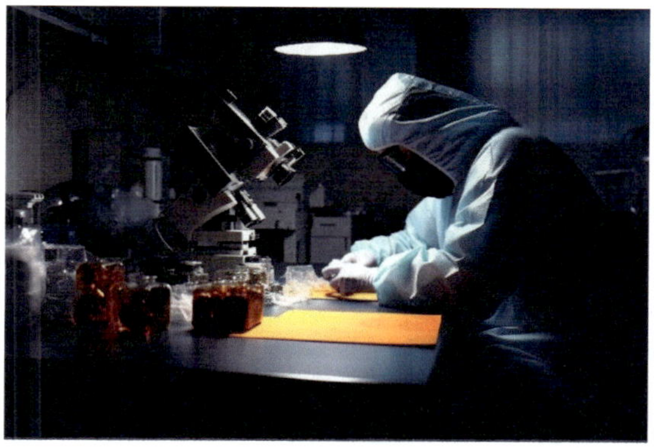

Figure 11.19. Forensic case verdicts really shape how people view both their doctors and our entire justice system.

Source: Fighter Law. (2024). *Forensic Scientist Analyzing Evidence.* https://www.fighterlaw.com/wp-content/uploads/2024/01/forensic-scientist-analyzing-evidence.jpg.

The very idea of what makes a professional practitioner ends up wedded to these decisions; negative media spins, for instance, can spark doubts among training house officers (and others) who witness unprofessional behavior firsthand (Noor et al., 2024). Even though most medicolegal reports tend to clear healthcare professionals - one study even noted that malpractice was absent in 98.2% of cases - it remains a real challenge to communicate these findings effectively to everyone. In most cases, this complex relationship between forensic outcomes and public perception necessitates a careful and thoughtful examination of ethical practices in the field.

11.4.6. Ethical Considerations in Wrongful Convictions

Wrongful convictions do not just hurt those directly targeted—they throw the whole criminal justice system into a kind of ethical tailspin. Forensic professionals, for instance, bear a heavy responsibility to keep their findings spot-on; even a tiny mistake can wreak havoc on an individual's life and disturb the wider community. In analytical chemistry, the call to adhere to strict ethical standards is clear—mistakes or shady practices can cause irreparable harm and hinder genuine justice (Bulska, 2024). Then there is the side of medical ethics and legal medicine, where, generally speaking, solid ethical guidelines are seen as key to managing the messiness of forensic work, a point underlined by several studies (Sharifi et al., 2022). In a nutshell, if forensic experts foster a genuine culture of accountability, they may significantly reduce the likelihood of wrongful convictions while preserving the core principles of justice.

11.4.7. Forensic Ethics in International Contexts

Nowadays, forensic ethics jumps over country lines, influencing practices in ways that are not easily boxed into one system. Take consent, confidentiality, and even how forensic evidence gets used—these ideas shift a lot depending on the local laws and customs, so what is accepted in one place might raise eyebrows in another. Forensic professionals often have to figure out these puzzles, balancing respect for traditions with legal expectations, which generally nudges them toward wanting one kind of universal ethical guide. Consider global health projects that report on disease burdens (Ferrari et al., 2024); here, ethical matters require careful handling so that interventions remain scientifically sound while also acknowledging cultural sensitivities. And as newer stuff like AI starts popping up in forensics, there is a real need to talk about transparency and bias—making sure that even when embracing fresh tech, everyone stays on the responsible side (Sallam, 2023).

11.4.8. Comparative Analysis of Ethical Standards Globally

Ethical norms vary a lot worldwide, and these differences really shape how medicine gets practiced, especially in forensic work (Figure 11.20). Often, this is not just random—it mostly stems from cultural, legal, and social influences that, in most cases, shape how ethical decisions are made. Take coercive practices like pushing for involuntary hospitalization, for example: in some regions, patient rights get almost exclusive focus, while in other areas, protecting the public is considered paramount (Chieze et al., 2021).

These mixed approaches, frankly, reflect just how tricky it is to keep medical integrity intact when crossing borders. And then there is the whole matter of new technology—advancements that help track perception and can clarify interactions in educational settings, yet they also stir up debates about consent and privacy in forensic contexts (Smirnova, 2023). When professionals in forensic medicine find themselves navigating these shifting ethical backdrops, it becomes pretty clear that leaning on a framework which weaves together all these varied concerns with basic humanitarian values is essential.

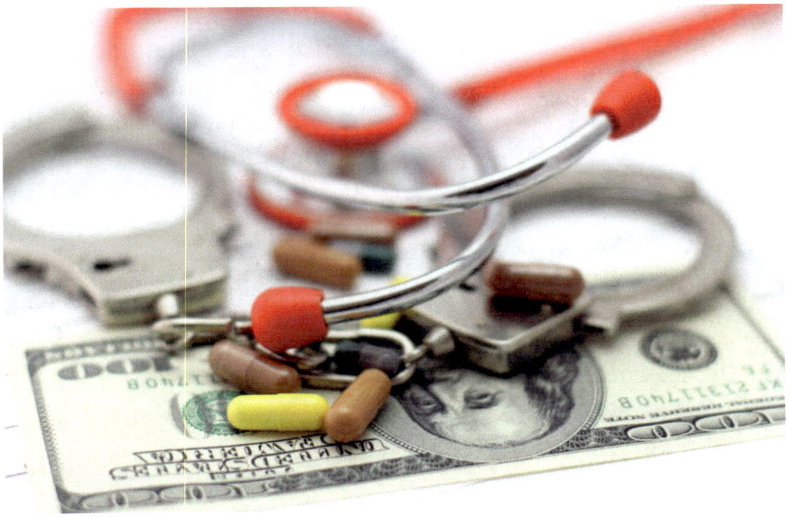

Figure 11.20. Ethical norms vary a lot worldwide, and these differences really shape how medicine gets practiced, especially in forensic work.

Source: iPleaders. (2019). *Forensic Science Under Criminal Law.* https://blog.ipleaders.in/wp-content/uploads/2019/06/images-10.jpg.

11.4.9. Recommendations Based on Case Study Findings

Forensic work tied up with medical ethics is not a neat, one-size-fits-all puzzle. Instead, a mix of ideas drawn from various case studies appears to be what is needed. For example, building trust in AI for health care may come down to simply talking more clearly and getting users more involved – recent findings (Starke et al., 2025) suggest that positive, down-to-earth interactions with these systems can really make a difference. Tackling the stubborn problem of burn fatalities requires prevention plans that take a close look at who gets hurt and how things go wrong; this can involve rethinking investigation protocols and raising public awareness about burn risks in home settings (Lama et al., 2024). All in all, these thoughts point to the need for a unified approach that weds the pace of modern tech with honest ethical insights and practical education – paving the way for a forensic practice that is more trustworthy and effective.

Test Your Knowledge

1 Was there any conflict of interest in the case? If so, how was it handled?

2 Did the forensic professional remain impartial, or was there evidence of bias?

SUMMARY

Forensic science is changing fast, and it is clear that sticking to solid medical ethics and good conduct really counts. The mix of healthcare and legal duties makes it necessary for forensic experts to think twice about how their choices affect both patients and the justice system—sometimes in ways you might not expect. A quick review of past missteps reveals that issues such as off-target prescriptions and inadequate treatment decisions can significantly disrupt lives in these cases (Berzina et al., 2025). It is also interesting to note that ethical training for many new healthcare pros is not always up to par; studies reveal notable gaps in the ethical know-how of those just starting out in the field (Jamal et al., 2024). By blending real-world experience with more traditional learning, the forensic community can boost its commitment to high standards and integrity, ensuring that justice gets done while keeping everyone's health and rights in check.

Medical ethics and professional duties in forensics often become intertwined, creating hurdles that are not always easy to navigate. Bias—often sneaking in subtly—shows up in forensic work, especially when technology takes the plunge into decision-making; this is not simply a neat swap of data for judgment. Organizations now struggle with using complex data methods, sometimes risking inadvertent harm to people or communities, which makes the entire process even more complicated. Look at the COVID-19 episode; it made it glaringly obvious how external shocks can upend care, particularly in mental health, leaving professionals to scramble under increased pressure. The stress, shifting work setups, and raw reality of the field have reshaped what ethical duty means for those in forensic medical practice, nudging us (in most cases) to demand clearer guidelines and firmer support systems for everyone involved (Foye et al., 2021; Schwartz et al., 2022).

KEY TERMS FROM THIS CHAPTER

- Analysis
- Credibility
- Education
- Personal bias
- Professional identity
- Technology
- Commitment
- Decision-making
- Fair
- Professional behavior
- Public trusts
- Training

CRITICAL THINKING QUESTIONS

1. **Which of the following principles is primarily concerned with ensuring that a forensic practitioner causes no harm to the patient or individual involved in an investigation?**
   a. Autonomy
   b. Non-maleficence
   c. Justice
   d. Beneficence
2. **In the context of forensic medicine, informed consent is most important for which of the following?**
   a. Reporting findings to law enforcement
   b. Performing a medicolegal autopsy
   c. Using a patient's blood sample for testing
   d. All of the above
3. **Which of the following best describes the ethical principle of confidentiality in forensic medicine?**
   a. Forensic doctors must never share any medical information
   b. Forensic doctors must share all medical information with the police
   c. Confidential information should be shared only with those legally authorized to receive it
   d. Forensic doctors can share information with family members of the deceased without permission
4. **What should a forensic professional do if they are pressured to provide a biased testimony in court?**
   a. Agree to the request to avoid legal consequences
   b. Refuse to testify
   c. Remain impartial and provide only factual information
   d. Alter the testimony to suit the needs of the defense or prosecution
5. **Which of the following best defines the dual loyalty ethical dilemma faced by forensic professionals?**
   a. Balancing professional duties with personal opinions
   b. Choosing between the legal system and healthcare interests
   c. Determining whether to prioritize patient care or law enforcement objectives
   d. Deciding whether to report a crime or keep it confidential

Short Answer Questions

1. What is the importance of medical ethics in forensic practice?
2. How does confidentiality apply to medicolegal cases?
3. When can a forensic doctor breach patient confidentiality legally?
4. What is informed consent, and why is it essential in forensic examinations?
5. How should a medical professional handle dual loyalty in custodial deaths or police cases?
6. What are the ethical responsibilities of a doctor during a medicolegal autopsy?
7. How does a forensic expert maintain professional impartiality during legal testimony?

Answers to Critical Thinking Questions

1. (b); 2. (d); 3. (c); 4. (c); 5. (c)

REFERENCES

1. Akbar, M. F., Tianwin, J., Devano, E., & Kartawiguna, D., (2024). Assessing the impact of medical ethics violations on the effectiveness of artificial intelligence in telemedicine. In *2024 12th International Conference on Cyber and IT Service Management (CITSM)*. https://www.semanticscholar.org/paper/1e18e8ae1fb252a9f8b7792bc3fb7ff75d730232 (accessed on 9th May 2025).
2. Ali, S., Abuhmed, T., El-Sappagh, S., Muhammad, K., Alonso, J. M., Confalonieri, R., Guidotti, R., et al. (2023). Explainable artificial intelligence (XAI): What we know and what is left to attain trustworthy artificial intelligence. *Information Fusion, 99*, 101805. https://doi.org/10.1016/j.inffus.2023.101805.
3. Anjum, N., Alshahrani, H., Shaikh, A., Mahreen-Ul-Hassan, M., Kiran, M., Raz, S., & Alam, A., (2025). Cyber-biosecurity challenges in next-generation sequencing: A comprehensive analysis of emerging threat vectors. *IEEE Access, 13*, 52006–52035. https://www.semanticscholar.org/paper/9645dfcdf3984098c659c194745929a2fa0d18c3 (accessed on 9th May 2025).
4. Berzina, A., & Pletenetska, A. O. (2025). Forensic medical and legal analysis of cases of improper performance of professional duties by medical employees, including incorrect prescription of medical products. *Polski Merkuriusz Lekarski: Organ Polskiego Towarzystwa Lekarskiego, 53*(1), 94–99. https://www.semanticscholar.org/paper/02401bff69d4348e778 6465ecfbfa5212ac70fa3 (accessed on 9th May 2025).
5. Bodinaku, B., Sula, G., & Zahaj, S., (2024). Ethics in conflict: Diverging views on unethical behavior among students and faculty in Albanian higher education. *Journal of Educational and Social Research*. https://www.semanticscholar.org/paper/e20baa79cae0d1cc63d1ff819c5fce7e9c1f1686 (accessed on 9th May 2025).
6. Bulska, E., (2024). From afar and from the inside: About the importance of ethics in the global world of science. *Brazilian Journal of Analytical Chemistry*. https://www.semanticscholar.org/paper/201a572f3cb68f4ece61c312d016c6117c9f0c77 (accessed on 9th May 2025).
7. Chatterjee, B., & Sarkar, J., (2012). Awareness of medical ethics among undergraduates in a West Bengal medical college. *Indian Journal of Medical Ethics, 9*(2), 93–100. https://www.semanticscholar.org/paper/2af400a8a252e8e73a91a5642ffca9d0dd085f10 (accessed on 9th May 2025).
8. Chieze, M., Clavien, C., Kaiser, S., & Hurst, S., (2021). Coercive measures in psychiatry: A review of ethical arguments. *Frontiers in Psychiatry, 12*. https://doi.org/10.3389/fpsyt.2021.790886.
9. Cortegiani, A., Battaglini, D., Amato, G., Behr, A., Donadello, K., Einav, S., Frigo, M. G., et al. (2024). Dissemination of clinical and scientific practice through social media: A SIAARTI consensus-based document. *Journal of Anesthesia, Analgesia and Critical Care, 4*. https://www.semanticscholar.org/paper/49ed71bdd9b4c507d8d621e8513ae88b3e55406e (accessed on 9th May 2025).
10. De Micco, F., Martino, F., & Campobasso, C. P. (2020). Ethical issues in age assessment by the third molar development. *Australian Journal of Forensic Sciences, 54*, 88–99. https://doi.org/10.1080/00450618.2020.1789220.
11. Ferrari, A. J., Santomauro, D., Aali, A., Abate, Y. H., Abbafati, C., Abbastabar, H., Abd ElHafeez, S., et al. (2024). Global incidence, prevalence, years lived with disability (YLDs), disability-

adjusted life-years (DALYs), and healthy life expectancy (HALE) for 371 diseases and injuries in 204 countries and territories and 811 subnational locations, 1990–2021: A systematic analysis for the Global Burden of Disease Study 2021. *The Lancet, 403*, 2133–2161. https://doi.org/10.1016/s0140-6736(24)00757-8.

12. Ford, G. G. (2000). *Ethical Reasoning in the Mental Health Professions*. https://www.semanticscholar.org/paper/f724f07cf84695de69caa36a2ca6cf0bc7afc251 (accessed on 9th May 2025).

13. Foye, U., Dalton-Locke, C., Harju-Seppänen, J., Lane, R., Beames, L., Vera, S. J. N., Johnson, S., et al. (2021). How has COVID-19 affected mental health nurses and the delivery of mental health nursing care in the UK? Results of a mixed-methods study. *Journal of Psychiatric and Mental Health Nursing, 28*, 126–137. https://doi.org/10.1111/jpm.12745.

14. Gooding, P., & Kariotis, T., (2021). Ethics and law in research on algorithmic and data-driven technology in mental health care: Scoping review. *JMIR Mental Health, 8*, e24668. https://doi.org/10.2196/24668.

15. Gundugurti, P. R., Bhattacharyya, R., Kondepi, S., Chakraborty, K., & Mukherjee, A., (2022). Ethics and law. *Indian Journal of Psychiatry, 64*, S7–S15. https://doi.org/10.4103/indianjpsychiatry.indianjpsychiatry_726_21.

16. Harabišová, M., (2018). *Medical Ethics in Dimensions*, 2018, 51–58. Matej Bel University in Banská Bystrica, https://www.semanticscholar.org/paper/7df6c5be5bf4f41ed406c4fce232d702caa12aba (accessed on 9th May 2025).

17. Hope, L., Anakwah, N., Antfolk, J., Brubacher, S. P., Flowe, H. D., Gabbert, F., Giebels, E., et al. (2021). Urgent issues and prospects at the intersection of culture, memory, and witness interviews: Exploring the challenges for research and practice. *Legal and Criminological Psychology, 27*, 1–31. https://doi.org/10.1111/lcrp.12202.

18. Jamal, S., Anwar, S., Anwar, F., Afraz, N., Idrees, H., Manzoor, I., Fayaz, S., et al. (2024). Awareness of medical ethics among undergraduates of physical therapy. *Journal of Health and Rehabilitation Research*. https://www.semanticscholar.org/paper/4b5fea8b8c1b064ea04a977c5da3fd51541dcdf7 (accessed on 9th May 2025).

19. Jaramillo-Rincón, S. X., Cortés, C. C., Contreras, V. L., Morales, P. K., & Nuñez, O. N., (2024). Crime scene simulation: A novel approach to forensic medicine education. *Voces y Silencios. Revista Latinoamericana de Educación*. https://www.semanticscholar.org/paper/698110b661e9a878150b4a2a383af6c736da5263 (accessed on 9th May 2025).

20. Jayalath, M., Nanayakkara, R., Jayasundara, K. M. P. D., Abeysekara, C. M., & Abeynayake, A. M. J. (2025). Are Sri Lankan allopathic medical practitioners ethical enough? A KAP survey in selected allopathic healthcare institutions in Sri Lanka. *Sri Lanka Journal of Health Research*. https://www.semanticscholar.org/paper/dd0fdff329cb72ce76ab56b3512e4839a3248e2f (accessed on 9th May 2025).

21. Karasik, N., (2023). Protecting the autonomy of patients with severe mental illness through psychiatric advance directive peer-facilitation. *Voices in Bioethics, 9*. https://doi.org/10.52214/vib.v9i.11800.

22. Kashefi, M. H., Bohlooli, N., Eskandari, K., & Emari, H., (2024). A holistic model of organizational trust with the approach of professional ethics in Iranian health system: A case study of the universities of medical sciences in Iran. *Research and Development in Medical Education*.

https://www.semanticscholar.org/paper/e0b4f77d39be25f1776db2625a6811ea04c3de09 (accessed on 9th May 2025).

23. Kitulwatte, I., & Edirisinghe, P., (2019). Ethical dilemmas in forensic medical practice. *Sri Lanka Journal of Forensic Medicine, Science & Law*. https://www.semanticscholar.org/paper/202e3bb7264f1408a7255ac718592de789910d20 (accessed on 9th May 2025).

24. Kling, D., Phillips, C., Kennett, D., & Tillmar, A., (2021). Investigative genetic genealogy: Current methods, knowledge and practice. *Forensic Science International Genetics, 52*, 102474. https://doi.org/10.1016/j.fsigen.2021.102474.

25. Lama, B., Gupta, V. P., & Thakuria, D., (2024). An autopsy-based study on the patterns of injuries of burn cases in Jorhat District, Assam. *Asian Journal of Pharmaceutical and Clinical Research*. https://www.semanticscholar.org/paper/338f9f6f78f7880aec5a9bc4939189d7fb90908e (accessed on 9th May 2025).

26. Mariani, M. M., Perez-Vega, R., & Wirtz, J., (2021). AI in marketing, consumer research and psychology: A systematic literature review and research agenda. *Psychology and Marketing, 39*, 755–776. https://doi.org/10.1002/mar.21619.

27. Mukesh, Y. (2022). New draft of National Medical Commission, Registered Medical Practitioner (Professional Conduct) Regulations, 2022: Critical analysis. *International Journal of Health Research and Medico-Legal Practice*. https://www.semanticscholar.org/paper/3a374d1daedc1d00575b9740d9ea19869ad94553 (accessed on 9th May 2025).

28. Noor, S., Aslam, F., Ejaz, A., Malik, A., Nasir, H., Awan, N., Khattak, I. Q., et al. (2024). Unprofessional behavior among house officers in Pakistan's public and private hospitals: Prevalence, perceptions, and participation. *Cureus, 16*. https://www.semanticscholar.org/paper/b15f7faa3a8f909c4aacf17c721ce16197a8d897 (accessed on 9th May 2025).

29. Novotný, R., Novotná, Z., Andraščíková, Š., & Smatana, J., (2024). Bioethics of pandemics and disasters within the context of public health ethics and ethics of social consequences. *Ethics & Bioethics, 14*, 72–79. https://www.semanticscholar.org/paper/d9822d39d6b010cc44e31992074fe2f311a37ae5 (accessed on 9th May 2025).

30. Olivier, M., (2016). On the morality of teaching students IT crime skills: Extended abstract. In *Proceedings of the Computer Science Education Research Conference 2016*. https://www.semanticscholar.org/paper/5431acfee7472338086a0b4bca4b651fc080b0e3 (accessed on 9th May 2025).

31. Pérez-Puentes, M. M., Sáez-Rodríguez, J., Girela-López, E., & Beltran-Aroca, C. M. (2024). Professional responsibility at the Institute of Legal Medicine and Forensic Sciences of Córdoba between 2012 and 2022. *Cuadernos de Medicina Forense*. https://www.semanticscholar.org/paper/45ae280f7233a28664a092d3c07eba759d13aef0 (accessed on 9th May 2025).

32. Ranade, N., & Saravia, M., (2024). Teaching AI ethics in technical and professional communication: A systematic review. *IEEE Transactions on Professional Communication 67*, 422–436. https://www.semanticscholar.org/paper/898d84785c6cad97f7b78b607d0418b7d6b49270 (accessed on 9th May 2025).

33. Razieva, D. B. (2025). Illegality as an element of disciplinary misconduct of medical workers. *Bulletin of the Institute of Legislation and Legal Information of the Republic of Kazakhstan*. https://www.semanticscholar.org/paper/b941b2da6da4e23deaef51874bfd4a021cdfc649 (accessed on 9th May 2025).

34. Rosenbaum, K. B., & Rosmarin, D., (2021). The boundaries of critiquing a colleague. *The Journal of the American Academy of Psychiatry and the Law, 49*, 470–472. https://www.semanticscholar.org/paper/9f216257071c65b974719bbd3781f8c5eea38b98 (accessed on 9th May 2025).

35. Sagan, S. D. (2016). Ethics, technology & war. *Daedalus, 145*, 6–11. https://doi.org/10.1162/daed_e_00407 (accessed on 9th May 2025).

36. Sallam, M., (2023). ChatGPT utility in healthcare education, research, and practice: Systematic review on the promising perspectives and valid concerns. *Healthcare, 11*, 887. https://doi.org/10.3390/healthcare11060887.

37. Sallam, M., (2023). The utility of ChatGPT as an example of large language models in healthcare education, research and practice: Systematic review on the future perspectives and potential limitations. *medRxiv*. Cold Spring Harbor Laboratory. https://doi.org/10.1101/2023.02.19.23286155.

38. Saputra, R., Zaid, M., Suwadi, P., Barkhuizen, J., & Tiolince, T., (2023). Reconstruction of chemical castration sanctions implementation based on the medical ethics code (Comparison with Russia and South Korea). *Lex Scientia Law Review, 7*, 61–118. https://doi.org/10.15294/lesrev.v7i1.64143.

39. Sarraf-Yazdi, S., Pisupati, A., Goh, C., Ong, Y. T., Toh, Y., Goh, S., & Krishna, L., (2024). A scoping review and theory-informed conceptual model of professional identity formation in medical education. *Medical Education*. https://www.semanticscholar.org/paper/49af5d403abb23fc69363c89d17b3a870ad194a3 (accessed on 9th May 2025).

40. Scheuerman, M. K., Hanna, A., & Denton, E., (2021). Do datasets have politics? Disciplinary values in computer vision dataset development. *Proceedings of the ACM on Human-Computer Interaction, 5*, 1–37. https://doi.org/10.1145/3476058.

41. Schwartz, R., Vassilev, A., Greene, K., Perine, L., Burt, A., & Hall, P., (2022). *Towards a Standard for Identifying and Managing Bias in Artificial Intelligence*. https://doi.org/10.6028/nist.sp.1270.

42. Senbekov, M., Saliev, T., Bukeyeva, Z., Almabayeva, A., Zhanaliyeva, M., Aitenova, N., Toishibekov, Y. M., et al. (2020). The recent progress and applications of digital technologies in healthcare: A review. *International Journal of Telemedicine and Applications, 2020*, 1–18. https://doi.org/10.1155/2020/8830200.

43. Shaikh, S. N., Abbas, U., Shah, T., Uqaili, A. A., Buksh, H. A., & Fatima, M., (2025). Self-assessment of medical ethics and professionalism: Comparison between preclinical and clinical medical students. *Journal of Medical Education and Curricular Development, 12*. https://www.semanticscholar.org/paper/5edc09f4ed479e5f297ef24796b784dff472b4e8 (accessed on 9th May 2025).

44. Shalaby, R., & Agyapong, V. I. O. (2020). Peer support in mental health: Literature review. *JMIR Mental Health, 7*, e15572. https://doi.org/10.2196/15572.

45. Sharifi, M., Ghadipasha, M., Shojaei, A., Nedjat, S., Rashidpouraie, R., Moosapour, H., & Tabatabaei, S. M. (2022). The ethical considerations in the main practices of the Iranian Legal Medicine Organization: A qualitative study. *International Journal of Medical Toxicology and Forensic Medicine*. https://www.semanticscholar.org/paper/ed4eb9ea2914b00298e9be217612b9b976aa02ff (accessed on 9th May 2025).

46. Shrivastava, S., & Suhoyo, Y., (2024). Educational framework to train undergraduate medical students in ethics and professionalism in India. *Journal of Medical Society*. https://www.semanticscholar.org/paper/718eb7250bda971b206edef6501b8603c4dcbe63 (accessed on 9th May 2025).
47. Simpson, S., Richardson, L., Pietrabissa, G., Castelnuovo, G., & Reid, C., (2020). Videotherapy and therapeutic alliance in the age of COVID-19. *Clinical Psychology & Psychotherapy, 28*, 409–421. https://doi.org/10.1002/cpp.2521.
48. Sivasamy, S., Patel, V. S., Prabhakaran, R., Dhandayuthapani, S., & Batra, J., (2024). Complexity, advances, adaptation, and shaping the future of medical ethics. *Santosh University Journal of Health Sciences*. https://www.semanticscholar.org/paper/a75303215f0e37ccb1807e53d57b1cfac3107078 (accessed on 9th May 2025).
49. Smirnova, Y. K. (2023). Application of eye-tracking technology dual eye tracking (DUET) in the study of cooperation between children with atypical development and adults in the learning process. *Forum, 1*, 98–99. https://doi.org/10.61365/forum.2023.078.
50. Starke, G., Gille, F., Termine, A., Aquino, Y. S. J., Chavarriaga, R., Ferrario, A., Hastings, J., et al. (2025). Finding consensus on trust in AI in health care: Recommendations from a panel of international experts. *Journal of Medical Internet Research, 27*. https://www.semanticscholar.org/paper/408c4479a10799d58237cca95a1a9760abe4f565 (accessed on 9th May 2025).
51. Stolte, F., Aleksandrova-Yankulovska, S., Thiemicke, P., Orzechowski, M., Schuetz, C., & Steger, F., (2024). Pediatric systemic inflammatory response syndrome (SIRS) and the development of patient-specific therapy: Ethical perspectives through experts' opinions. *Frontiers in Public Health, 12*. https://www.semanticscholar.org/paper/c35e7f900f9b3d6c8fd9ffb7fa29ee4a15c97c7f (accessed on 9th May 2025).
52. Stoyanova, M., Nikoloudakis, Y., Panagiotakis, S., Pallis, E., & Markakis, E., (2020). A survey on the Internet of Things (IoT) forensics: Challenges, approaches, and open issues. *IEEE Communications Surveys & Tutorials, 22*, 1191–1221. https://doi.org/10.1109/comst.2019.2962586.
53. Ugleva, A. V., Shilova, V. A., & Karpova, E. A. (2024). Index of "ethicality" of AI systems in medicine: From theory to practice. *Ethical Thought*. https://www.semanticscholar.org/paper/b2b864eb3df9e4d69a33398b93e6666fedf6cc32 (accessed on 9th May 2025).
54. Van, V. R., (2025). Redefining intelligence: Collaborative tinkering of healthcare professionals and algorithms as hybrid entity in public healthcare decision-making. *AI & Society*. https://www.semanticscholar.org/paper/819cddddd52215ebd7fcd70a0be7f7e08a02dfc1 (accessed on 9th May 2025).
55. Veale, M., & Zuiderveen Borgesius, F., (2021). Demystifying the draft EU Artificial Intelligence Act—Analyzing the good, the bad, and the unclear elements of the proposed approach. *Computer Law Review International, 22*, 97–112. https://doi.org/10.9785/cri-2021-220402.
56. Wang, Y., Pan, Y., Yan, M., Su, Z., & Luan, T. H. (2023). A survey on ChatGPT: AI-generated contents, challenges, and solutions. *IEEE Open Journal of the Computer Society, 4*, 280–302. https://doi.org/10.1109/ojcs.2023.3300321.
57. Waseem, S., Khalid, S., Zaheer, S., Ahmed, R., Zahid, P., Ullah, M., & Sajjad, A., (2024). Perceptions of medical ethics and professionalism among practicing physicians of Azad Jammu and Kashmir: A mix-method study of ethical dilemmas. *Kashf Journal of Multidisciplinary Research*.

https://www.semanticscholar.org/paper/c6e64b327251a17d83a767df3355ef6a53f886c2 (accessed on 9th May 2025).

58. Yiğitcanlar, T., Desouza, K. C., Butler, L., & Roozkhosh, F., (2020). Contributions and risks of artificial intelligence (AI) in building smarter cities: Insights from a systematic review of the literature. *Energies, 13*, 1473. https://doi.org/10.3390/en13061473.

59. Zeitlyn, D., (2012). Anthropology in and of the archives: Possible futures and contingent pasts. Archives as anthropological surrogates. *Annual Review of Anthropology, 41*, 461–480. https://doi.org/10.1146/annurev-anthro-092611-145721.

60. Zhang, Z., Al Hamadi, H., Damiani, E., Yeun, C. Y., & Taher, F., (2022). Explainable artificial intelligence applications in cyber security: State-of-the-art in research. *IEEE Access, 10*, 93104–93139. https://doi.org/10.1109/access.2022.3204051.

CONSENT IN MEDICAL PRACTICE

12

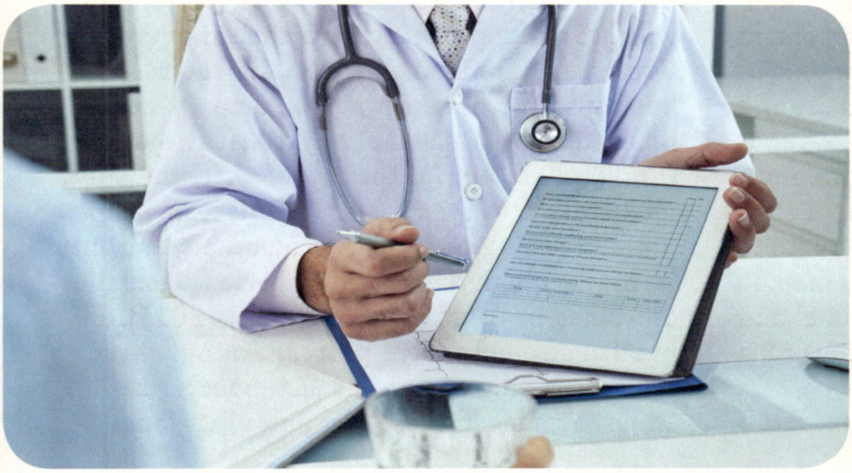

LEARNING OBJECTIVES

After studying this chapter, you will be able to:

1. Understand the legal framework of consent in forensics.
2. Explain ethical considerations in obtaining consent.
3. Identify challenges in obtaining consent in forensic settings.
4. Know the role of forensic practitioners in consent.

Introduction

Medical ethics today is not straightforward at all—especially when you mix in forensic work, where legal stuff and medical care often get tangled together. Doctors, for instance, have this tricky double role; they need to deliver solid health care and, at the same time, make sure people's rights are looked after, which, in many cases, boils down to getting genuine, informed consent. It is a real challenge to work out how to do a deep, proper exam while still letting patients call the shots, and the sensitive nature of forensic cases makes it even messier sometimes. Recognizing this delicate juggle not only raises ethical standards but also helps build that crucial trust in our healthcare systems. When ideas about consent shift—especially in the forensic arena—it is essential, generally speaking, to examine how consent is handled and regulated in these specialized situations. And with technology and AI moving so fast, they bring along both new chances and fresh headaches for people in the field (Ali et al., 2023; Zeppenfeld et al., 2022).

Definition of Consent in Medical Practice

Consent is a key pillar in ethical healthcare—it protects a patient's right to decide and preserves their dignity (Figure 12.1). In forensic medicine, however, this idea gets a bit tangled, mixing deep investigations with the simple need for personal choice. In most cases, being informed means patients get all the details about any procedure, from potential risks to potential benefits, so they really know what to expect rather than just feeling pushed into a decision. Zeppenfeld et al. (2022) show that as our understanding of consent shifts, so too can how much trust and involvement patients have—especially when it comes to tricky areas like mental health. Plus, when you add in peer support services (PSSs), as Shalaby et al. (2020) point out, real-life experiences can help clear things up, making the concept of consent feel more personal and naturally guiding forensic practices toward a kinder, more respectful approach.

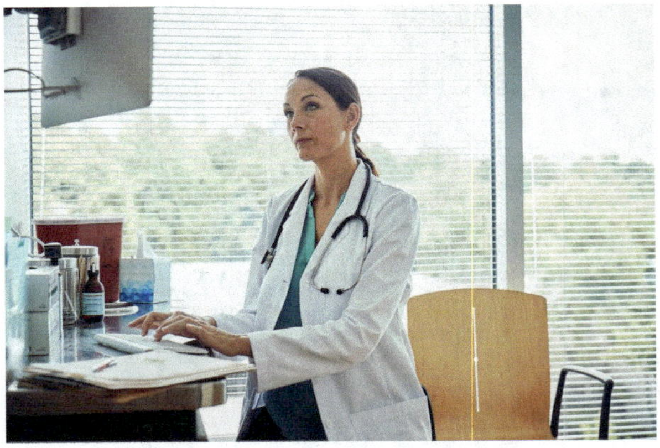

Figure 12.1. Consent is a key pillar in ethical healthcare.

Source: Adobe Inc. (n.d.). *Adobe Acrobat Resources.* https://www.adobe.com/acrobat/resources/media_1ad38e88ca15c434183ec26357d4cf974a3c6f10d.jpeg?width=1200&format=pjpg&optimize=medium.

Importance of Consent in Forensic Settings

Working in forensic cases is not simple. Getting clear, upfront consent—especially from folks who have been sidelined—is really important. Professionals in these fields often face tough ethical puzzles, struggling to delve into details without compromising someone's freedom. In forensic mental health, there's evidence, generally speaking, that when patients get a say, intervention strategies work better. You will hear occupational therapists in everyday forensic talks stressing the need for choices that line up with what each person actually needs; this really drives home why consent matters (Craik et al., 2007). On top of that, the way medico-legal experts see victims can shape the support given during evaluations and, in turn, affect both the victim's experience and the outcomes in court (McMillan et al., 2015). All in all, a strong consent process not only keeps things ethically sound but also boosts patient empowerment in these complex situations

Historical Context of Consent in Medicine

Medicine's past reveals a tumultuous journey when it comes to respecting people's choices, with significant consequences that even surface in forensic cases. In the earlier days, patients were hardly ever asked what they wanted—decisions were made without their say, and sadly, this often led to misuse and abuse, mostly hitting those already pushed aside. Around the mid-1900s, with a growing clamor for human rights and ethical behavior, folks generally started insisting that patients deserve a voice. Cultural norms were shifting, and with that change came a new look at what it means to truly give consent—trust between doctors and patients started to really matter. Clinical research moved forward, and legal rules changed, too, so informed consent began to mean more than just a form; it required honest, clear talk about risks and benefits. Lately, debates about gender and sexual health—especially when young people are involved—have nudged us into rethinking old, tired ideas about consent. In most cases, everyday attitudes about violence and coercion complicate matters further, leaving us to grapple with what consent should really mean in the messy world of forensic medicine (Hlavka, 2014; Reed et al., 2016).

Ethical Considerations Surrounding Consent

At the crossroads of medicine and forensic work, issues of consent naturally bubble up as a major concern. Patients must understand what giving their consent actually involves—especially if their personal information might be used in investigations. When you factor in vulnerable groups, things get even complex; their ability to choose freely can be hampered, so extra care tends to be needed. .

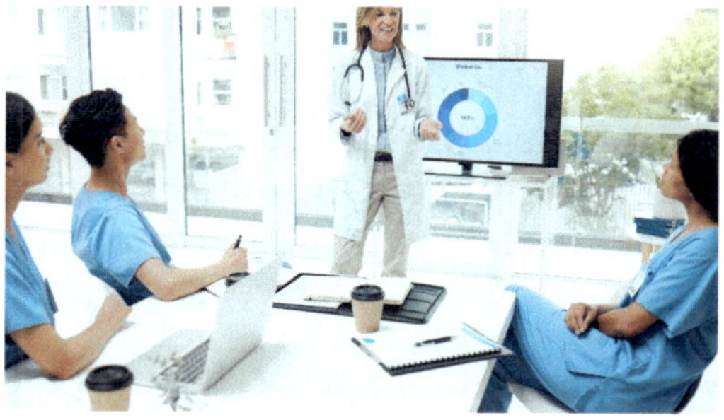

Figure 12.2. Patients must really get what giving their okay actually involves—especially if their personal info might wind up being used in investigations.

Source: Mādavi. (2024). *Untitled Design 11-1.* https://madavi.co/wp-content/uploads/2024/04/Untitled-design-11-1.jpg.

With digital progress and IoT devices constantly gathering data (often in unexpected ways), understanding consent becomes a whole new challenge—without clear-cut rules, that fragile boundary between privacy and forensic interest can easily blur (Stoyanova et al., 2020). Generally speaking, solving these ethical puzzles is not just about blindly following old-school consent guidelines; we also need to craft flexible, sometimes even slightly imperfect frameworks that shield individuals while still allowing forensic inquiries to move forward, thus preserving both ethical values and judicial integrity (Zeppenfeld et al., 2022) (Figure 12.2)

Legal Implications of Consent in Forensics

Consent lies at the center of forensic work, and its legal connections are becoming increasingly tangled. Rapid technological advances make personal and genetic data far easier to access – but they also raise the chances for misuse. In most cases, standards like the General Data Protection Regulation (GDPR) show that consent is not just a procedural box to tick; it is essential for handling data ethically and legally, especially when it involves identifying individuals in forensic settings (Shabani et al., 2019). When it comes to particularly sensitive information, such as genomic details, the extra ethical burden on practitioners means stricter oversight and more robust consent measures are needed to ward off potential harm (Seshadri et al., 2019). All in all, a solid grasp of both legal rules and ethical guidelines helps professionals navigate these murky waters, ensuring that consent remains a fundamental part of forensic medical practice.

12.1. The Legal Framework of Consent in Forensics

Learning Outcome

1. Understand the overview of consent laws in medical practice;
2. Know the differences between informed consent and implied consent;
3. Explain the role of state and federal regulations;
4. Describe case law influencing consent in forensics;
5. Focus on consent in relation to minors and vulnerable populations;
6. Know exceptions to consent requirements in forensic settings;
7. Describe documentation and record-keeping for consent;
8. Identify consequences of lack of consent in forensic cases;
9. Learn international perspectives on consent laws.

Legal frameworks and informed consent often get tangled up in forensic settings. In this area, it is not merely about individual choice—consent reaches into wider social issues too. The idea of protecting patients' rights is evident, even when forensic exams introduce a range of complex legal details.

Take Article 21 of the Indian Constitution, for instance (Mahani et al., 2024); it basically signals that informed consent is vital in intense medical situations like forensic assessments. It is not just about listing facts clearly—what really matters is that the agreement is given freely. Also, as mentioned in Tsyganova (2024), if explicit consent is not available, healthcare professionals need to keep detailed records to comply with legal requirements. All in all, these rules back up our ethical standards and help shed light on just how central consent is in the forensic world.

12.1.1. Overview of Consent Laws in Medical Practice

Modern healthcare places a strong emphasis on informed consent—it is not just a legal formality, but a genuine commitment to respecting patient autonomy and upholding ethical standards (Figure 12.3). Instead of simply following rules, patients are expected to have a clear picture of what a treatment involves, including its risks and benefits; this idea stems from a mix of laws and past legal decisions that, in many cases, insist on enough detail to truly guide choice.

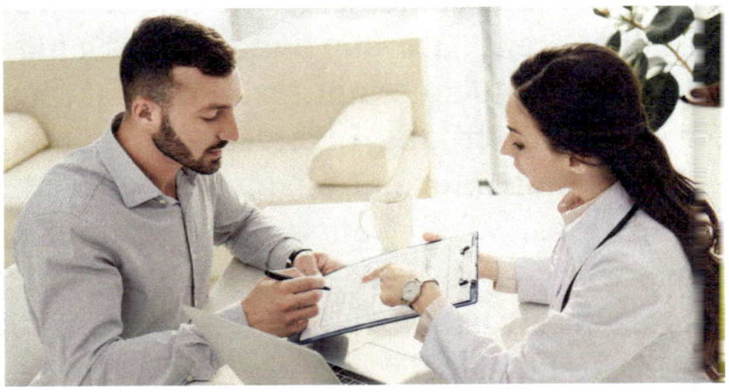

Figure 12.3. Modern healthcare leans hard on informed consent.

Source: RVO Health. (2019). *Patient and Doctor Signing Document.* https://media.post.rvohealth.io/wp-content/uploads/2019/10/Patient_Doctor_Signing_1200x628-facebook.jpg.

In forensic settings, things tend to get even trickier and the stakes higher—consent here can affect not only individual care but also public safety and legal responsibility. For instance, as forensic experts increasingly use cutting-edge tools like Investigative Genetic Genealogy (Kling et al., 2021), the challenge of securing clear, informed consent deepens, calling for a better understanding of the legal frameworks that underlie patient rights. Similarly, when explainable AI steps into forensic work, transparency over how decisions are made becomes all the more crucial (Ali et al., 2023). Generally speaking, these evolving tools and complex rules mean that the concept of informed consent is more nuanced and, frankly, a bit more complicated than it used to be.

12.1.2. Differences Between Informed Consent and Implied Consent

Deciphering consent is a serious business in such areas as medicine, and it feels particularly so in forensic work – where the entire process can be quite messy. Informed consent tends to be presented as a straightforward deal: patients are presented with all the information they require regarding risks, benefits, and other options before anything can proceed. Implied consent, however, tends to emerge more organically—frequently from circumstances or even just a patient's behavior, without the benefit of a formal ritual. This dichotomy truly highlights why maintaining patient control and a shared decision-making atmosphere is so essential both ethically and in terms of compliance. For the most part, providing informed consent is all about patients being right there with their medical decisions, contemplating those choices based on their own objectives and values (Perrenoud et al., 2015). However, sometimes implied consent can cause its own set of problems, particularly when a patient's understanding of what is occurring is uncertain, resulting in potential ethical concerns (Research in Implementation Science and eHealth, 2021). Ultimately, recognizing these discrepancies is paramount within forensic medical environments, as how consent is managed can influence not just treatment outcomes but legal outcomes as well.

12.1.3. Role of State and Federal Regulations

Consent in forensic medicine is tangled in a messy mix of state and federal rules that often do not mesh smoothly (Figure 12.4). Federal guidelines typically outline broad parameters for healthcare consent, while state laws often add specific stipulations that vary significantly, resulting in a patchwork of regulations. Generally speaking, these rules are meant to create consistency; instead, they sometimes give rise to unexpected ethical challenges in forensic work. Doctors find themselves juggling different obligations depending on their jurisdiction—this can lead to genuine confusion. On top of that, rapid advancements in artificial intelligence are stirring up debates about trust and fairness in data usage (Schwartz et al., 2022). In most cases, initiatives like the AI Act in Europe suggest that solid enforcement measures are needed to keep pace with these emerging technologies (Veale et al., 2021). Ultimately, having a clear, unified framework is crucial for ensuring that informed consent in forensic medical practice remains both ethical and truly understood.

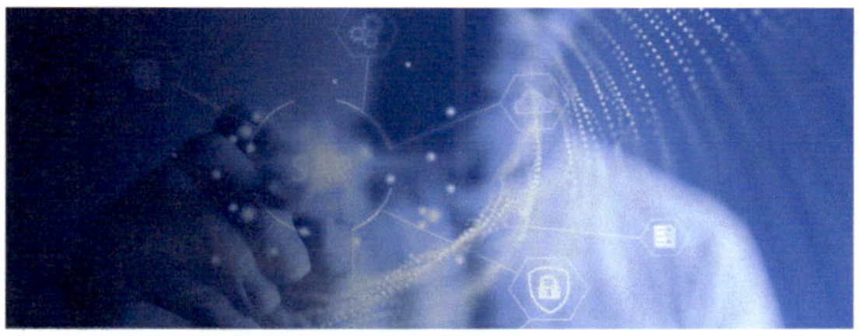

Figure 12.4. Consent in forensic medicine is tangled in a messy mix of state and federal rules.

Source: New Era Technology. (2024). *SAP Intelligent Application Managed Services (iAMS) Blog Background Image.* https://digital.neweratech.com/hubfs/New%20Era%20Microsite/Articles/sap_iams_blog_bg.jpg.

12.1.4. Case Law Influencing Consent in Forensics

Case law and the need for clear consent mix together in ways that really shape the ethics in forensic medicine. Landmark rulings have established guidelines that not only outline individual rights but also remind forensic experts of their responsibilities in safeguarding those rights. Take the case where courts insist on informed consent—especially when it comes to intimate examinations or genetic tests, meaning doctors must point out any potential risks and side effects; it is not merely a box-checking exercise. This approach makes the process feel genuine, building a solid trust between patients and their healthcare providers. Generally speaking, as new rulings emerge and legal standards shift (sometimes in unexpected ways), forensic pros are continually nudged to update their practices in line with the latest advances in science and technology (Vishnopolska et al., 2018; Zeppenfeld et al., 2022).

12.1.5. Consent in Relation to Minors and Vulnerable Populations

Today's forensic medicine scene shows that consent issues for minors and other at-risk folks are not as straightforward as one might hope (Figure 12.5).

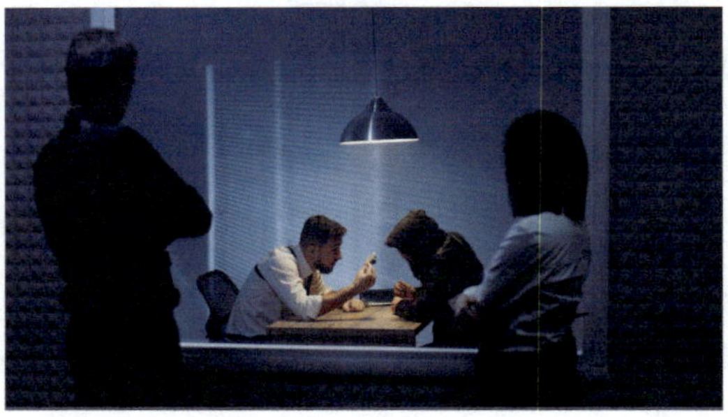

Figure 12.5. Today's forensic medicine scene shows that consent issues for minors and other at-risk folks are not as straightforward as one might hope.

Source: Cato Institute. (2024). *Police Interrogation.* https://www.cato.org/sites/cato.org/files/styles/optimized/public/2024-08/police-interrogation-cropped.jpg?itok=dQ1exrub.

Generally speaking, many of these individuals might not fully get what participating in a medical evaluation implies; they can miss out on grasping all the consequences. It is not just about handing over the complete procedure details—there is also a real need to keep their rights and overall well-being front and center. In many sensitive cases, involving matters of parental permission or legal guardianship only muddies the waters further, as guardians' priorities may not always align with what the minors truly need.

Recent research (Kling et al., 2021) reminds us that we urgently need better systems designed to safeguard these groups while keeping the consent process both clear and respectful of individual choice. And given today's social worries—especially with the lingering effects of the COVID-19 crisis—it seems even more vital to adopt flexible, sometimes imperfect, ways of communicating that help cut through misinformation and ease public anxiety (Saleem et al., 2020).

12.1.6. Exceptions to Consent Requirements in Forensic Settings

Forensic work often starts with the idea of informed consent, yet in practice, that expectation frequently runs into notable exceptions. Sometimes, when law enforcement is involved, the drive for justice tends to push aside the usual consent procedures—an occurrence that stirs up quite a bit of controversy. Take, for example, situations where authorities access genetic samples from hospitals without obtaining a patient's consent; such moves raise deep ethical concerns.

This pattern not only puts the privacy of sensitive medical information at risk, but it can also undermine trust in healthcare institutions, making people wary of seeking necessary care (Brown et al., 2024). Meanwhile, new tech like artificial intelligence and even human microchipping is wedded into forensic procedures, forcing us, in most cases, to rethink what consent really means. Overall, these developments seem to blur boundaries and call for an honest, careful look at our ethical standards.

12.1.7. Documentation and Record-Keeping for Consent

Consent documentation is a real linchpin in forensic medicine (Figure 12.6). It not only backs up patient rights but also serves as a crucial part of our legal and ethical responsibilities—especially when disputes end up in court. Keeping detailed records lowers the risk of mixed-up details during treatment or exams, which, in most cases, helps everyone stay accountable.

Digital technology is not standing still, and as it changes rapidly, ensuring that consent files remain both complete and secure is becoming increasingly challenging. New rules like those laid out in the AI Act (Schwartz et al., 2022; Veale et al., 2021) generally nudge us toward smarter ways of handling data, since even a hint of bias can sometimes creep into digital consent processes. All in all, a flexible, robust documentation system is not just a nice-to-have; it is absolutely necessary for upholding both ethical standards and legal compliance in this field.

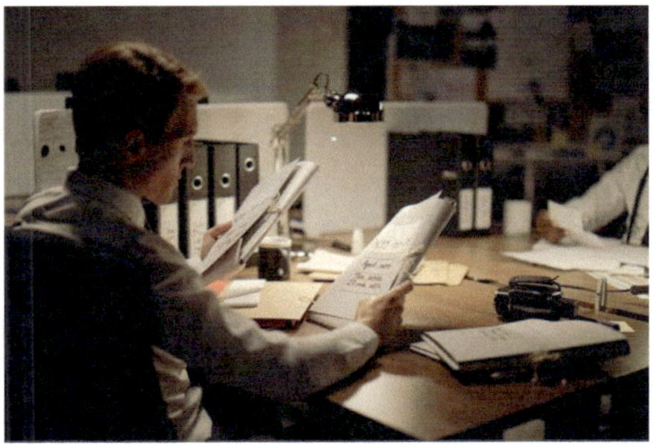

Figure 12.6. Consent documentation is a real linchpin in forensic medicine.

Source: Splunk Inc. (2024). *Forensic Investigator Role*. https://www.splunk.com/content/dam/splunk-blogs/images/en_us/2024/10/forensic-investigator-role2.jpeg.

12.1.8. Consequences of Lack of Consent in Forensic Cases

Forensic medicine is a complex area where obtaining consent can lead to significant legal, ethical, and personal complications. Not getting that clear permission does not just dent the trust in medical practice—it can also throw off the strength of the evidence gathered. You see, when consent is ignored, legal challenges often follow: evidence might be tossed aside and practitioners left facing potential liabilities, which slowly chips away at public confidence in our healthcare system. It is well known that ethical guidelines encourage us to respect individual autonomy; consider cases where patients were subjected to invasive procedures without their knowledge or consent. Studies show, in most cases, that these oversights ripple far beyond legal issues, affecting psychological well-being and even family dynamics, and ultimately making us question the whole moral base of forensic practices (Lechien et al., 2020; Zeppenfeld et al., 2022).

12.1.9. International Perspectives on Consent Laws

Examining consent laws worldwide reveals, in most cases, a complex blend of cultural practices, legal regulations, and the evolving nuances of medical ethics. Often, these variations do not just mirror different ideas about personal freedom and privacy; they also end up affecting how forensic medicine is practiced. Take the rapid rise of tech – especially with the Internet of Things (IoT) – which in many cases brings about unexpected hurdles for gathering and analyzing digital evidence; this newer landscape tends to muddle traditional consent protocols and stokes fresh concerns about privacy and security (Stoyanova et al., 2020). In parallel, changes in how mental and behavioral disorders are classified – as seen in the World Health Organization's recent revisions generally hint that our understanding of consent is always evolving, with notable impact on healthcare in forensic settings. All in all, these global viewpoints make it increasingly clear that we need to craft unified legal standards that prioritize informed consent, even as medical practices and societal values shift at a rapid pace (Reed et al., 2016) (Figure 12.7).

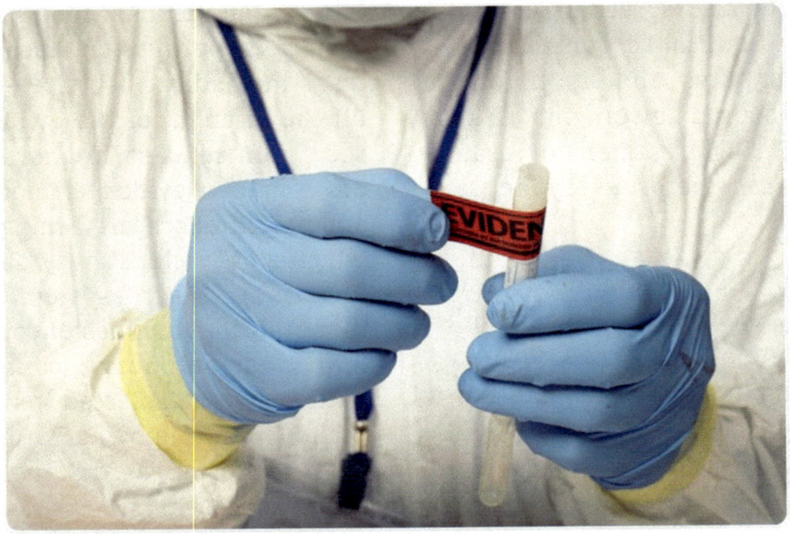

Figure 12.7. International perspectives on consent laws in forensic medicine.

Source: Shutterstock. (2020). *Businessman Working on Laptop with Financial Chart.* https://d2jx2rerrg6sh3.cloudfront.net/image-handler/picture/2020/5/shutterstock_366037751.jpg.

Test Your Knowledge

1. What legal requirements must be fulfilled for obtaining consent for a forensic medical examination?
2. In what circumstances can informed consent be legally overridden or waived in forensic practice?

12.2. Ethical Considerations in Obtaining Consent

Learning Outcome

1. Understand autonomy and patient rights;
2. Explain the role of coercion and undue influence;
3. Identify ethical dilemmas in emergency situations;
4. Balance public safety and individual rights;
5. Know the impact of cultural differences on consent;
6. Describe ethical training for forensic practitioners;
7. Focus on the role of ethics committees in consent issues;
8. Know case studies highlighting ethical challenges;
9. Discuss future ethical considerations in forensic consent.

Forensic work in medical practice pushes us to rethink how consent is handled. Securing vital evidence often becomes a balancing act—a tug-of-war between gathering critical details and honoring a person's right to choose.

Things get even murkier when vulnerable populations or situations where informed consent is less than robust enter the picture. In such cases, it is not just about laying out all the facts clearly, but also about reassuring everyone that their rights and dignity won't be overlooked, at least in most instances.

Digital forensics, which usually involves sifting through personal data, adds another layer of concerns about privacy and data security. Ultimately, addressing these ethical challenges is crucial for establishing trust and ensuring that forensic investigations adhere to proper standards (Stoyanova et al., 2020; Zeppenfeld et al., 2022).

12.2.1. Autonomy and Patient Rights

Patient choice stands at the heart of forensic medicine, where the tug-of-war between personal rights and society's wider needs can get pretty tangled (Figure 12.8). People should be the ones making decisions about their own treatment—especially when legal matters might be in play—rather than simply following preset rules. Ensuring that consent remains genuine means patients maintain tight control over their health details and any potential legal exposure, which generally protects them from undue coercion. When these safeguards slip, it opens the door to pressures that chip away at trust not only in forensics but even in mental health care settings (Sashidharan et al., 2019). Ultimately, every patient carries the inherent right to say yes or no to treatment, a principle that should be woven into everyday clinical practice to honor true human dignity and autonomy (Lechien et al., 2020).

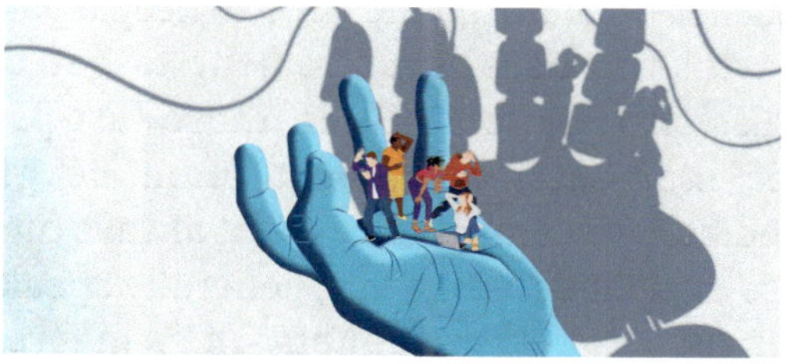

Figure 12.8. People should be the ones making decisions about their own treatment—especially when legal matters might be in play—rather than simply following preset rules.

Source: Freedom House. (2023). *Freedom on the Net 2023: The Repressive Power of Artificial Intelligence.*

12.2.2. The Role of Coercion and Undue Influence

Patient autonomy in healthcare does not always play out as planned—it often collides with the heavy influence of coercion in forensic settings. In many cases, forced measures like mandatory psychiatric hospitalizations show how individuals can end up subtly steered into decisions that, in effect, chip away at their freedom. Recorded experiences generally suggest that such pressures are harmful, sparking ethical questions about the claimed benefits even when the supporting science is fairly thin (Hofstad et al., 2022). There are also marked variations from one region to another, which hint at a patchwork approach in how compulsory hospitalizations are enforced (Hofstad et al., 2021). All in all, this uneven situation suggests that we need to take a closer, more nuanced look at what drives these coercive practices—since they not only cast doubt on genuine consent but also muddy the ethical waters of medical care in forensic contexts.

12.2.3. Ethical Dilemmas in Emergency Situations

When emergencies hit and time is scarce, doctors and nurses sometimes run into ethical headaches—balancing the need to keep a patient safe with the usual requirement to get clear permission (Figure 12.9). In those fast-paced, hectic moments, care must often be given immediately, meaning there is not always time to secure explicit consent; this, generally speaking, leaves room for ethical doubts. Then, in forensic cases where patients might be incapacitated or just not cooperating, the tug-of-war between respecting a person's choice and the pressing need for urgent treatment becomes even messier. The clash between legal mandates and good ethical sense can leave many healthcare providers feeling genuinely torn up inside; studies (Liberati et al., 2021) even show that mental health workers often end up stressed when forced to make such tough calls. Knowing the guidelines—such as those set out by the Indian Psychiatric Society—might seem to offer a clear map; however, the unpredictable chaos of real emergencies often makes it difficult to adhere to these rules exactly (Gundugurti et al., 2022).

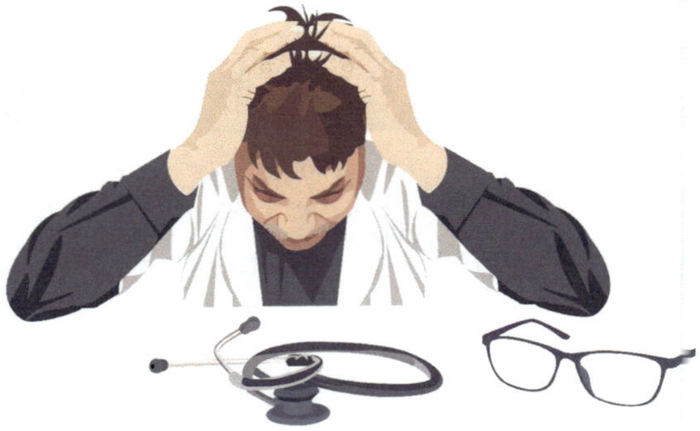

Figure 12.9. When emergencies hit and time is scarce, doctors and nurses sometimes run into ethical headaches—balancing the need to keep a patient safe with the usual requirement to get clear permission.

Source: Getty Images. (2023). *Frustrated.* https://media.npr.org/assets/img/2023/08/01/gettyimages-1340951348_custom-f663b142674bc1c2875186224c7437104608107a.jpg.

12.2.4. Balancing Public Safety and Individual Rights

Public safety and individual rights can get pretty tangled—especially when forensic work depends so much on medical consent. Forensic teams nowadays are increasingly accessing genetic and medical records, and this practice sparks numerous ethical debates on how to balance community safety with respect for personal freedoms. In a look at the issue, de Groot et al. (Samuel, 2021) point out that sticking strictly to an individual consent model in forensic genetics falls short; they argue we really need to widen the conversation to include the communal ripple effects data use can have. You can spot a similar vibe in talks over mental health laws, where there is a push to honor patients' rights even though public safety—especially in forensic psychiatry (Elahai, 2021)—remains a top concern. All in all, finding a fair mix means not only keeping individual rights intact but also being committed to the welfare of the community and clear, ethical practices.

12.2.5. The Impact of Cultural Differences on Consent

In forensics, culture drives how consent is understood in ways you might not immediately expect. Cultural norms—which, in many cases, vary wildly—shape people's ideas about what giving consent really means, often resulting in miscommunications during medical care. Sometimes, decision-making is seen as a family duty rather than a personal right, and that twist can blur the clarity of informed consent. Shared decision making (SDM) shows up as a promising idea in healthcare; however, its rollout, generally speaking, hits snags when deep-rooted cultural differences come into play, making the issue as much about social nuances as about technical procedures (Figure 12.10). While SDM is often touted for its role in enhancing patient outcomes, its practical application can falter due to these cultural gaps. Ultimately, if we want consent to be more than just a ticked box, we really must address these cultural layers and ensure that the process is both truly informed and respected (Slade, 2017; Zeppenfeld et al., 2022).

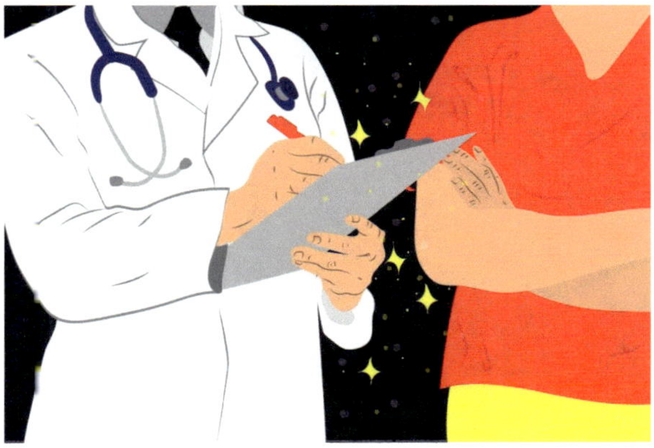

Figure 12.10. Shared decision making (SDM) shows up as a promising idea in forensics.

Source: Mad in America. (2020). *Shared Decision Making.* https://www.madinamerica.com/wp-content/uploads/2020/12/shared-decision-making.jpg.

12.2.6. Ethical Training for Forensic Practitioners

Forensic medical work relies on solid ethical training—it is something that professionals just cannot ignore. Cases often get messy, especially when patients struggle with serious mental health challenges, and suddenly sorting out consent becomes front and center. Good ethics not only keep the public safe but also help practitioners avoid getting tangled up in legal issues if things go sideways. In many instances, there is a growing suggestion to try out restorative justice approaches—even though their use in forensic settings is still finding its footing. Generally speaking, some recommendations lean toward integrating restorative justice awareness into routine training, urging a closer examination of whether a patient can truly give informed consent rather than merely assessing whether they might benefit (Drennan et al., 2021). Plus, offering peer support services (PSSs) seems to boost open dialogue and understanding, which, in turn, can lead to more genuinely informed consent and better patient outcomes (Shalaby et al., 2020).

12.2.7. The Role of Ethics Committees in Consent Issues

Forensic medical practice can be challenging when it comes to handling consent, and ethics committees often play a key role in ensuring everything remains ethical and on track (Figure 12.11). They are usually the ones sifting through how consent is gathered, weighing patient autonomy against legal demands while also considering how forensic findings might affect someone's life. In most cases, these committees adhere to established guidelines—such as those outlined in the Helsinki Declaration—to safeguard participants' rights and well-being (Kazitskaya et al., 2021). They also take care to make sure that everything about the consent process is clearly documented and communicated, which really helps build trust between doctors and patients. It is not just about ticking legal boxes; their involvement helps promote a culture of accountability and ethical care, especially in those delicate forensic situations (Lechien et al., 2020). All in all, their advice and oversight tend to sharpen up how consent is handled, boosting the overall quality of forensic medical services.

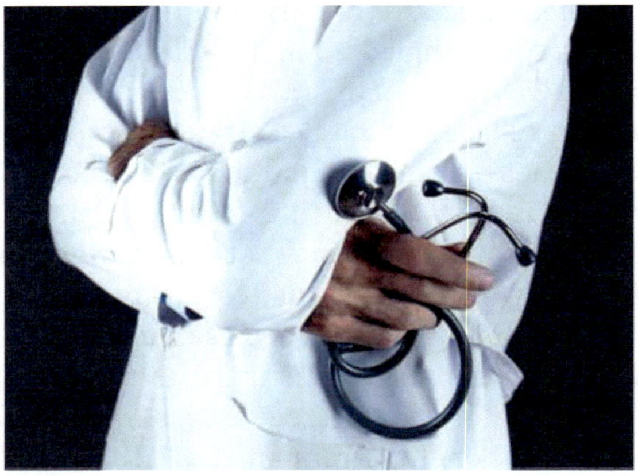

Figure 12.11. Forensic medical practice can be tricky when it comes to handling consent, and ethics committees tend to jump in as key players in keeping everything ethical and on track.

Source: Scholastica. (2022). *Scholastica Logo.* https://s3.amazonaws.com/production.scholastica/article/36539/medium/photo-1625134673337-519d4d10b313?1655743557.

12.2.8. Case Studies Highlighting Ethical Challenges

Forensic medicine's ethical challenges are not always cut and dry—I mean, you really have to dig into various case studies to catch the full picture. Sometimes, skipping clear, informed consent stirs up both legal headaches and moral muddles, especially when the sensitive stuff is on the line. And when mental health issues mix with forensic evaluations, getting a proper consent gets even more dicey, since folks might be too vulnerable to fully grasp what is going on. For example, there's evidence that adding PSSs can improve the chat between patients and healthcare providers; in many cases, though, some studies show effects that are nearly neutral, which could end up wasting resources. Plus, as Zeppenfeld et al. (2022) point out, consent really becomes a tougher nut to crack in places where mental health is not well handled—this all signals a real need for better frameworks in forensic medicine to make sure that consent stays both informed and voluntary, much like the ongoing debates around PSSs in healthcare suggest.

12.2.9. Future Ethical Considerations in Forensic Consent

Forensic medicine is advancing at breakneck speed, and this advancement has complicated the concept of informed consent somewhat. New technology—such as genetic testing and even computerized data gathering—challenges us to think anew about how individual privacy and public confidence interplay, usually with surprises.

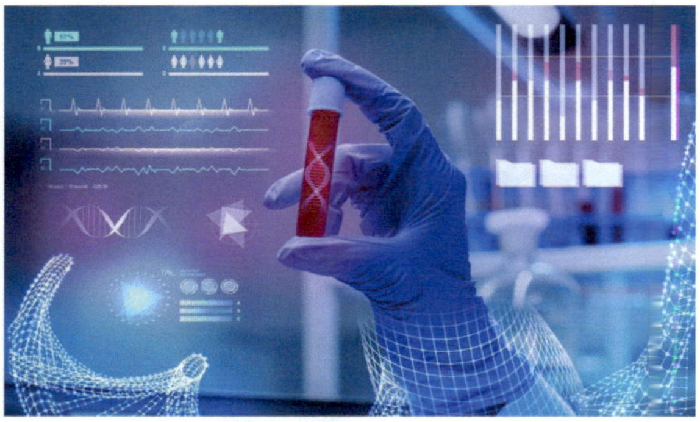

Figure 12.12. New tech—like genetic tests and even digital data collection—push us to reconsider how personal privacy and public trust come into play, often in ways that catch us off guard.

Source: Indian Retailer. (2023). *Biotechnology Specialist Conducting Experiments in a Laboratory.*

ALRC Report 96, for example, overall observes that we require clear ground rules to deal with genetic information; if our consent procedures falter, the consequences are dire (Opeskin et al., 2025). Meanwhile, combining bioethics with international criminal law introduces additional layers of complexity—particularly when corporate liability emerges in messy situations such as genetic exploitation or organ trafficking (Long et al., 2017). Ultimately, implementing a system that relies on openness and genuinely respects individual autonomy could very well be the most effective means by which forensic medicine can forge through these difficulties without compromising patient care and overall public trust (Figure 12.12).

Test Your Knowledge

1. In what ways can cultural sensitivity impact the process of obtaining consent for forensic procedures?
2. How should a forensic practitioner handle a situation where the patient cannot give consent (e.g., unconscious, mentally ill, or deceased)?

12.3. Challenges in Obtaining Consent in Forensic Settings

Learning Outcome

1. Identify situations where consent may be difficult to obtain;
2. Know the role of mental health in consent capacity;
3. Discuss the impact of trauma on consent comprehension;
4. Focus on language barriers and informed consent;
5. Describe the influence of power dynamics in forensic settings;
6. Learn strategies for improving consent processes;
7. Know the role of technology in facilitating consent;
8. Learn case examples of consent challenges in forensics;
9. Address consent challenges.

Consent in forensic settings is not a straightforward affair—it is a complex mix of legal, ethical, and medical concerns that often complicate the entire process. Sometimes, practitioners run into people who are pretty vulnerable or just under too much pressure, making it tricky for them to really grasp what they are agreeing to. The situation gets even murkier when factors like mental fitness and a slightly coercive atmosphere are thrown into the mix. Healthcare providers, who sometimes double as legal agents, can find themselves in sticky situations that may compromise the authenticity of consent. Research (Zeppenfeld et al., 2022) indicates that many individuals misinterpret the meaning of their consent, highlighting a notable gap in understanding within these forensic environments. All of this generally suggests that clearer, straightforward guidelines and a more open style of communication are needed to tackle the many, layered challenges involved in obtaining valid consent in forensic settings (Khalil et al., 2020).

12.3.1. Situations Where Consent May Be Difficult to Obtain

In tense, complex medical situations, getting proper consent can really be a headache. Emergencies often leave patients unable to speak up about what they need, so doctors end up navigating a maze of both ethical and legal issues—sometimes relying on advance directives or turning to a surrogate decision-maker. For instance, in a critical oncology case, the physician is compelled to expedite a necessary intervention while also respecting the patient's previously expressed wishes (Research in Implementation Science and eHealth, 2021). The risks that come with some treatments only complicate things further, especially when patients, already on edge, struggle to keep up with the details. Research generally shows that the heavy blend of technical jargon and complex explanations can leave patients more confused than informed (Hoes et al., 1995). All in all, these consent situations call for a kind of careful, if somewhat messy, balancing act that keeps patient welfare and ethical obligations squarely in mind (Figure 12.13).

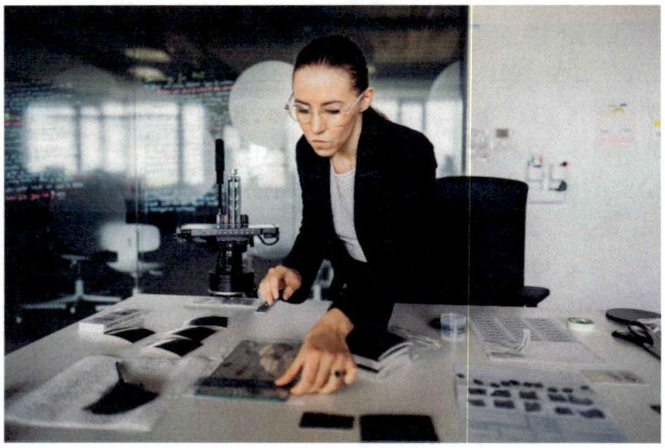

Figure 12.13. There may be some situations where consent may be difficult to obtain.

Source: Innovatrics. (2023). *Biometric Technology in Action.*

12.3.2. The Role of Mental Health in Consent Capacity

Consent in forensic medicine is not a simple process—it is tangled up with mental health. People with mental health challenges often find that their emotional and thinking skills are not up to speed when it comes to making choices about their treatment. Sometimes, various psychiatric issues muddle a person's judgment or insight, which in turn makes giving clear consent even trickier. PSSs, which have been on the rise recently, remind us that folks should feel they have got a say in understanding their rights and choosing their care (Shalaby et al., 2020). Generally speaking, integrating mental health factors into the legal and medical framework not only supports individual autonomy but also helps address the gaps left by inadequate support systems, ultimately improving the consent process in forensic settings (Zeppenfeld et al., 2022).

12.3.3. Impact of Trauma on Consent Comprehension

Forensic medical consent is not a straightforward matter—trauma often muddles how patients absorb information (Figure 12.14). When someone undergoes a traumatic experience, it tends to throw off basic mental skills like memory, attention, and even decision-making, leaving them more susceptible to undue influence during those pivotal moments when they are asked to agree. This is not merely an incidental occurrence; trauma's impact on thinking can make it tough for individuals to process details clearly, sometimes even paving the way for coercion or manipulative tactics. Health professionals, in most cases, need to be extra mindful of these vulnerabilities and adjust their approach by relying on clear, plain language and genuine emotional support. Some experts suggest that adding PSSs could offer a helpful boost in understanding for patients dealing with trauma, potentially easing some of the strain on our healthcare systems (Shalaby et al., 2020). All in all, ensuring that consent maintains its ethical and meaningful role in forensic practice means keeping a close eye on these psychological challenges (Lechien et al., 2020).

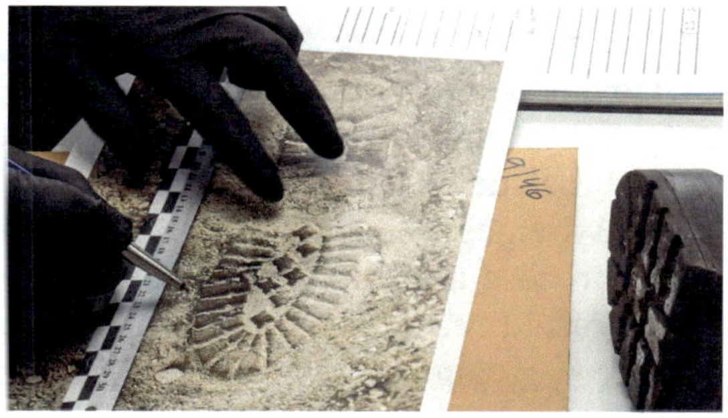

Figure 12.14. Trauma's impact on thinking can make it tough for individuals to process details clearly, sometimes even paving the way for coercion or manipulative tactics.

Source: Bangor University. (2024). *Port 99.* https://www.bangor.ac.uk/sites/default/files/styles/16x9_1920w/public/2024-06/port_99.jpg?h=b692b260&itok=YFVdnvOI.

12.3.4. Language Barriers and Informed Consent

Clear, direct communication sits at the heart of medicine—especially in forensic contexts where getting true, informed consent is absolutely vital. Language differences often block a full understanding of medical procedures and muddle what consent really means. Sometimes, the added pressure of tangled legal and ethical responsibilities forces forensic practitioners to work even harder to be clear. In most cases, studies show that as traditional teaching methods fade away, fresh and inventive approaches pop up; these tend to boost engagement but also spotlight fresh hurdles when trying to explain complex ideas (Khalil et al., 2020). I also see that involving peers with real-life experience in mental health support can sometimes patch up communication gaps, even if the outcomes on resource use can be all over the place (Shalaby et al., 2020). So, dealing with language barriers is not just a minor detail in getting consent—it is a key step in making sure everyone truly gets their rights and responsibilities in a forensic setting.

12.3.5. The Influence of Power Dynamics in Forensic Settings

Grasping how power shifts in forensic settings matters—a lot, really—especially when it comes to how people end up giving consent (Figure 12.15). Often, those in charge turn out to be professionals like forensic examiners or even law enforcement, and this can create a subtle, unspoken push for agreement. In many cases, individuals facing forensic exams may feel that they have little choice; they worry that saying no could lead to unwanted consequences. This situation challenges the whole idea of voluntary consent and, frankly, raises some ethical alarms given that many people in the legal system are already in pretty vulnerable spots. In most cases, you have to consider how these power gaps drain consent of its real meaning, which ties into broader legal and ethical debates about truly informed decision-making in fields like medicine (Ali et al., 2023). Additionally, it highlights the importance of clear protocols—ones that foster open and balanced conversations during these assessments—so that, ultimately, consent emerges as a genuine, informed choice rather than something reluctantly given under pressure (Zeppenfeld et al., 2022).

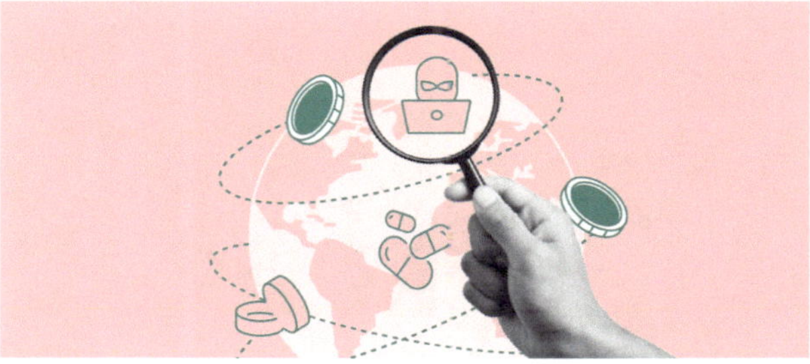

Figure 12.15. Grasping how power shifts in forensic settings matters—a lot, really—especially when it comes to how people end up giving consent.

Source: Chainalysis. (2024). *Public Key Episode 137: The Cyber Avengers.* https://www.chainalysis.com/wp-content/uploads/2024/11/episode-137-website-graphic.png.

12.3.6. Strategies for Improving Consent Processes

Improving consent in forensic medicine is not about following one textbook rule—it means mixing a few smart ideas together. First off, patients need real clarity right from the start: instead of burying details in long-winded legal language, standard consent forms break down what a procedure involves and what choices lie ahead, so folks really get their rights and the possible outcomes. Digital tools, such as online consent platforms, can also streamline the process and reduce errors (Khalil et al., 2020). It helps, too, when patients feel free to ask questions; a relaxed, open atmosphere can clear up doubts almost as they come up. Equally important is giving medical personnel hands-on training about the ins and outs—and even the ethical side—of informed consent (Zeppenfeld et al., 2022). All in all, putting these pieces together results in a clearer, more flexible, and truly patient-focused approach to consent in forensic settings.

12.3.7. The Role of Technology in Facilitating Consent

Technology is changing medicine in unexpected ways—especially in forensic environments—by transforming how patients give consent (Figure 12.16). Digital platforms break complicated info into bite-sized pieces, which lets healthcare providers explain what is going on in terms anyone can grasp, ensuring patients know their rights and what procedures involve. Generally speaking, innovations like telehealth not only open up access to specialized care but also give patients the opportunity to be more involved in decision-making, fostering a genuine sense of autonomy. PSSs, for example, have noted that mixing in real lived experiences can enrich the consent process, building trust and clear, honest communication between care professionals and patients (Shalaby et al., 2020). Additionally, using electronic health records streamlines document keeping so that consent is not just informed but also verifiable under medical ethics (Zeppenfeld et al., 2022). All in all, blending technology with consent practices ends up boosting the quality of care in forensic practice.

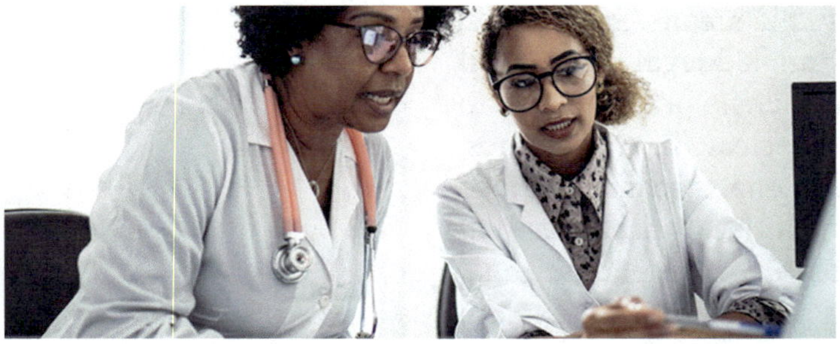

Figure 12.16. Technology is changing medicine in unexpected ways—especially in forensic environments—by transforming how patients give consent.

Source: Avantor. (n.d.). *How Technology is Shaping the Future of Clinical Trials.* https://occapi.avantorsciences.com/medias/HowTechnologyIsShapingTheFutureOfClinicalTrials1920x750.jpg?context=bWFzdGVyfGltYWdlc3wxNDExODJ8aW1hZ2UvanBlZ3xhR1EwTDJnNFlTODVOakE1TVRreU9UWTBNVEkyTDBodmQxUmxZMmh1YjJ4dlozbEpjMU5vWVhCcGJtZFVhR1ZHZFhSMWNtVlBaa05zYVc1cFkyRnNWSEpwWVd4ek1Ua3lNRWcxTmpBdWFuQm58YjhlMWNkODE5ZjczZTExNmYxYmU3Y2MxZDVhMzYzMDUwM2Y0YzgxODZkMWFiZGU5ZjVhNjIzOTgxOGViOWFlYg.

12.3.8. Case Examples of Consent Challenges in Forensics

Consent in forensic medical practice can get downright messy when real cases are considered. Looking at examples reveals that, with survivors of sexual violence, the need for internal vaginal exams—even though these exams are key for gathering evidence—can feel alarmingly invasive and might even lead to further trauma if survivors are not fully informed or feel a bit pressured (Ritchie et al., 2025). In another scenario, when forensic procedures are part of immigrant policing, things get even knotty: psychological evaluations and various medical assessments are conducted without always having crystal-clear agreements on what happens with the information collected (Zhang et al., 2024). In most cases, these moments highlight a pressing need to continually revisit and update consent practices, ensuring that individual rights remain protected as forensic evidence collection becomes increasingly complex.

12.3.9. Recommendations for Addressing Consent Challenges

Consent in medical care, especially in forensic contexts, is not a one-size-fits-all matter—it is nuanced and requires a mix of recommendations aimed at upholding ethics and protecting vulnerable individuals (Figure 12.17). One promising tactic is to focus less on whether a patient might benefit from an intervention and more on whether they are truly ready and able to give consent, since this approach picks up on the subtle twists of individual mental health situations (Drennan et al., 2021). Open, unforced communication can also help restore trust between providers and patients, ensuring that the decision to proceed is both informed and voluntary. Training healthcare workers in restorative justice practices adds yet another angle, arming them with practical tools to navigate ethical dilemmas while keeping patient rights at the forefront (Zeppenfeld et al., 2022). In the end, these ideas work together to mend the gaps in current consent processes and steer us toward a healthcare system that genuinely respects every person's dignity.

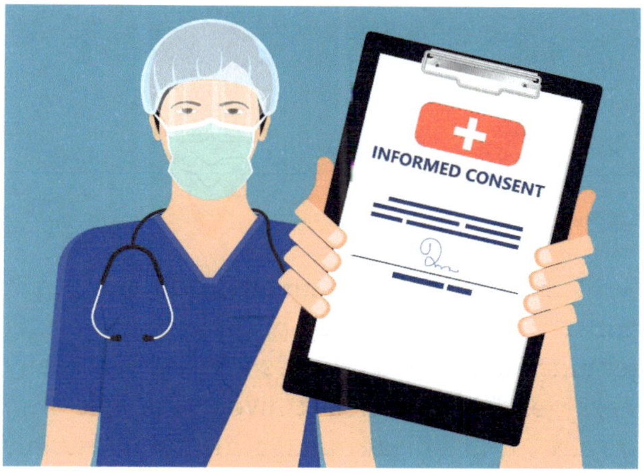

Figure 12.17. Consent in medical care, especially in forensic contexts, is not a one-size-fits-all matter.

Source: Smith, J. (2023). Innovative technology in clinical trials. *Clinical Research Journal.*

Test Your Knowledge

1. What challenges arise when obtaining consent from minors for forensic procedures, and how can these challenges be ethically addressed?
2. In cases of death investigation, what difficulties may arise when trying to obtain consent for an autopsy from grieving or emotionally distressed family members?

12.4. The Role of Forensic Practitioners in Consent

Learning Outcome

1. Know responsibilities of forensic medical examiners;
2. Focus on training and education on consent issues;
3. Understand the communication skills necessary for obtaining consent;
4. Build trust with patients and families;
5. Explain the importance of clear explanations of procedures;
6. Describe involvement of legal counsel in consent discussions;
7. Collaboration with law enforcement and legal entities;
8. Discuss continuous professional development on consent;
9. Describe advocacy for patient rights in forensic contexts.

Forensic experts in medicine do more than run technical tests. They grapple with getting genuine consent—a process that can get really messy, especially when it involves people who are already at a disadvantage, like crime victims or those with limited capacity. Their know-how helps keep a person's right to decide front and center, even when unusual challenges pop up in forensic settings. In most cases, these professionals end up juggling ethical demands for patient independence with the strict legal rules that steer forensic work. This balancing act typically requires a solid understanding of both legal norms and ethical ideals; consider digital forensics, where a flawed consent process can directly impact evidence admissibility and erode public trust in forensic methods (Stoyanova et al., 2020). At the end of the day, their role turns out to be vital in upholding respect for individual rights while still ensuring that the forensic process remains sound (Abiodun et al., 2019).

12.4.1. Responsibilities of Forensic Medical Examiners

Forensic medical examiners juggle a mix of duties that bridge the worlds of medicine and law (Figure 12.18). They do not just run detailed health checks; they also collect evidence all while making sure individual rights—especially when it comes to consent—are respected. Because their work is so delicate, these professionals often find themselves wrestling with ethical puzzles. In most cases, if someone can give permission, examiners ensure that it happens, but there are also times—like when someone is dealing with mental illness or is not fully capable—when proper consent just is not there. You might notice, as some literature points out (Shalaby et al., 2020; Zeppenfeld et al., 2022), that a gap is widening between communities handling mental health issues and the healthcare providers looking after them. Effective, sometimes even conversational, communication, along with a clear sense of ethical duty, really can make or break trust and integrity in the forensic medical field.

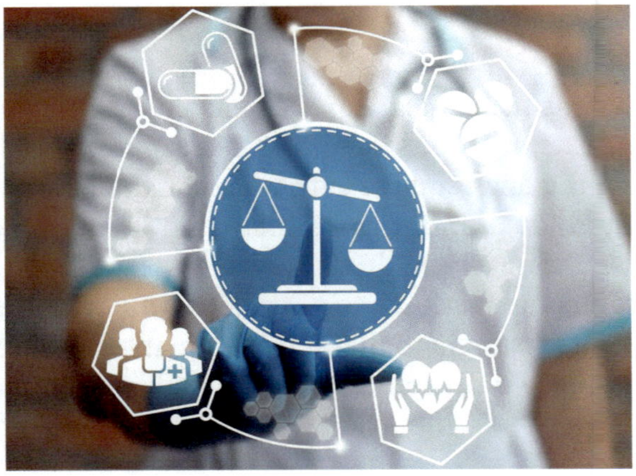

Figure 12.18. Forensic medical examiners juggle a mix of duties that bridge the worlds of medicine and law.

Source: Médecins Sans Frontières. (2024). *Medical Professionals Providing Aid in a Conflict Zone.*

12.4.2. Training and Education on Consent Issues

These days, consent training in healthcare – especially when it comes to forensic work – is more crucial than ever. Many professionals find themselves tangled in ethical challenges with vulnerable populations, so getting clear, informed consent is not just a legal formality but also a matter of understanding subtle cultural and psychological factors. Training now goes beyond dry legal definitions; it digs into real-life scenarios, often using case studies and hands-on simulations to bring the concept to life. In most cases, educators combine these approaches in ways that feel both practical and somewhat unpredictable, allowing students to grasp the true complexities of consent. As we have seen with public health hurdles like the COVID-19 pandemic, there is a growing push for flexible, adaptive teaching methods that help everyone keep pace with shifting standards in medical ethics (Brassett et al., 2020; Zeppenfeld et al., 2022).

12.4.3. Communication Skills Necessary for Obtaining Consent

Clear communication is crucial when asking for consent, and this is especially true within forensic medicine, where matters can feel exceptionally delicate (Figure 12.19). Health professionals often find themselves in intricate conversations, balancing strict legal duties with the emotional needs of patients and their families, sometimes even juggling unexpected turns in the dialogue. Instead of getting lost in convoluted jargon, they benefit from speaking in plain language and truly listening—this not only makes the details easier to grasp but also creates a space where trust and openness can naturally develop. They also need to show genuine empathy, since, in most cases, the circumstances around forensic evaluations can be both overwhelming and unsettling. When providers place the patient at the center, they ensure that everyone receives the information they need, while also empowering individuals to feel in control in situations that might otherwise seem disempowering. All these challenges, in a way, stress the ongoing need for regular, sometimes even rigorous, communication training to maintain both ethical standards and personal autonomy, as noted in ongoing discussions within related fields (Naveed et al., 2015; Zeppenfeld et al., 2022).

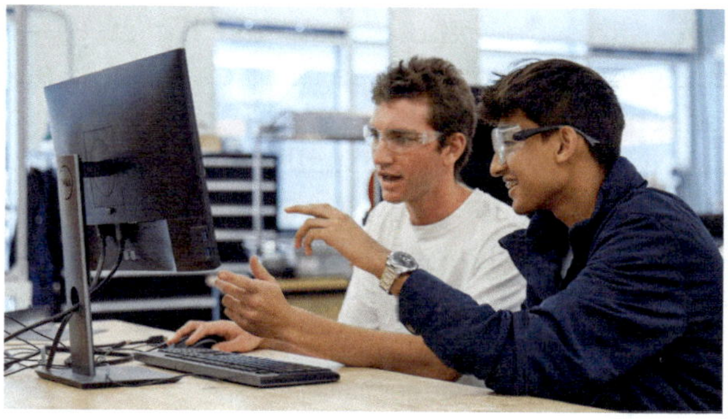

Figure 12.19. Clear communication is crucial when asking for consent, and this is especially true within forensic medicine, where matters can feel exceptionally delicate.

Source: Summer Discovery. (2024). *Summer Discovery Course Banner.*

12.4.4. Building Trust with Patients and Families

Building a genuine connection between doctors and patients makes a huge difference—even more so when legal issues complicate things, as in forensic settings. Trust really forms the base for this bond, letting everyone chat openly and share decisions, which is key to obtaining proper informed consent. In one palliative care study, it was generally noted that clearer talk and closer teamwork among care providers help boost trust with patients and their families (Tan et al., 2021). In forensic medicine, patients can feel especially vulnerable when legal complexities come into play with their care. The findings also suggest that keeping the link between family physicians and patients strongly calls for a bit of system flexibility and some targeted educational outreach on the benefits of available care options, ultimately building a trust-based framework that eases the entire consent process (Tan et al., 2021).

12.4.5. The Importance of Clear Explanations of Procedures

In forensic medicine, a clear rundown of procedures does more than just list steps—it changes how patients see their own rights and consent. Doctors who explain each phase of a forensic evaluation usually build trust and, generally speaking, help people feel more in control of decisions about their health and legal matters.

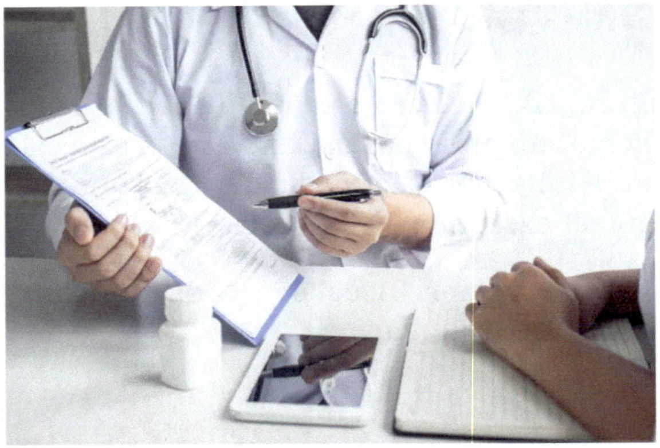

Figure 12.20. Doctors who explain each phase of a forensic evaluation usually build trust and, generally speaking, help people feel more in control of decisions about their health and legal matters.

Source: Pyramids Global. (2023). *Patient Confidentiality in Healthcare.*

It matters a lot in delicate situations, where outcomes can involve not only legal issues but also personal challenges. Honestly, when procedures are laid out plainly, the risk of mix-ups drops—kind of similar to the push for transparency in AI decision-making discussions (Ali et al., 2023). Sticking to simple, unpretentious communication lets patients weigh both the benefits and potential risks, and often this leads to a better overall experience with their care (Zeppenfeld et al., 2022) (Figure 12.20).

12.4.6. Involvement of Legal Counsel in Consent Discussions

Consent discussions in forensic medicine are not always straightforward—they often get messy enough that a lawyer's input becomes necessary to sort out the tangled ethical and legal issues. Generally speaking, having a legal expert nearby helps doctors follow the law while also keeping a sharp eye on patients' rights, especially in situations where historical wrongs or the needs of vulnerable groups come into play. This type of legal backup not only clarifies what consent truly means, but it also resolves potential conflicts and ensures that all details about treatment choices and risks are properly explained. In some cases, having legal counsel present in the room makes it easier to discuss those complex situations involving involuntary consent, particularly in forensic settings where patients may be incapacitated or otherwise unable to give informed consent. All in all, this teamwork—though a bit unconventional at times—builds a stronger ethical foundation for practice, emphasizing patient autonomy and clear decision-making, which, in most cases, aligns well with the evolving standards of care in the field (Glick, 2023; Lee, 2024).

12.4.7. Collaboration with Law Enforcement and Legal Entities

Medical work and law enforcement meet in a space that is anything but simple—a kind of delicate dance that demands careful balancing of ethics and justice. Sometimes, especially in forensic settings where consent is crucial, it is not enough to simply check boxes; both parties must agree on what sharing sensitive details truly means. Doctors and legal experts end up talking—sometimes in a roundabout, informal way—to figure out exactly how patient's rights are protected, even when law enforcement needs access for investigations (Figure 12.21). Generally speaking, this process forces everyone to face tricky ethical questions about divulging private medical information, particularly when police or detective work steps in. In many cases, keeping these interactions as open and transparent as possible, though a bit rough around the edges, helps ease worries about bias and breaches of privacy. When practices are explained clearly—and, admittedly, not always perfectly—accountability gets a boost, and public trust often follows suit. All in all, this mix of different voices and perspectives underscores why a multi-disciplinary approach in forensic medicine remains so essential (Ali et al., 2023; Schwartz et al., 2022).

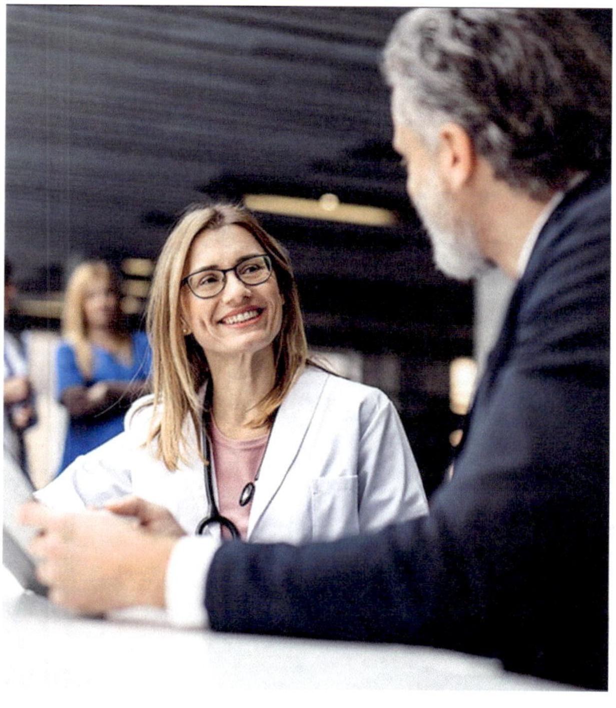

Figure 12.21. Doctors and legal experts end up talking—sometimes in a roundabout, informal way—to figure out exactly how patient's rights are protected, even when law enforcement needs access for investigations.

Source: Grant Thornton UK LLP. (n.d.). *Doctors in a Healthcare Setting*. https://www.grantthornton.co.uk/contentassets/c0a96bb626084d3c84bb94c75bafad49/589x658-doctors.jpg.

12.4.8. Continuous Professional Development on Consent

Forensic medicine is evolving fast, and practicing continuous professional development (CPD) really makes a difference when it comes to understanding consent. Doctors—caught in the messy maze of informed consent with its legal twists and ethical turns—rely on ongoing training to pick up on the finer points that crop up in forensic work. Different laws and ever-changing patient rights mean that clinicians have to be sharp not only technically but also ethically. Programs like hands-on workshops and even certification courses help share the know-how, getting professionals ready to handle those tricky consent issues. This increased awareness builds stronger bonds with patients and underpins trustworthy forensic practices, ultimately leading, in most cases, to better health outcomes at the unpredictable intersection of medicine and law (Kooij et al., 2018; Zeppenfeld et al., 2022).

12.4.9. Advocacy for Patient Rights in Forensic Contexts

Patient rights in forensic scenarios hinge on understanding the messy ethical issues around asking for consent. In mental health care—especially in settings tangled with forensic scrutiny—coercion sometimes shows up and chips away at a patient's freedom, stirring up real human rights and ethical debates. Public safety concerns often push security to the forefront, leaving individual freedoms in the background. There is a growing call for treatment that leans more on genuine agreement—a sign that psychiatry might need a bit of a cultural makeover where oppressive tactics get dropped in favor of respecting core human rights (Sashidharan et al., 2019). Furthermore, this shift must be accompanied by modern advances in psychiatric methods, such as the biopsychosocial approach, which aims to encompass all aspects of patient care while also addressing the gaps in current practices (Stein et al., 2022). Without this kind of determined advocacy, there is a risk that the real, respectful connection with patients in forensic settings will just fall by the wayside (Figure 12.22).

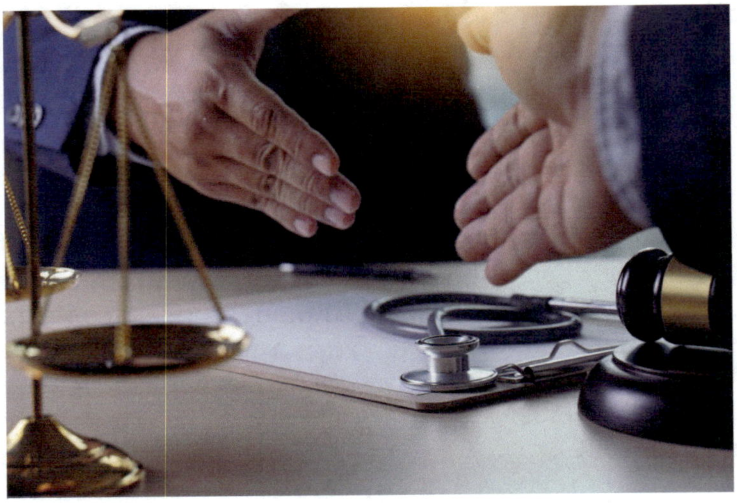

Figure 12.22. Advocacy for patient rights in forensic.

Source: AIHCP. (2024). *Depositphotos_203776390_S.* https://aihcp.net/main/wp-content/uploads/2024/02/Depositphotos_203776390_S.jpg.

Test Your Knowledge

1. What are the core responsibilities of a forensic practitioner in obtaining informed consent?
2. How should a forensic practitioner explain the purpose and scope of a procedure to ensure valid consent?

SUMMARY

Consent in forensic medicine is a messy business—patients' rights can easily get lost in a jumble of rigid rules and expectations. Doctors often find themselves balancing strict legal demands with their own gut feelings about what's right, so making sure patients know exactly what is happening really comes first. Some recent findings (Ha et al., 2025) hint that a straightforward, down-to-earth chat between providers and patients is key—especially when procedures are extra delicate in forensic situations. And then there is the social media twist, where spreading medical information can become problematic; in such cases, practices backed by solid scientific evidence should clearly take precedence over self-promotion (Cortegiani et al., 2024). When patient choice is truly respected, it not only adds credibility to forensic practices but also builds stronger public trust in our healthcare systems. In most cases, keeping everyone well-informed through ongoing, sometimes imperfect but honest, education about consent remains absolutely essential.

Consent and forensic medicine mix together in ways that can really complicate things. At the heart of it, informed consent means that patients must grasp exactly what they are signing up for—no fluff—whether it is about a medical treatment or the legal fallout of their decisions. This clarity turns even more crucial in forensic settings where even small misunderstandings can upend someone's entire life. New technology—think AI and cloud computing—is now in the picture, and in most cases, it stirs up fresh concerns about privacy and whether our consent still retains its original meaning. Recent research hints that a shift toward genuine openness and a bit more trust-building may be just what is needed to defend patient rights and keep personal data safe. All in all, tackling these issues, rather than in bits and pieces, seems essential as forensic practices wedded to old principles adjust to our fast-changing technological world (Ahmad et al., 2021; Ali et al., 2023).

KEY TERMS FROM THIS CHAPTER

- Artificial intelligence
- Consistency
- Evaluations
- Forensic assessments
- Jurisdiction
- Public safety
- Confusion
- Ethical standards
- Fairness
- Informed consent
- Law
- Transparency

CRITICAL THINKING QUESTIONS

1. **In forensic medicine, informed consent means:**
   a. The patient's family must give consent for any medical examination
   b. The individual must understand the purpose, risks, and benefits of the procedure before agreeing
   c. Consent is not required for autopsies or post-mortem examinations
   d. Consent is only required for routine medical procedures, not for forensic investigations
2. **When can a forensic doctor legally conduct an autopsy without the consent of the deceased's family?**
   a. If the family provides verbal consent
   b. When the death is suspected to be suspicious, and the autopsy is ordered by the police or court
   c. If the deceased had signed a consent form prior to death
   d. Only when a hospital requires an autopsy for medical reasons
3. **Which of the following factors must be evaluated to determine an individual's capacity to consent to a forensic examination?**
   a. The individual's age
   b. The individual's understanding of the procedure and its consequences
   c. The individual's physical strength
   d. The individual's previous criminal history
4. **In forensic practice, informed consent is NOT required for which of the following situations?**
   a. Post-mortem examination of a body
   b. A psychiatric evaluation ordered by the court
   c. Routine blood tests in a suspected case of substance abuse
   d. Forensic medical examination of a living patient with an injury following assault
5. **In cases of sexual assault, consent for a forensic examination must include which of the following?**
   a. Only a verbal agreement from the patient
   b. A detailed written form explaining the examination process, its purpose, and the potential outcomes
   c. Consent from law enforcement without involving the patient
   d. Consent for police questioning, not the medical examination

Short Answer Questions

1. What are the key components of informed consent in forensic medical practice?
2. Why is informed consent particularly important during a medicolegal autopsy?

3. How does the principle of autonomy relate to obtaining consent from patients in forensic medicine?
4. Under what circumstances can consent be waived or overridden in forensic medical practice?
5. How should a forensic practitioner handle situations where consent cannot be obtained due to the patient being unconscious or deceased?
6. What role does capacity to consent play in forensic evaluations, especially with mentally ill individuals or minors?
7. How can forensic practitioners ensure that consent is voluntary and not coerced in legal or custodial settings?

Answers to Critical Thinking Questions

1. (b); 2. (b); 3. (b); 4. (a); 5. (b).

REFERENCES

1. Abiodun, O. I., Kiru, M. U., Jantan, A., Omolara, A. E., Dada, K. V., Umar, A. M., Linus, O. U., et al. (2019). Comprehensive review of artificial neural network applications to pattern recognition. *IEEE Access, 7*, 158820–158846. https://doi.org/10.1109/access.2019.2945545.
2. Ahmad, W., Rasool, A., Javed, A. R., Baker, T., & Jalil, Z., (2021). Cyber security in IoT-based cloud computing: A comprehensive survey. *Electronics, 11*, 16. https://doi.org/10.3390/electronics11010016.
3. Ali, S., Abuhmed, T., El–Sappagh, S., Muhammad, K., Alonso, J. M., Confalonieri, R., Guidotti, R., et al. (2023). Explainable artificial intelligence (XAI): What we know and what is left to attain trustworthy artificial intelligence. *Information Fusion, 99*, 101805. https://doi.org/10.1016/j.inffus.2023.101805.
4. Brassett, C., Cosker, T., Davies, D. C., Dockery, P., Gillingwater, T. H., Lee, T. C., Milz, S., et al. (2020). COVID-19 and anatomy: Stimulus and initial response. *Journal of Anatomy, 237*, 393–403. https://doi.org/10.1111/joa.13274.
5. Brown, T., Duensing, S., & Wong, B., (2024). Forensic genetics in the shadows. *Journal of Law and the Biosciences, 11*. https://www.semanticscholar.org/paper/564691848bc5d39082e78559e9ea5970c0a2f9bc (accessed on 9th May 2025).
6. Cortegiani, A., Battaglini, D., Amato, G., Behr, A., Donadello, K., Einav, S., Frigo, M. G., et al. (2024). Dissemination of clinical and scientific practice through social media: A SIAARTI consensus-based document. *Journal of Anesthesia, Analgesia and Critical Care, 4*. https://www.semanticscholar.org/paper/49ed71bdd9b4c507d8d621e8513ae88b3e55406e (accessed on 9th May 2025).
7. Craik, C., & Stewart, P., (2007). *Occupation, Mental Illness and Medium Security: A Study of Occupational Engagement in Two Forensic Regional Secure Units*. https://core.ac.uk/download/334187.pdf (accessed on 9th May 2025).
8. Drennan, G., & Swanepoel, F., (2021). Restorative justice practice in forensic mental health settings: Bridging the gap. *The International Journal of Restorative Justice, 5*, 168–191. https://doi.org/10.5553/tijrj.000103.
9. Elahai, I., (2021). Effectiveness of structured teaching program on knowledge regarding legal issues in mental health among GNM 2nd year students in selected nursing school of Jaipur: A pre-experimental study. *IJCRT, 9*, 950–958. https://www.semanticscholar.org/paper/61addbb1ef23d1cb6e77d4b900737f7d852a9d03 (accessed on 9th May 2025).
10. Giulia, L. E., Richards, N., Willars, J., Scott, D. A., Boydell, N., Parker, J., Pinfold, V., et al. (2021). A qualitative study of experiences of NHS mental healthcare workers during the COVID-19 pandemic. *BMC Psychiatry, 21*. https://doi.org/10.1186/s12888-021-03261-8.
11. Glick, S., (2023). Ethical need for a fertility decision-aid for transgender adults of reproductive age. *Voices in Bioethics*. https://www.semanticscholar.org/paper/372df8fe029a0cedb5b7b3fc6a40199dea5dbbe5 (accessed on 9th May 2025).
12. Gundugurti, P. R., Bhattacharyya, R., Kondepi, S., Chakraborty, K., & Mukherjee, A., (2022). Ethics and law. *Indian Journal of Psychiatry, 64*, S7–S15. https://doi.org/10.4103/indianjpsychiatry.indianjpsychiatry_726_21.

13. Ha, S., Seon, C., Hong, J., Goo, B., Kim, E., Lee, S., Lyou, M. S., et al. (2025). Evaluating the safety of thread-embedding acupuncture: Protocol for a multi-center, prospective, observational study in clinical practice. *Healthcare, 13.* https://www.semanticscholar.org/paper/56db1bbdbd2fff2a74d865f45d324007012cf4d8 (accessed on 9th May 2025).

14. Hlavka, H. R. (2014). Normalizing sexual violence. *Gender & Society, 28*, 337–358. https://doi.org/10.1177/0891243214526468.

15. Hoes, A., Grobbee, D., Lubsen, J., Veld, A., Does, E., & Hofman, A., (1995). Diuretics, β-blockers, and the risk for sudden cardiac death in hypertensive patients. *Annals of Internal Medicine, 123*, 481–487. https://www.semanticscholar.org/paper/6e2097d7dd2bd114a0deee4d14118be819f5cb09 (accessed on 9th May 2025).

16. Hofstad, T., Rugkåsa, J., Ose, S. O., Nyttingnes, O., & Husum, T. L. (2021). Measuring the level of compulsory hospitalization in mental health care: The performance of different measures across areas and over time. *International Journal of Methods in Psychiatric Research, 30.* https://doi.org/10.1002/mpr.1881.

17. Kazitskaya, A. S., Bondarev, O. I., Bugaeva, M. S., Zhukova, A. G., & Yadykina, T. K. (2021). Morphometric and genetic studies of the mechanisms of damage to the cardiovascular system in Kuzbass miners with dust lung pathology. *Russian Journal of Occupational Health and Industrial Ecology, 61*, 611–619. https://doi.org/10.31089/1026-9428-2021-61-9-611-619.

18 Khalil, R., Mansour, A., Fadda, W. A., Almisnid, K., Aldamegh, M. S., Al-Nafeesah, A., Alkhalifah, A., et al. (2020). The sudden transition to synchronized online learning during the COVID-19 pandemic in Saudi Arabia: A qualitative study exploring medical students' perspectives. *BMC Medical Education, 20.* https://doi.org/10.1186/s12909-020-02208-z.

19 Kling, D., Phillips, C., Kennett, D., & Tillmar, A., (2021). Investigative genetic genealogy: Current methods, knowledge and practice. *Forensic Science International: Genetics, 52*, 102474. https://doi.org/10.1016/j.fsigen.2021.102474.

20. Kooij, J. J. S., Bijlenga, D., Salerno, L., Jaeschke, R., Bitter, I., Balázs, J., Thome, J., et al. (2018). Updated European consensus statement on diagnosis and treatment of adult ADHD. *European Psychiatry, 56*, 14–34. https://doi.org/10.1016/j.eurpsy.2018.11.001.

21. Lechien, J. R., Chiesa-Estomba, C. M., Hans, S., Barillari, M. R., Jouffe, L., & Saussez, S., (2020). Loss of smell and taste in 2013 European patients with mild to moderate COVID-19. *Annals of Internal Medicine, 173*, 672–675. https://doi.org/10.7326/m20-2428.

22. Lee, Y., (2024). Consciously choosing unconsciousness. *Voices in Bioethics.* https://www.semanticscholar.org/paper/b549afbb3983ab2a3151e51ce7ae296948448179 (accessed on 9th May 2025).

23. Long, R., (2017). *Bioethics, Complementarity, and Corporate Criminal Liability.* https://core.ac.uk/download/131213205.pdf (accessed on 9th May 2025).

24. Mahani, A., & Zadu, R., (2024). The role of consent in Indian judiciary: Implications for cancer treatment practices. *Indian Journal of Forensic and Community Medicine.* https://www.semanticscholar.org/paper/639270c91e18a61f76de252d87dac89880e137f7 (accessed on 9th May 2025).

25. McMillan, L., & White, D., (2015). "Silly girls" and "nice young lads": Vilification and vindication in the perceptions of medico-legal practitioners in rape cases. *Feminist Criminology, 10*(3), 279–298. https://core.ac.uk/download/293879559.pdf (accessed on 9th May 2025).

26. Muhammad, N., Ayday, E., Clayton, E. W., Fellay, J., Gunter, C. A., Hubaux, J. P., Malin, B., et al. (2015). Privacy in the genomic era. *ACM Computing Surveys, 48*, 1–44. https://doi.org/10.1145/2767007.

27. Opeskin, B., Weisbrot, D., & Breen, K., (2025). *Essentially Yours: The Protection of Human Genetic Information in Australia*. https://core.ac.uk/download/pdf/30672952.pdf (accessed on 9th May 2025).

28. Perrenoud, B., Velonaki, V. S., Bodenmann, P., & Ramelet, A., (2015). The effectiveness of health literacy interventions on the informed consent process of health care users: A systematic review protocol. *JBI Database of Systematic Reviews and Implementation Reports, 13*, 82–94. https://www.semanticscholar.org/paper/915e4caa185e4cace1517ed0b2188ea213006949 (accessed on 9th May 2025).

29. Reed, G. M., Drescher, J., Krueger, R. B., Atalla, E., Cochran, S. D., First, M. B., Cohen-Kettenis, P. T., et al. (2016). Disorders related to sexuality and gender identity in the ICD-11: Revising the ICD-10 classification based on current scientific evidence, best clinical practices, and human rights considerations. *World Psychiatry, 15*, 205–221. https://doi.org/10.1002/wps.20354.

30. Research In Implementation Science And eHealth (2021). *Computer-Based Decision Tools for Shared Therapeutic Decision Making in Oncology: A Systematic Review (Preprint)*. https://www.semanticscholar.org/paper/927ee4f29eacc593ca61501b2e67918ee99670ec (accessed on 9th May 2025).

31. Ritchie, J., & Doherty, M., (2025). Medico-legal evidence: Survivor relational autonomy and informed consent in sexual assault examinations. *Feminist Legal Studies*. https://www.semanticscholar.org/paper/c150896543196de6c1bf209411c7d766a146966b (accessed on 9th May 2025).

32. Sadykov, M. B., Begaliyev, Y., Bakhteev, D., Kaziyeva, A. N., & Khussainov, O. B. (2024). On the application of artificial intelligence and chipping of persons in forensic medicine: Review. *Russian Journal of Forensic Medicine*. https://www.semanticscholar.org/paper/f25dda1e34ca8e08950226e8f3d6e7ee3db7a602 (accessed on 9th May 2025).

33. Sallam, M., Dababseh, D., Yaseen, A., Al-Haidar, A., Ababneh, N. A., Bakri, F. G., & Mahafzah, A., (2020). Conspiracy beliefs are associated with lower knowledge and higher anxiety levels regarding COVID-19 among students at the University of Jordan. *International Journal of Environmental Research and Public Health, 17*, 4915. https://doi.org/10.3390/ijerph17144915 (accessed on 9th May 2025).

34. Samuel, G., (2021). Investigative genetic genealogy: Can collective privacy and solidarity help? *Journal of Medical Ethics, 47*, 796, 797. https://www.semanticscholar.org/paper/bcb11df5768672f5b9cbd20e36e546f54555787b (accessed on 9th May 2025).

35. Sashidharan, S. P., Mezzina, R., & Pūras, D., (2019). Reducing coercion in mental healthcare. *Epidemiology and Psychiatric Sciences, 28*, 605–612. https://doi.org/10.1017/s2045796019000350.

36. Schwartz, R., Vassilev, A., Greene, K., Perine, L., Burt, A., & Hall, P., (2022). *Towards a Standard for Identifying and Managing Bias in Artificial Intelligence*. https://doi.org/10.6028/nist.sp.1270.

37. Seshadri, S., & Ramaswamy, S., (2019). Clinical practice guidelines for child sexual abuse. *Indian Journal of Psychiatry, 61*, 317. https://doi.org/10.4103/psychiatry.indianjpsychiatry_502_18.

38. Shabani, M., & Marelli, L., (2019). Re-identifiability of genomic data and the GDPR. *EMBO Reports, 20*. https://doi.org/10.15252/embr.201948316.

39. Shalaby, R., & Agyapong, V. I. O. (2020). Peer support in mental health: Literature review. *JMIR Mental Health, 7*, e15572. https://doi.org/10.2196/15572.

40. Slade, M., (2017). Implementing shared decision making in routine mental health care. *World Psychiatry, 16*, 146–153. https://doi.org/10.1002/wps.20412.

41. Stein, D. J., Shoptaw, S., Vigo, D., Lund, C., Cuijpers, P., Bantjes, J., Sartorius, N., et al. (2022). Psychiatric diagnosis and treatment in the 21st century: Paradigm shifts versus incremental integration. *World Psychiatry, 21*, 393–414. https://doi.org/10.1002/wps.20998.

42. Stoyanova, M., Nikoloudakis, Y., Panagiotakis, S., Pallis, E., & Markakis, E., (2020). A survey on the Internet of Things (IoT) forensics: Challenges, approaches, and open issues. *IEEE Communications Surveys & Tutorials, 22*, 1191–1221. https://doi.org/10.1109/comst.2019.2962586.

43. Tan, A., Spice, R., & Sinnarajah, A., (2021). Family physicians supporting patients with palliative care needs within the patient medical home in the community: An appreciative inquiry study. *BMJ Open, 11*. https://www.semanticscholar.org/paper/7a127de75f805a676738cea93815352e654e701a (accessed on 9th May 2025).

44. Tsyganova, O. A. (2024). *Providing Medical care Without Patient or Legal Representative's Consent, and Patient Refusal of Medical Intervention: Regulatory Framework and Legal Practice*. Russian Family Doctor. https://www.semanticscholar.org/paper/98d8a0c4855698bf956385a768f79792afb0380c (accessed on 9th May 2025).

45. Veale, M., & Zuiderveen, B. F., (2021). Demystifying the draft EU artificial intelligence act—Analyzing the good, the bad, and the unclear elements of the proposed approach. *Computer Law Review International, 22*, 97–112. https://doi.org/10.9785/cri-2021-220402.

46. Vishnopolska, S., Turjanski, A. G., Herrera Piñero, M., Groisman, B., Liascovich, R., Chiesa, A., & Martí, M. A. (2018). Genetics and genomic medicine in Argentina. *Molecular Genetics & Genomic Medicine, 6*, 481–491. https://doi.org/10.1002/mgg3.455.

47. Zeppenfeld, K., Tfelt-Hansen, J., Riva, M., Winkel, B. G., Behr, E. R., Blom, N. A., Charron, P., et al. (2022). 2022 ESC guidelines for the management of patients with ventricular arrhythmias and the prevention of sudden cardiac death. *European Heart Journal, 43*, 3997–4126. https://doi.org/10.1093/eurheartj/ehac262.

INDEX

J

K

L

M

N

O

P

R

S

T

U

V

W

X

Z